《(英汉对照)精编实用中医文库》

编纂委员会

总　主　编　陈凯先　李其忠(执行)　何星海
编　　　委(按姓氏笔画为序)
马烈光　何建成　余小萍　沈雪勇
张婷婷　陈红风　陈德兴　赵　毅
郭　忻　黄　平　虞坚尔　詹红生
缪晚虹

编译委员会

总　主　译　施建蓉　胡鸿毅　徐　瑶(执行)
编　译　者(按姓氏笔画为序)
朱爱秀　杨　渝　肖元春　张忆萍
诸建民　黄国琪　董　晶　韩丑萍

《中医内科学》

主　　　编　余小萍
副　主　编　窦丹波　柳　文　周家俊
主　　　译　张忆萍

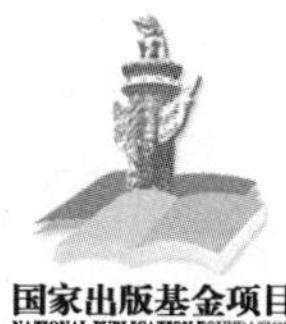

An Intensively Compiled Practical English-Chinese Library of Traditional Chinese Medicine

(英汉对照)精编实用中医文库

Chief General Compilers CHEN Kaixian LI Qizhong(Executive) HE Xinghai

总主编 陈凯先 李其忠(执行) 何星海

Chief General Translators SHI Jianrong HU Hongyi XU Yao(Executive)

总主译 施建蓉 胡鸿毅 徐 瑶(执行)

Internal Medicine of Traditional Chinese Medicine

中医内科学

Chief Compiler **YU Xiaoping**

Chief Translator **ZHANG Yiping**

主编 余小萍

主译 张忆萍

上海浦江教育出版社(原上海中医药大学出版社)

Shanghai Pujiang Education Press (Former Shanghai University of TCM Press)

An Intensively Compiled Practical English-Chinese Library of Traditional Chinese Medicine

Compilation Board of the Library

Chief General Compilers CHEN Kaixian LI Qizhong(Executive) HE Xinghai

Members(Listed in the order of the number of strokes in the Chinese names)

MA Lieguang	HE Jiancheng	YU Xiaoping	SHEN Xueyong
ZHANG Tingting	CHEN Hongfeng	CHEN Dexing	ZHAO Yi
GUO Xin	HUANG Ping	YU Jian'er	ZHAN Hongsheng
MIAO Wanhong			

Compilation and Translation Committee of the Library

Chief General Translators SHI Jianrong HU Hongyi XU Yao(Executive)

Translators(Listed in the order of the number of strokes in the Chinese names)

ZHU Aixiu	YANG Yu	XIAO Yuanchun	ZHANG Yiping
ZHU Jianmin	HUANG Guoqi	DONG Jing	HAN Chouping

Internal Medicine of Traditional Chinese Medicinee

Chief Compiler YU Xiaoping

Deputy Chief Compilers DOU Danbo LIU Wen ZHOU Jiajun

Chief Translator ZHANG Yiping

Foreword

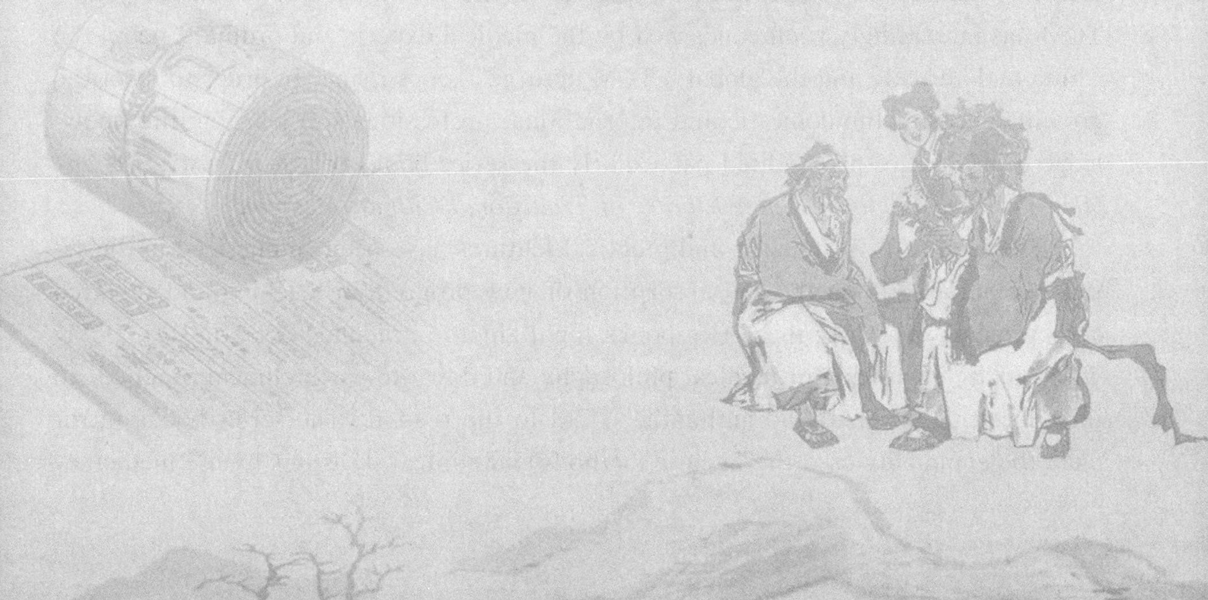

With the traditional medical philosophy and clinical experience as the principal body, the science of Traditional Chinese Medicine (TCM) is a comprehensive subject to study the rules of life activities and the disease prevention, diagnosis, treatment, rehabilitation as well as healthcare. The science of TCM has a long history of development and belongs to a summary of experiences that Chinese nation has fought against diseases for over several thousand years, is also an important component part of Chinese outstanding traditional culture and has contributed greatly to the healthcare undertaking and development of Chinese nation.

By increasing enhancement of modern living standard, change of living modes and acceleration of ageing process, the chronic diseases represented by tumors, cardiovascular diseases and diabetes become gradually the important factors in impacting the health of mankind, but TCM presents the better therapeutic effects. Nowadays, the modern medical mode of "society-psychology-biology" has been advocated in medical science, changing from the medical idea of "disease treatment" to "health promotion". The more and more patients in China and abroad have chosen natural and low side-effect Chinese herbal medicine for their problems. With the changes in medicine modes and in spectrum of diseases in the recent several dozens of years, TCM has increasingly been concerned by the medical experts and ordinary people in China and abroad, and the global " TCM upsurge" keeps rising. In order to meet the growing needs of the domestic and international professionals in learning the knowledge of TCM, we have edited particularly the series books of *An Intensively Compiled Practical English-Chinese Library of Traditional Chinese Medicine*.

The scientific, systematic and practical features have been emphasized in the series books. Based upon the full absorption of new progress in teaching and research achievements of TCM, the series books highlight the academic essentials of TCM, with precise exposition of medical philosophy and down-to-earth clinical practice, to introduce the "original and authentic" TCM to the readers. The series books introduce the commonly used therapeutic methods and clinical skills in Chinese medicine, by the clinically encountered and frequently seen diseases and the relevant ailments predominantly effective by Chinese medical therapies.By studying the series books, the readers can learn the knowledge and techniques of TCM on gradual progress and become proficient gradually in TCM.

The series books highlight "the precise features in three aspects" —capable in authors, refined in contents and accurate in translation. The majority of the authors of the series books are senior experts from the related faculties of Shanghai University of Traditional Chinese Medicine. The translator team is composed of the senior teachers with plentiful expertise in translation of TCM from international education college and foreign language center of Shanghai University of Traditional Chinese Medicine. In order to meet the needs of the readers in China and abroad, the basic and clinical core contents are selected and the latest research achievements are consulted based upon the principle "to seek its essentials but its completion" in the series books.

The series books can satisfy the beginners with certain knowledge of English language in studying TCM systematically and can also be used as the textbooks for education of TCM and pharmacy for foreign students. We sincerely hope the publication of the series books plays its promoting role for TCM going to the world.

Editors

June, 2017

中医学是以传统医学理论与实践经验为主体，研究人体生命活动规律和疾病预防、诊断、治疗、康复以及保健的一门综合性学科。中医学历史悠久，源远流长，是中华民族几千年来同疾病作斗争的经验总结，也是中国传统文化的重要组成部分，长期以来为中国人民的健康保健事业和民族繁衍作出了巨大的贡献。

随着现代生活水平的不断提高、生活方式的改变以及老龄化进程的加快，以肿瘤、心血管疾病和糖尿病等为代表的慢性病日渐成为影响人类健康的重要因素，而中医药显示了良好的治疗效果。当今的医学倡导“社会—心理—生物”的现代医学模式，医学理念从“疾病治疗”向“健康促进”转变，国内外越来越多的患者选择天然、毒副作用低的中医药治疗疾病。近几十年来，随着医学模式的转变和疾病谱的改变，中医学日益引起越来越多的海内外医学专家和普通民众的关注，全球性的“中医热”正在持续升温。为了满足海内外人士日益高涨的学习中医学知识的需求，我们特地编撰了《（英汉对照）精编实用中医文库》丛书。

本丛书注重“三性”——科学性、系统性、实用性。丛书在充分吸取近年中医教学、科研进展的基础上，突出中医学术精华，理论阐述准确、临床切合实际，向读者介绍“原汁原味”的中医学；丛书介绍中医学常用的治疗方法和临床技能，所涉及的病证均为临床常见病、多发病和中医优势病种。丛书的13个分册涵盖了中医基础与临床的主干课程，通过阅读本丛书，读者可以由浅入深、循序渐进地学习中医药知识和技能。

本丛书突出“三精”——作者精干、内容精炼、翻译精准。丛书的中文作者绝大部分为上海中医药大学各相关教研室的资深专家，翻译团队由上海中医药大学国际教育学院和外语中心具有丰富的中医药学翻译经验的骨干教师组成。为了适合海内外读者的需求，丛书本着“求其精而不求其全”的原则，选取了基础和临床的核心内容，翻译上参考了最新的研究成果。

本丛书既可满足具有一定英语水平的初学中医者系统学习中医所用，也可供中医药留学生教育作为教材使用，衷心希望本丛书的出版在中医药走向海外进程中发挥应有的推动作用。

编者

2017年6月

Note for Compilation

编写说明

Internal Medicine of Traditional Chinese Medicine (TCM) is a clinic discipline based on TCM theories, focusing on etiology and pathogenesis of internal diseases and treatment principles by pattern identification. Moreover, it is also the basis of study and research work of other TCM-related clinic subspecialties.

The textbook here consists of two parts: a general introduction and specific discussions.The introduction has two chapters, of which the first introduces the classification, nomination and characteristics of internal diseases in TCM and the second focuses on the treatment procedures and fundamental principles of internal diseases in TCM. Specific discussions is divided into seven chapters, respectively lung system diseases, heart system diseases, spleen system diseases, liver system diseases, kidney system diseases, diseases of qi, blood and body fluid, and diseases of body parts and meridians. Forty common clinical internal diseases are discussed in order of basic concepts, key etiology and pathogenesis, and pattern identification, among which pattern identification is the core, subdivided into keys points of pattern identification and therapeutic methods of different patterns (manifestation, therapeutic method, formula and herbs, and modification).

中医内科学是以中医学理论为指导，阐述内科病证的病因病机及其辨证论治规律的一门临床学科。它既是一门临床专业学科，又是学习和研究中医其他临床学科的基础。

本教材设总论和各论。总论分二章，第一章介绍中医内科疾病分类、命名及其特点；第二章介绍中医内科病证的诊治步骤和基本要求。各论分七章，按肺系病证、心系病证、脾系病证、肝系病证、肾系病证、气血津液病证、肢体经络病证的顺序排列，分别介绍了 40 个临床常见病证的基本概念、主要的病因病机和辨证论治。其中以辨证论治为重点，分别按辨治要点、分型论治（证候、治法、方药和加减）。

Contents

目　录

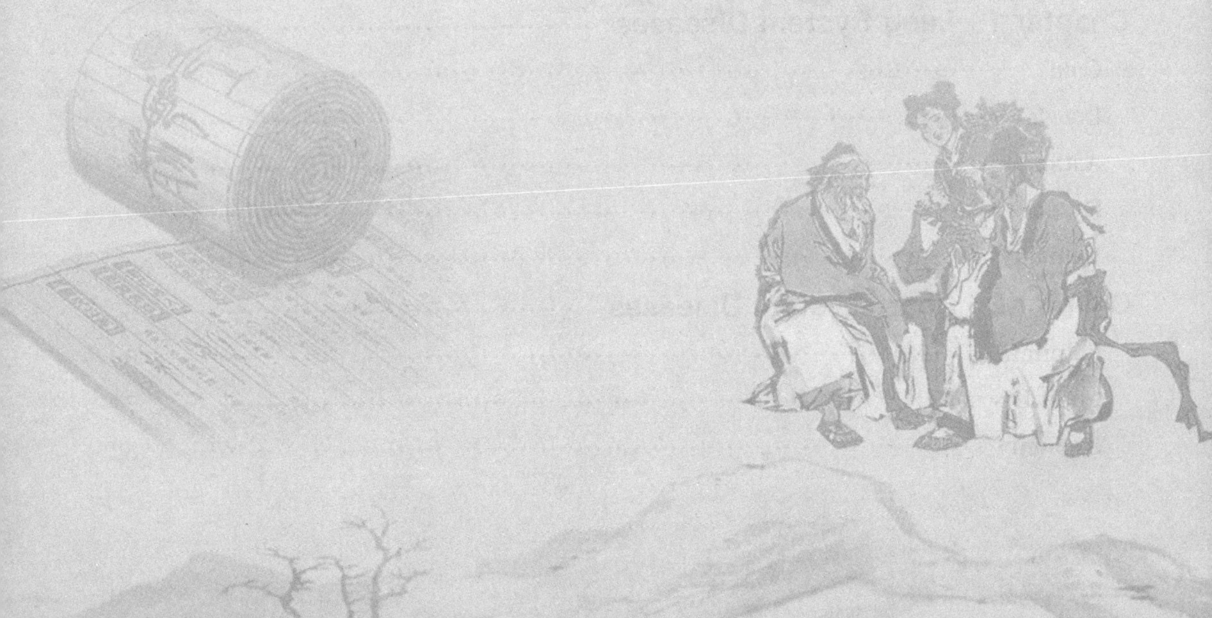

General Introduction

Chapter 1 Classification, Nomination and Characteristics of Internal Diseases in TCM ······ (3)

Section 1 Classification of Internal Diseases in TCM ······ (3)

Section 2 Nomination of Internal Diseases in TCM ······ (4)

Section 3 Characteristics of Internal Diseases in TCM ······ (5)

Chapter 2 Diagnostic Procedures and Fundamental Requirements of Internal Diseases in TCM ······ (7)

Section 1 Diagnostic Procedures of Internal Diseases in TCM ······ (7)

Section 2 Fundamental Requirements of Treatment on Internal Diseases in TCM ······ (8)

Section 3 Treatment Principles of Internal Diseases in TCM ······ (11)

Specific Discussions

Chapter 1 Lung System Diseases ······ (16)

Cold ······ (16)

Cough ······ (24)

Asthma ······ (35)

Dyspnea ······ (44)

Hemoptysis ······ (54)

Chapter 2 Heart System Diseases ······ (60)

Palpitation ······ (60)

Chest Discomfort ······ (71)

Insomnia ······ (82)

总 论

第1章 中医内科疾病分类、命名及其特点 …… (3)

第1节 中医内科疾病分类 …… (3)

第2节 中医内科病证的命名 …… (4)

第3节 中医内科病证的特点 …… (5)

第2章 中医内科病证的诊治步骤和基本要求 …… (7)

第1节 中医内科病证的诊治步骤 …… (7)

第2节 中医内科病证的诊治基本要求 …… (8)

第3节 中医内科病证的治疗原则 …… (11)

各 论

第1章 肺系病证 …… (16)

感冒 …… (16)

咳嗽 …… (24)

哮病 …… (35)

喘证 …… (44)

咳血 …… (54)

第2章 心系病证 …… (60)

心悸 …… (60)

胸痹 …… (71)

不寐 …… (82)

Epilepsy .... (91)
Dementia .... (99)
Chapter 3 Spleen System Disease .... (108)
Stomachache .... (108)
Vomiting .... (117)
Abdominal Pain .... (128)
Diarrhea .... (138)
Dysentery .... (149)
Constipation .... (160)
Hematemesis .... (170)
Hemafecia .... (174)
Chapter 4 Liver System Diseases .... (181)
Hypochondriac Pain .... (181)
Jaundice .... (189)
Tympanites .... (198)
Headache .... (209)
Vertigo .... (219)
Stroke .... (227)
Goiter .... (240)
Chapter 5 Kidney System Diseases .... (249)
Edema .... (249)
Stranguria Syndrome .... (261)
Bloody Urine .... (270)
Long Bi .... (275)
Impotence .... (285)
Chapter 6 Diseases of Qi, Blood, and Body Fluid .... (292)
Obstruction of Dampness .... (292)
Depressive Disorder .... (298)
Consumptive Thirst .... (307)
Abnormal Perspiration (Sweating) .... (317)

痫病 …… (91)

痴呆 …… (99)

第 3 章　脾系病证 …… (108)

胃痛 …… (108)

呕吐 …… (117)

腹痛 …… (128)

泄泻 …… (138)

痢疾 …… (149)

便秘 …… (160)

吐血 …… (170)

便血 …… (174)

第 4 章　肝系病证 …… (181)

胁痛 …… (181)

黄疸 …… (189)

鼓胀 …… (198)

头痛 …… (209)

眩晕 …… (219)

中风 …… (227)

瘿病 …… (240)

第 5 章　肾系病证 …… (249)

水肿 …… (249)

淋证 …… (261)

尿血 …… (270)

癃闭 …… (275)

阳痿 …… (285)

第 6 章　气血津液病证 …… (292)

湿阻 …… (292)

郁证 …… (298)

消渴 …… (307)

汗证 …… (317)

Fever Due to Internal Injury ······ (323)
Consumptive Disease ······ (331)
Chatper 7 Diseases of Body Parts and Meridians ······ (346)
Bi Syndrome ······ (346)
Flaccidity Syndrome ······ (358)
Tremor ······ (367)
Lumbago ······ (375)

内伤发热 …………………………………………………………………… (323)
虚劳 ……………………………………………………………………… (331)
第7章 肢体经络病证 ……………………………………………… (346)
痹证 ……………………………………………………………………… (346)
痿证 ……………………………………………………………………… (358)
颤证 ……………………………………………………………………… (367)
腰痛 ……………………………………………………………………… (375)

General Introduction

Internal Medicine of Traditional Chinese Medicine (TCM) is a clinical subspecialty based on Traditional Chinese Medicine theory, dealing with the etiology and pathogenesis of internal diseases and the principles of treatment by pattern identification with traditional Chinese materia herbs. It is guided by physiologic and pathologic theories of Traditional Chinese Medicine on zang-fu organs, meridians and collaterals, qi, blood and body fluid, featured by treatment according to pattern identification. Internal Medicine of TCM is the basis of TCM clinical subspecialty.

中医内科学是运用中医学理论阐述内科病证的病因病机及辨证论治规律，并以中医药治疗为主的一门临床学科。它以中医脏腑、经络、气血津液等生理病理学说为指导，辨证论治为特点，既是一门临床专业课，也是临床其他各科的基础。

Chapter 1 Classification, Nomination and Characteristics of Internal Diseases in TCM

第1章 中医内科疾病分类、命名及其特点

Section 1 Classification of Internal Diseases in TCM

第1节 中医内科疾病分类

Internal diseases in TCM come in great variety and wide coverage. Etiologically, they are categorized into exogenous diseases and miscellaneous endogenous diseases. Exogenous diseases are acute heat diseases caused by six climatic and epidemic exogenous pathogenic factors, including exogenous febrile diseases, wind-warm diseases, fever diseases in summer, damp fever, which are usually treated according to theories of six meridians, defensive qi, nutrient blood and *san jiao*. Endogenous diseases are, otherwise, caused by improper diet, internal injuries and changes of emotions and minds, which are usually treated according to pathological changes and features of dysfunction of zang-fu organs, meridians and collaterals, qi, blood and body fluid. We will classify exogenous diseases and endogenous diseases in zang-fu organs into seven categories:

中医内科疾病病种多，范围广。按病因可以分为外感时病和内伤杂病两大类。外感疾病是由外感六淫及戾气所致，包括伤寒、风温、暑温、湿温等急性热病，常按六经、卫气营血和三焦理论进行辨证论治。内伤病证多由饮食、劳伤、情志等所伤，包括脏腑、肢体经络、气血津液诸病，主要根据脏腑、经络、气血津液失常的病理变化及病机特点进行辨证论治。本书是在病因分类的基础上，以脏腑分类为主导，将伤寒、温病以外的外感病证和内伤杂病分为七大类即肺系病

lung system diseases, heart system diseases, spleen system diseases, liver system diseases, kidney system diseases, diseases of qi, blood and body fluid, and diseases of body parts and meridians.

证、心系病证、脾胃系病证、肝胆病证、肾系病证、气血津液病证、肢体经络病证。

Section 2 Nomination of Internal Diseases in TCM

第 2 节 中医内科病证的命名

Internal diseases are usually named from etiology, pathogenesis, pathological production, pathological location, main symptom and physiological signs. For example, stroke, is named in terms of etiology; depressive disorder, Bi syndrome are named in terms of pathogenesis; retention of phlegm and fluid are named in terms of pathological production; coughing, dyspnea, vomiting, diarrhea and vertigo are named in terms of main symptoms; jaundice, edema and tympanites are named in terms of physiological signs. In thousands of years, herbsl practice, this traditional way of nomination has been settled down and gradually become a systematic knowledge with corresponding disease names of etiology and pathogenesis, clinical characteristics, diseases identification, pathological changes and development, detailed treatment, formulae, prevention and prognosis, which provides a useful guidance for clinical practice.

中医内科病证的命名原则主要是以病因、病机、病理产物、病位、主症、体征为依据。如以病因命名的有中风、中暑、虫证等;以病机命名的有郁证、痹证、厥证等;以病理产物命名的有痰饮等;以病位命名的有胸痹、肺痈、肺痨等;以主症命名的咳嗽、喘证、呕吐、泄泻、眩晕等;以主要体征命名的黄疸、积聚、水肿、鼓胀等。在几千年的医疗实践过程中,这种传统的命名方法已具有确定的含义,在中医内科学术理论的指导下,逐步形成了与病名相应的病因病机、临床特点、类证鉴别、发展演变、转归预后的系统认识,以及辨证论治的具体治法、方药和预防调护,这些知识有效地指导着临床。

Section 3 Characteristics of Internal Diseases in TCM

第3节 中医内科病证的特点

1 Characteristics of Exogenous Diseases

Exogenous diseases are seasonal and acute diseases caused by exogenous pathogenic factors like the six climatic pathogenic factors and epidemic pathogenic factors invading the body via skin, hair, mouth and nose. When epidemic and infectious pathogenic factors are involved, such diseases are infectious and epidemic. Take acute jaundice as an example, which is caused by exogenous infectious damp-heat and develops quickly into the inside shortly after some temporary symptoms. The heat evil goes so intense as to captivate the *san jiao* and even invade the nutritious blood and endanger the heart and liver. For its acuteness, it can become regionally epidemic and infectious.

1 外感时病的特点

中医内科外感时病的病因为六淫、戾气等外邪，发病常与季节有关，起病较急，病邪多由皮毛、口鼻而入，由表传里。多具有季节性、传变性，若兼夹戾气、疫毒，则具有传染性、流行性。如急性黄胆型肝炎病因为外感湿热疫毒，发病急骤，初起虽有短暂表证经过，但邪毒迅即由表入里，而致热毒炽盛，充斥三焦，甚则深入营血，内陷心肝，其来势凶猛，传变迅速，可呈区域性流行，互相传染。

2 Characteristics of Miscellaneous Endogenous Diseases

Endogenous diseases are due to improper diet, tiredness and injuries of emotions and minds. It is characterized by its complicacy of multiple factors, zang fu organs and complexity of different diseases and syndromes. Imbalance of qi, blood, yin and yang of the zang qi is the major cause of miscellaneous endogenous diseases. In the disease development, more than one zang organs are usually attacked and even fu organs could be endangered, with which, a second attack by exogenous pathologic factors or co-existence of different pathogenic

2 内伤杂病的特点

内伤杂病多由饮食、劳倦、情志所伤所致，其特点是多因素相加、多脏腑相关、多病性复合、多病证杂见，其基本病机为脏腑气血阴阳失调。在病情演变过程中，往往病及多脏，且可脏病及腑，或因复感外邪，或因多种病理因素的产生，而出现寒热虚实错杂的证候，并可多病重叠。如喘证病因有外感、

factors can result in complicate syndrome of cold with heat, deficiency with excess and co-existence of different diseases. For example, dyspnea can be caused by exogenous or endogenous pathogenic factors and can come in deficiency or excess pathologically. It could be triggered and worsened by many factors. During continuous onsets, asthenia of healthy qi is invaded by pathogenic factors and retention of cold transforms into heat, which leads to the symptoms of cold outside while heat inside and excess of *shang jiao* (upper jiao) while deficiency of *xia jiao* (xia jiao). As coughing continues, it will lead to dyspnea as well as phlegm and fluid incubated in the lung when lung is deficient of healthy qi and stops distributing body fluid which further results in the retention of fluid and phlegm. In the end, cough, phlegm and dyspnea co-exist.

内伤两端,病理性质有虚实两类,可由多种因素诱发和加重,在反复发作过程中,常因正虚感邪、寒郁化热,而表现表寒里热、上盛下虚的证候;咳嗽久延,可以致喘,亦可因肺虚气不布津,停而为饮,聚而成痰,导致痰饮伏肺,而见咳、痰、喘并存。

Chapter 2 Diagnostic Procedures and Fundamental Requirements of Internal Diseases in TCM

第2章 中医内科病证的诊治步骤和基本要求

Section 1 Diagnostic Procedures of Internal Diseases in TCM

第1节 中医内科病证的诊治步骤

The diagnostic procedures can be summarized as "combined use of the four diagnostic methods", "investigating causes and examining pathological mechanism", "analyzing pathological mechanism", "deciding on treatment" and "selecting formulae and giving prescriptions".

中医内科疾病的诊治步骤可以归纳为四诊合参、求因审机、分析病机、确立治法和选方遣药。

1 Combined Use of Four Diagnostic Methods

Inspection, listening and smelling examination, inquiry and palpation are the first stepsto know about the etiology, characteristics, symptoms, previous treatment and outcomes, which is the premise for further diagnosis and treatment. The truthfulness of collected information by the four methods is very critical for pattern identification. Meanwhile, focusing on important information is also very important.

1 四诊合参

首先要通过望、闻、问、切四诊,对患者作仔细的诊查,了解患者的发病原因、病史特点、临床表现、诊治经过及结果。全面收集患者的临床资料,这是诊治疾病的前提。四诊资料是否准确,关系到辨证准确与否。同时还要做到重点突出,四诊合参,为辨证提供必要的依据。

2　Investigating Causes and Examining Pathological Mechanism

Every internal disease takes on different clinical symptoms and doctors have to analyze the symptoms and signs to speculate on the causes, pathogenesis, nature, location of diseases, target on the essence and give treatment accordingly.

2　求因审机

内科病证有各自的临床特点，通过分析患者的症状、体征来推求病因、病机、病性、病位，抓住病证的实质，治疗也有了更强的针对性。

3　Deciding on Treatment

The principles and methods of treatment should be based on pattern identification, focusing on the etiology and pathogenesis.

3　确立治法

确立治法即根据辨证的结果确立相应的治疗原则和方法，立法要紧扣病因病机。

4　Selecting Formulas and Herbs

Formulas and Herbs should be chosen according to treatment methods based on pattern identification and make sure the chosen formulas and herbs are right for the disease. Dosage and compatibility of materia herbs should be adjusted according to the very diseases concerned.

In sum, the diagnostic procedures mentioned above exemplifies the unity of "pathogenesis", "methods", "formulas" and "materia medica" in pattern identification.

4　选方遣药

选方即根据辨证立法来选择适当的治疗方剂，做到"方证相应"。遣药即在选定方剂的基础上确定药物的剂量、配伍，针对具体病情随症加减，灵活应用方剂。

总之，以上的诊治步骤体现的了辨证论治的"理、法、方、药"的统一。

Section 2　Fundamental Requirements of Treatment on Internal Diseases in TCM

第 2 节　中医内科病证的诊治基本要求

1　Emphasis on the Whole-and-parts Relationship

The human body is an organic holistic system in which the five zang organs as the center, along with

1　重视整体和局部的关系

人体是以五脏为中心，配合六腑，通过经络系统，联

the six fu organs, through the meridians and collaterals connect with the five body constituents, the five sense organs, the nine orifices and the limbs and bones. Pathological changes in parts are part of the pathological changes in the whole body. Therefore, when selecting formulas, doctors should pay attention to the parts as well as the whole body. Doctors should regulate the whole to promote the recovery of the body parts and in the end to restore the balance between yin and yang.

合五体、五官、九窍、四肢百骸而组成的有机联系的整体系统，局部病变是整体病理反应的一部分，因此立法选方，既要注意局部，更须重视整体，应通过整体调节以促进局部病变的恢复，使阴阳达到相对平衡。

2 Know about the Characteristics of Disease Pathogenesis

Internal diseases in TCM have theirown clinical characteristics and pathological changes. There fore, doctors have to know about pathogenesis characteristics of different disease to ensure the efficiency of the following treatment. Exogenous diseases should be categorized and treated in light of the theories of the six meridians, guarding healthy qi and nurturing blood and the *san jiao*. Miscellaneous endogenous diseases should be treated based on pattern identification in categories of zang-fu organs diseases, qi-blood-fluid diseases or limb-meridian diseases. Take lung system diseases for instance. Doctors should know that the pathological characteristics is that the lung qi has failed to disperse and has descended. Therefore, doctors should try to restore the the lung's physiological function of controling qi and breathing. Spleen system diseases are due to the obstruction of zhong jiao (zhong jiao) qi ascending and descending to the meridians so the treatment should be restoring spleen's function of controling transportation, transformation and clear awaying

2 掌握病证的病机特点

中医内科病证，有着各自的临床特点和病机变化。掌握不同的病机特点，有利于准确的诊治。外感时病应按六经、卫气营血和三焦进行证候归类和施治。内伤杂病主要按脏腑病证、气血津液病证和肢体经络病证来进行辨证论治。如肺系病证，应按肺气失于宣发肃降之病机特点进行辨证论治，以复肺主气、司呼吸的生理功能。脾胃系病证，主要按中焦气机升降失常之病机特点进行辨证论治，以复脾胃主运化、升清降浊的生理功能。心系病证应按血脉运行障碍和神明失司之病机特点进行辨证论治，以复心主血脉和心主神明的生理功能。肝系病证主要按肝气疏泄不畅、肝阳

the turbid. Heart diseases should be focused on restore heart's function of controling the blood vessels and mind based on pattern identification of blood circulation obstacles and loss of mind and consciousness. Liver system diseases have the characteristics of unsuccessful dispelling of liver qi, excessive ascending of liver yang, liver wind agitation. Therefore, the treatment should enable liver to dispel, store blood and nourish the tendons. Kidney system diseases are due to the deficiency of kidney yin and kidney yang. Thence, the treatment should restore kidney's function of controling growth, development, reproduction, bones and marrow. Diseases of qi, blood, body fluid, limbs, meridians and collaterals should be treated according to cold and heat, excess and deficiency as well as association with zang-fu organs.

升发太过、肝风内动等病机特点进行辨证论治，以复肝主疏泄、藏血濡筋等生理功能。肾系病证主要按肾阴、肾阳不足的病机特点进行辨证论治，以复肾主生长、发育、生殖、主骨、生髓等生理功能。气血津液病证、肢体经络病证应按其寒热虚实、隶属脏腑的不同进行辨证。

3　Combination ofPattern Identification and Disease Identification

When treating internal diseases, doctors should not only differentiate syndromes but also identify the diseases. Disease identification is to have a longitudinal knowledge about how the disease starts and develops, which helps to grasp the fundamental pathological changes in its development. Pattern identification is to have a lateral knowledge about one particular stage during the development so as to find out the major conflicts and minor conflicts of a certain disease under certain circumstances. Disease identification is a way to recognize and handle the fundamental conflicts in a certain disease while pattern identification is a way to recognize and handle the major conflicts in a certain disease. Therefore,

3　辨证与辨病相结合

中医内科临证时既要辨证，亦要辨病。辨病是对疾病的发生、发展全过程的纵向认识，有助于抓住贯穿于整个疾病过程中证的基本病理变化；辨证是对疾病发生、发展过程中某一阶段的横断面认识，便于找出发生于特定个体某一疾病在其所处一定条件下的主要矛盾和矛盾的主要方面。辨病论治，是认识和解决某一疾病过程中基本矛盾的手段；辨证论治，是认识和解决某一疾病过程

disease identification and pattern identification is mutually supportive and inseparable. Only when disease identification and pattern identification are integrated can doctors have a clear awayer picture of the nature of the disease.

中主要矛盾的手段。因此辨病与辨证是相辅相成的，在辨证的基础上辨病，在辨病的同时辨证，辨证与辨病相结合，有利于对疾病性质的全面准确认识。

Section 3 Treatment Principles of Internal Diseases in TCM

第3节 中医内科病证的治疗原则

1 Examining the Symptom and Speculating on the Pathogenesis

Examining thesymptoms and speculating on the pathogenesis is to analyze the complicated symptoms and signs in a holistic and dynamic manner; to summarize and speculate on the possible causes and the pathological mechanism; and finally, give the right treatment. As long as the major conflicts are known, it is easy to see through the complicacy. Typical examples are treating the same disease with different therapeutic methods and treating different diseases with the same therapeutic method. The former means different diseases when they have the same pathologic changes and same symptoms can be treated with the same therapeutic methods. Take retention of urine and enuresis for example. Though clinically they are different, they can be caused by kidney deficiency. Therefore, both diseases can be treated with *Golden Chamber Kidney Qi Pills* (Jin Kui Shen Qi Wan) to warm kidney and strengthen

1 审证求机论治

审证求机就是要整体和动态地去分析疾病的各种复杂的征象，综合归纳推论出疾病发生发展的原因、病变的机制，从疾病的本质入手，从根本上加以治疗。只要解决了疾病的主要矛盾和关键环节，一切复杂问题就会迎刃而解。如同病异治和异病同治则是审证求机论治的体现。异病同治是指不同的疾病，若出现相同的病理变化，即形成相同的证候时，可以采取相同的治法。如癃闭和遗尿虽系两种临床表现截然不同的疾病，但皆可因肾虚引起，故皆可予金匮肾气丸温肾助阳，癃闭病可借金匮

yang. As for retention of urine, *Golden Chamber Kidney Qi Pills* (Jin Kui Shen Qi Wan) can help bladder to restore its function of steaming and transformation while for enuresis, *Golden Chamber Kidney Qi Pills* (Jin Kui Shen Qi Wan) can restore kidney qi and consolidate it.

肾气丸恢复膀胱气化功能，遗尿病则可借金匮肾气丸恢复肾气的固摄作用。

2 Distinguishing the Secondary and the Primary Symptoms; Distinguishing Acute Diseases and Chronic Diseases

The secondary symptoms and the primary symptoms are relative concepts and they indicate the major and minor conflicts during the pathological development. The primary symptoms are the major conflicts while the secondary symptoms, minor conflicts. For example: healthy qi is the primary and pathogenic qi is the secondary; causes are the primary while symptoms are the secondary; previous diseases are the primary while new diseases are the secondary; exterior diseases are the secondary while interior diseases are the primary; acute diseases are the secondary while chronic diseases are the primary. Disease usually go through a very complicated process in which pathogenic qi and healthy qi, excess and deficiency rival against each other; causes and symptoms can be acute or chronic; new diseases comes before the former is cured; exterior symptoms and interior symptoms co-exist. So, doctors have to make sure of the primary and the second symptoms, of its acuteness and chronicness to adopt the methods of "treatment focusing on relieving the secondary symptoms if it is acute and treatment focusing on relieving the primary symptoms if it is chronic" and "treatment focusing on relieving both

2 明辨标本缓急

标和本是一个相对的概念，它主要说明病变过程中矛盾的主次关系。本是事物的主要矛盾，标是事物的次要矛盾。如：正气与邪气，则正气为本，邪气为标；病因与症状，则病因为本，症状为标；先病与后病，则先病为本，后病为标；表病与里病，则里病为本，表病为标；病情的缓急，则急者为标，缓者为本。疾病的发生发展过程极其复杂，常常有邪正盛衰、病因病证缓急、旧病未愈新病又起、表证与里证同在等问题，在临证时必须分清疾病的标本主次、轻重缓急，而采取"急则治其标，缓则治其本"和"标本同治"的方法进行治疗，这就是明辨标本缓急治疗原则。在标本俱急的情况下，必须采取标本同治的原则。

the primary and the secondary symptoms". In case the primary and secondary symptoms are both acute, doctors should focus on relieving both of them.

3 Treating Diseases in a Specific Way

The origin and development of diseases are influenced by many factors such as weather, climate, region, environment and especially, patients' particular physical conditions. Therefore, all those factors should be taken into consideration and give proper treatments. That is called treatment in a specific way including considering the season, the location and the patients.

3 顺应异法方宜

疾病的发生、发展受多方面因素影响，如时令气候、地理环境等，尤其是患者的个体体质因素对疾病影响更大。因此，在治疗疾病时，必须根据季节、气候、地区、患者的体质、年龄等不同特点而选用适宜治疗方法，这就是顺应异法方宜的治疗原则，具体包括因时制宜、因地制宜、因人制宜三个方面。

4 Adjusting the Balance of the Whole

To adjust the balance of the whole, doctors should begin from adjusting yin and yang, and then restore and establish the balance between them by eliminating the excess and replenishing the deficiency. To eliminate the excess of yin and yang, doctors can use the methods of warming, clear awaying, excreting, purging. To replenish the deficiency of yin and yang, doctors should make sure of replenishing yin or replenishing yang.

To adjust the balance of the whole body also requires a proper implementation of different treating measures and formulas to prevent new imbalance. For example, when attacking the pathogenic factors, make sure not to hurt the healthy factors; when replenishing deficiency, make sure to eliminate the pathogenic factors; when clear awaying a-

4 调节整体平衡

调节整体平衡，可以从调整阴阳入手，恢复和建立相对平衡的阴阳关系，不外去其有余，补其不足两个方面。去其有余，即去其阴阳之偏盛，有温、清、利、下等各种具体治法；补其不足，即补其阴阳之偏衰，有补阴与补阳之不同。

调节整体平衡，还要求对各种治疗措施和方药的运用都适可而止，不可矫枉过正，以防机体出现新的不平衡。如攻邪时须注意勿伤正，补虚时注意勿留邪，清热注意不要伤阳，散寒注意不

way heat, make sure to protect yang; when dispersing cold, make sure to no not to hurt yin; when invigorating the spleen, make sure to protect the stomach.

要伤阴,补脾注意不要碍胃等。

5 Paying Attention to Regulating and Nursing

Appropriate regulation and nursing helps to restore healthy qi and dispelp athogenic qi and speed up the recovery. On the contrary, neglect in this respect will not only hinder the recovery but also lead to relapse due to improper diet and tiredness. Therefore, doctors should pay attention to regulation and nursing.

Regulation and nursing includes diet nursing, life nursing, mental nursing and herbstion nursing. All these should be under the guidance of pattern identification. Besides, mental nursing should not be overlooked because a good spirit helps recovery. Also inappropriate food and drink should be paid attention to. Along with herbstion, acupuncture and needling, tuina, cupping and hot herbsted compress can be administrated to strengthen curative effects.

5 重视调摄护理

恰当的调护,有利于正气的恢复、邪气的祛除和促进患者早日康复。忽视调摄护理,不仅会延误康复时间,还会出现“食复”、“劳复”等情况,以致病情反复。因此,必须重视调摄护理。

调摄护理的内容十分丰富,如饮食护理、生活护理、精神护理、服药护理等。这些护理措施同样是以辨证论治为指导的,因此也当辨证施护,随证而异。此外,还应重视精神护理,使患者保持心情舒畅;在饮食护理方面要注意忌宜;在配合药物治疗时,可加用如针灸、推拿、拔火罐、熨法等其他治疗护理方法,以增强治疗效果。

Specific Discussions

各论

Chapter 1 Lung System Diseases

第1章 肺系病证

Cold

感　冒

Cold is acommon exogenous disease caused by lung's failure to disperse and cleanse and disharmony between Wei (Defensive) Qi and exterior. Its clinical symptoms are stuffy nose, running nose, sneezing, coughing, headache, aversion to cold, fever, discomfort all around and floating pulse.

感冒是感受触冒风邪导致肺失宣肃，卫表不和的常见外感疾病，临床以鼻塞、流涕、喷嚏、咳嗽、头痛、恶寒、发热、全身不适、脉浮为其特征。

1　Etiology and Pathogenesis

1　病因病机

The six exogenous climatic pathogenic factors, along with epidemic infectious pathogenic factors take the advantage of body's defensive weakness to attack the lung, Wei (Defense) Phase, skin and hair, resulting in the lung's failure to disperse and cleanse and disharmondy of Wei (Defense) Phase and exterior.

外感六淫、时行疫毒，乘人体御邪能力不足之时，侵袭肺卫皮毛，以致肺失宣肃，卫表失和。

1.1　The Six Climatic Pathogenic factors and Infectious Pathogenic factors Attacks the Body

1.1　外感六淫、疫毒，侵袭人体

Of the six climatic pathogenic factors, the pathogenic wind is the leading cause, along with seasonal qi, attacks the human body and presents different symptoms. For instance, when wind-cold attacks, skin and hair block up and the lung qi fails

外感六淫以风邪为主因，在不同季节与当令之气相合伤人，而表现不同。常见风寒外袭，皮毛闭塞，肺气失宣；或风热犯表，皮毛疏泄

to be dispersed; or when wind-heat attacks the exterior, skin and hair discharge unsuccessfully and the lung fails to cleanse. In summer, it is often the case that wind and summer-heat along with dampness fail the lung to clear away and the spleen to transport. In autumn, wind-dryness attacks the exterior and the lung fluid is injured. But when epidemic and infectious pathogenic factors prevail, the situation can be worse and undecided and the diseases will be infectious or epidemic in any season.

不畅，肺失清肃；夏季多为风暑夹湿，卫表不和，肺气不清，脾胃失运；秋季常见风燥袭表，肺津受损。时行疫毒伤人，则病情重而多变，相互传染，广泛流行，不限于季节。

1.2 The Exogenous Pathogenic Factors invade when Healthy Qi Weakens, Wei (Defensive) Qi and Exterior Collapses due to improper life styles

People get cold when their lifestyles and dressing are impropriate, or when they are overtired and the healthy qi is consumed and injured, or when they do not adjust to climatic changes because at that time, the muscular striae of the skin loosens and the Wei (Defensive) Qi and the exterior weaken and the exogenous pathogenic factors invade. Those who were born with defects and not well regulated, who are old and weak, who are ill for long time and who are seriously injured, are easy to be affected by pathogenic factors due to weakness of the Wei (Defensive) Qi and the exterior. When cold last for a long time, it is known as cold due to weakness. Those who have had lung diseases and the lung Wei (Defense) Phase is poor in regulation are also prone to be affected by exogenous pathogenic factors. At that time, endogenous disease and exogenous diseases trigger each other.

1.2 生活起居失当，正气亏虚，卫表不固，外邪乘袭

若生活起居不当，衣着失宜；或劳作过度，正气耗伤；或气候变化，失于调节，以致腠理不密，卫表不固，外邪乘袭，遂致感冒。若先天不足，后天失调，或年老体衰，或久病、重病损伤，体质虚弱，卫表不固，稍有不慎，极易感邪，或感冒后迁延不已，缠绵难愈，则称之为虚体感冒。其他如肺经素有旧疾，肺卫调节功能低下，也易感受外邪，内外相引发病。

Pathological location of cold lies in Wei (Defensive) Qi, the exterior and lung. The pathogenic

感冒的病位在卫表肺系，外邪或从口鼻而入，或从

factors attack the lung-wei via nose and mouth, skin and hair, resulting in the disharmony between Wei (Defensive) Qi and the exterior and the lung's failure to disperse and cleanse. During the pathological development, symtoms might change. For example, if wind-cold is depressed and transformed into heat or if cold has transformed into heat before the exogenous cold is solved, then it will present the symptoms of simultaneous occurrence of cold and heat. If cold due to wind-heat or summer-heat dampness fails to be treated timely and correctly, congestion of interior heat will be generated. Those who are weak when they get cold are difficult to recover and prone to relapse.

皮毛内侵,侵犯肺卫,卫表不和,肺失宣肃。在病程中各证型可发生演变,如风寒郁而化热,或外寒未解而内已化热形成寒热错杂证;或风热、暑湿感冒失治误治,导致内热壅盛。虚体感冒者常缠绵难愈,反复不已。

2 Syndrome Differentiation and Treatment

2 辨证论治

2.1 Key Points of Syndrome Differentiation

2.1 辨治要点

To treat cold, doctors have to first distinguish cold due to wind-cold from cold due to wind-heat. To distinguish these two types of cold, doctors should identify how they are aversive to cold, how high the fever is, whether they sweat or not, have sore throat or not, and characteristics of their tongue and pulse. If it is cold in summer, doctors should distinguish whether it is due to the excess of summer-heat or the excess of summer-dampness. If it is cold due to weakness, doctors should know which the primary is and which the secondary is, pathogenic factors, healthy factors, deficiency and excess. Also along with clinical examinations, make sure there are no other diseases.

感冒首辨风寒与风热,主要从恶寒发热轻重,有汗无汗,有无咽痛及舌脉特点来辨别。暑月感冒辨暑热偏重与暑湿偏重,虚体感冒辨邪正虚实的主次,同时应结合临床辅助检查,以除外其他疾病。

In terms of treatment, doctors should start from relieving the exterior symptoms. Wind-cold syndromes should be relieved by sweating with pun-

治疗上当因势利导,从表而解。风寒证治以辛温发汗,风热证治以辛凉清解,暑

gent and warm herbs while wind-heat syndrome should be relieved by clear awaying with pungent and cold herbs. Syndromes of summer-heat with dampness can be treated by clear awaying the summer heat and relieving the exterior. If the symptoms of cold or heat are not evident, use pungent and moderate herbs. If there is alternate occurrence of cold and heat, treat by warming and clear awaying together. For those who have food retention, add some herbs of promoting digestion and for those with phlegm dampness, resolve the dampness and eliminate phlegm. Invigorating and astringent herbs should be avoided usually in case the pathogenic factors cannot be eliminated except for those who have cold due to weakness and whose healthy qi needs strengthening and deficiency needs replenishing. Those with cold due to weakness must not be force to sweat with very pungent and dispersing herbs because in such a way, the healthy qi will be serious injured. Therefore, herbs of invigorating the healthy qi can be used along with dispersing herbs to strengthen the heatlhy qi as well as reach the pathogenic factors. If the pathogenic factors are so serious as to invade inside, attacking the lung and transmit reversely into the pericardium, the patients should be treated according to syndrome differentiation and Treatment of epidemic febrile disease.

湿证治以清暑解表。若寒热之象不显，可选辛平之剂；寒热错杂，可温清并施；夹食滞者，加消导之品；夹痰湿者，应化湿祛痰；除虚体感冒兼顾扶正补虚以外，一般忌用补敛之品以防留邪。虚体感冒临证治疗不可过于辛散，强发其汗，重伤正气，应扶正达邪，在疏散药中酌加补正之品。若感邪较重化热入里犯肺，逆传心包，当以温病辨治原则处理。

2.2 Therapeutic Methods for Different Patterns

2.2 分型论治

2.2.1 Syndromes of the Exterior Restrained by Wind-cold

2.2.1 风寒束表证

Manifestations: Great aversion to cold, low fever, no sweat, headache, sore limbs and joints, heavy nasal sound or sneeze due to itch in the nose with clear away thin discharge sometimes, itch in

证候：恶寒重，发热轻，无汗，头痛，肢节酸疼，鼻塞声重或鼻痒喷嚏，时流清涕，咽痒，咳嗽，痰稀薄色白，口

the throat, cough, white thin phlegm, no thirst or preference to hot for drinks, white thin moist tongue fur, tense floating pulse.

不渴或渴喜热饮。舌苔薄白而润,脉浮紧。

Treatment: To relieve the exterior with pungent and warm herbs.

治法: 辛温解表。

Formulas and Herbs: *Herba Schizonepetae and Saposhnikoviae Radix Reaching Exterior Decoction* (Jing Fang Da Biao Tang), usually composed of *Schizonepetae Herba* (Jing Jie), *Saposhnikoviae Radix*(Fang Feng), *Perillae Folium*(Zi Su Ye), *Angelicae Dahuricae Radix*(Bai Zhi), *Zingiberis Rhizoma Recens* (Sheng Jiang), *Shallots* (Cong Tou).

方药: 荆防达表汤。常用荆芥、防风、苏叶、白芷、生姜、葱头疏风散寒。

Modification: For cold-wind complicated with dampness, heavy headache, sore muscles and joints and white thick tongue fur, dispel wind, disperse cold and eliminate dampness with *Schizonepetae Herba and Saposhnikoviae Radix Detoxifying Power* (Jing Fang Bai Du San); for severe exterior cold, great pain in the head and body, no sweating, use *Ephedrae Herba Decoction* (Ma Huang Tang) to disperse cold to relieve the exterior; for hidden dampness in the center, abdominal fullness and distention, poor appetite, loose stool, white thick tongue fur, add *Atractylodis Rhizoma* (Cang Zhu), *Magnoliae Officinalis Cortex* (Hou Pu), *Pinelliae Rhizoma* (Ban Xia) to resolve dampness and harmonize the center.

加减: 若风寒夹湿,头痛重,肌肉关节酸痛,苔白腻者,用荆防败毒散疏风散寒祛湿;若表寒重,头身痛,憎寒发热,无汗者,用麻黄汤散寒解表;若湿邪蕴中,脘痞,食少,便溏,苔白腻者,加苍术、厚朴、半夏化湿和中。

2.2.2 Syndromes of Wind-heat Attacking the Exterior

2.2.2 风热犯表证

Manifestations: Fever, slight aversion to cold, obstructed sweating, distending pain in the head, red face, cough, sticky or yellow phlegm, dry throat or swollen tonsils, stuffy nose with yellow turbid discharge, thirst, yellowish white thin tongue fur with red tongue tips and sides, rapid floating

证候: 身热较著,微恶风,汗出不畅,头胀痛,面赤,咳嗽,痰黏或黄,咽燥,或咽喉乳蛾红肿疼痛,鼻塞,流黄浊涕,口干欲饮。舌苔薄白微黄,舌边尖红,脉浮数。

pulse.

Treatment: To relieve the exterior with pungent and cool herbs.

治法: 辛凉解表。

Formulas and Herbs: *Lonicera and Forsythia Powder* (Yin Qiao San), usually composed of *Forsythiae Fructus* (Lian Qiao), *Sojae Semen Praeparatum* (Dan Dou Chi), *Menthae Haplocalycis Herba* (Bo He), *Lophatheri Herba* (Dan Zhu Ye), *Platycodi Radix*(Jie Geng)and *Glycyrrhizae Radix et Rhizoma* (Gan Cao) to relieve the exterior with pungent and cool medica; *Lonicerae Japonicae Flos*(Jin Yin Hua), *Phragmitis Rhiamoma* (Lu Gen) and *Amomi Fructus*(Niu Bang Zi) to clear heat and detoxify.

方药: 银翘散。常用连翘、淡豆豉、薄荷、淡竹叶、桔梗、甘草辛凉解表;金银花、芦根、牛蒡子清热解毒。

Modification: For wind-heat attacking the exterior, retention of lung qi, with symptoms of headache and fever, no or little sweating and slight aversion to cold, cough and dry throat, restlessness and thirst, use Chinese Green Onion Stalk, *Sojae Semen Praeparatum* and *Platycodi Radix Decoction* (Cong Chi Jie Geng Tang); for predominant lung heat constrained by wind-cold, heat blocked by cold, with symptoms of disturbing heat and aversion to cold, little sweating, cough with short breath, thick phlegm, coarse throat, use *Ephedra, Apricot, Gypsum Fibrosum and Liquorice Decoction* (Ma Xing Shi Gan Tang); for infectious cold due to febrile heat, with symptoms of high fever and great aversion to cold, ache in the head and body, swollen throat and tonsil, cough with ranting, add *Isatisdis Folium* (Da Qing Ye), *Taraxaci Herba* (Pu Gong Ying) and *Paridis Rhizoma* (Cao He Che) to clear away heat and detoxify.

加减: 若风热袭表,肺气不宣者,头痛身热,微寒无汗,或有汗不多,咳嗽咽干,心烦口渴,用葱豉桔梗汤清宣解表;若肺热素盛,风寒外束,热为寒遏,烦热恶寒,少汗,咳嗽气急,痰稠,声哑者,可用麻杏石甘汤,内清肺热,外散表寒;时行感冒热毒较盛,壮热恶寒,头痛身痛,咽喉肿痛,咳嗽气粗,配大青叶、蒲公英、草河车等清热解毒。

2.2.3 Syndromes of Summer-Heat and Dampness Attacking the Exterior

Manifestations: Fever, slight aversion to wind, heavy or sore limbs, heavy and distending sensation of the head, cough with sticky phlegm, turbid nasal discharge, restlessness, thirst or sticky in the mouth, thirst but no desire for drink, suppression in the chest and abdominal fullness and, nausea, loose stool, scanty reddish urine, yellow thin tongue fur, soft floating pulse.

Treatment: To clear away the summer-heat and eliminate the dampness to relieve the exterior.

Formulas and Herbs: *Newly Added Moslae Herba Drink*(Xin Jia Xiang Ru Yin), usually composed of *Lonicerae Japonicae Flos* (Jin Yin Hua), *Forsythiae Fructus* (Lian Qiao), *Nelumbinis Folium*(He Ye) fresh, *Phragmitis Rhiamoma* (Lu Gen) fresh to clear away the summer-heat; *Moslae Herba* (Xiang Ru) to enable sweating; and *Magnoliae Officinalis Cortex* (Hou Pu), *Lablab Semen Album* (Bai Bian Dou) to transform the dampness and harmonize the center.

Modification: For predominance of summer-heat, add *Coptidis Rhizoma* (Huang Lian), *Gardeniae Fructus* (Zhi Zi), *Scutellariae Radix* (Huang Qin), *Artemisiae Annuae Herba* (Qing Hao) to clear away and purge the summer-heat; for Wei (Defensive) Qi and the exterior trapped by dampness and heavy limb soreness, add *Pogostemonis Herba* (Huo Xiang), *Eupatorii Herba* (Pei Lan) to relieve the exterior; for predominance of dampness, with symptoms of sticky in the mouth, suppression in the chest and abdominal distention, abdominal fullness and loose stool, add *Atractylodis Rhizoma*

2.2.3 暑湿伤表证

证候: 身热,微恶风,汗少,肢体酸重疼痛,头昏重胀痛,咳嗽痰黏,鼻流浊涕,心烦口渴,或口中黏腻,渴不多饮,胸闷脘痞,泛恶,腹胀,大便溏,小便短赤。舌苔薄黄而腻,脉濡数。

治法: 清暑祛湿解表。

方药: 新加香薷饮。常用金银花、连翘、鲜荷叶、鲜芦根清暑解热;香薷发汗解表;厚朴、白扁豆化湿和中。

加减: 若暑热偏盛,加黄连、栀子、黄芩、青蒿清暑泄热;若湿困卫表,肢体酸重疼痛较甚,加藿香、佩兰等芳化宣表;若里湿偏盛,口中黏腻,胸闷脘痞,腹胀便溏,加苍术、白豆蔻、半夏、陈皮和中化湿;小便短赤加滑石、甘草、赤茯苓清热利湿。

(Cang Zhu), *Amomi Fructus Rotundus(Dou Kou)*, *Pinelliae Rhizoma* (Ban Xia), *Citri Reticulatae Pericarpium* (Chen Pi) to harmonize zhong jiao and resolve the dampness; for scanty and reddish urine, add *Talcum* (Hua Shi), *Glycyrrhizae Radix et Rhizoma* (Gan Cao) and *Poria* (Fu Ling) to clear away the heat and excrete dampness.

2.2.4 Syndromes of Cold due to Qi Deficiency

Manifestations: Great aversion to cold, fever, no sweat, headache and discomfort in the body, cough, white phlegm, too weak to cough up phlegm, weak and tired all the time, short breath and no desire to talk, relapse; pale tongue and thin tongue fur; weak floating pulse.

Treatment: To invigorate qi to relieve the exterior.

Formulas and Herbs: *Codonopsis Radix and Perillae Foliume* Drink (Shen Su Yin), usually composed of *Codonopsis Radix* (Dang Shen), *Glycyrrhizae Radix et Rhizoma* (Gan Cao), *Poria* (Fu Ling) to invigorate and strengthen the healthy qi and *Perillae Folium* (Zi Su Ye), *Puerariae Lobatae Radix* (Ge Gen), *Puerariae Lobatae Radix* (Qian Hu) to disperse the wind to relieve the exterior; *Pinelliae Rhizoma* (Ban Xia), *Citri Reticulatae Pericarpium* (Chen Pi), *Aurantii Fructus* (Zhi Qiao) and *Platycodi Radix* (Jie Geng) to disperse lung qi, resolve phlegm and stop coughing.

Modification: For great aversion to cold, low fever, cold limbs, low voice, pale and plump tongue, deep weak fine pulse, which is affection by exogenous factors due to yang deficiency, use *Rebuilding Powder* (Zai Zao San) to strengthen yang to relieve the exterior; for spontaneous perspira-

2.2.4 气虚感冒证

证候: 恶寒较甚,发热,无汗,头痛身楚,咳嗽,痰白,咯痰无力,平素神疲体弱,气短懒言,反复易感。舌淡苔白,脉浮而无力。

治法: 益气解表。

方药: 参苏饮。常用党参、甘草、茯苓补气扶正;苏叶、葛根、前胡疏风解表;半夏、陈皮、枳壳、桔梗宣肺化痰止咳。

加减: 若恶寒重,发热轻,四肢欠温,语音低微,舌质淡胖,脉沉细无力,为阳虚外感,用再造散助阳解表。平时自汗,易反复感冒者,可常服玉屏风散以益气固表,以

tion, ready to catch colds, use regularly *Jade screen Powder* (Yu Ping Feng San) to consolidate qi and strengthen the exterior.

防感冒。

2.2.5 Syndromes of Cold Due to Yin Deficiency

Manifestations: Fever, slight aversion to wind and cold, little sweating, dizziness, restless, thirst, dry cough and little phlegm; red tongue with little tongue fur; deep fine pulse.

Treatment: To nourish yin to relieve the exterior.

Formulas and Herbs: *Modified Polygonatum Decoction* (Jia Jian Wei Rui Tang), usually composed of *Polygonati Odorati Rhizoma* (Yu Zhu) to nourish yin and replenish the source of sweat; *Sojae Semen Praeparatum* (Dan Dou Chi), *Menthae Haplocalycis Herba* (Bo He), *Bulbus Allii Fistulosi* (Cong Bai), *Platycodi Radix* (Jie Geng) to disperse the exterior and pathogenic factors; *Cynanchi Atrati Radix et Rhizoma* (Bai Wei) to clear away the heat and harmonize yin, *Glycyrrhizae Radix et Rhizoma* (Gan Cao) and *Jujubae Fructus* (Da Zao) to moist and harmonize the center.

Modification: For predominance of yin deficiency, thirst and dry throat, add *Glehniae Radix* (Bei Sha Shen), *Ophiopogonis Radix* (Mai Men Dong) to nourish yin and produce body fluid; for predominance of blood deficiency, paleness, light lip and nail color and fine pulse, add *Rehmannia Radix* (Di Huang) and *Angelicae Sinensis Radix* (Dang Gui) to nourish yin and nourish blood.

2.2.5 阴虚感冒证

证候：身热，微恶风寒，少汗，头昏，心烦，口干，干咳少痰。舌红少苔，脉细数。

治法：滋阴解表。

方药：加减葳蕤汤。常用玉竹滋阴以资汗源；淡豆豉、薄荷、葱白、桔梗疏表散邪；白薇清热和阴；甘草、大枣甘润和中。

加减：若阴虚明显，口渴咽干，加沙参、麦门冬滋阴生津；若血虚明显，面色无华，唇甲色淡，脉细，加地黄、当归滋阴养血。

Cough

Cough is due to lung's failure to disperse resul-

咳　嗽

咳嗽是指肺失宣降，肺

ting in the upward flow of lung qi and cough with sound, phlegm and sputum. It is an independent diseases as well as a main symptom of lung diseases.

气上逆作声,咯吐痰液而言,既是独立的病证,又是肺系疾病的主要症状之一。

1 Etiology and Pathogenesis

1 病因病机

Cough can be divided into exogenous cough and endogenous cough. The former is due to lung's being attacked by six climaticed exogenous factors and the latter, due to dysfunction of zang-fu organs and lung's being attacked by exogenous pathogenic factors. Regardless of exogenous factors or endogenous factors, both of them can disenable the lung to disperse and lung qi flow upward causing cough.

咳嗽的病因有外感、内伤两大类,外感咳嗽为六淫外邪侵袭肺系;内伤咳嗽为脏腑功能失调,内邪干肺。无论邪从外入,或是自内而发,均可引起肺失宣肃,肺气上逆作咳。

1.1 Six Climatic Exogenous Factors Attacking the Lung

1.1 外感六淫,侵袭肺系

Extreme weather with irregular cold and heat resulting in dysfunction of Wei (Defensive) Qi's can make it possible for the exogenous pathogenic factor attacks the lung through nose, mouth, skin and hair, disenabling the lung to disperse and resulting in cough. Or inhalation of smog and smelly gases depresses the lung qi and brings about the lung's failure to disperse, causing cough.

天气冷热失常,卫外功能失调,六淫之邪从口鼻或皮毛入内,侵袭肺系,肺失宣肃为咳。或吸入烟尘、异味气体,肺气被郁,肺失宣肃为咳。

1.2 Uncontrolled Diet and Turbid Phlegm Attacking the Lung

1.2 饮食不节,痰浊犯肺

Uncontrolled diet or excessive eating, drinking and smoking scorches the lung and the stomach. Too much pungent, spicy, greasy, sweaty, hot food result in dampness and phlegm while too raw cold food hurts the stomach and the spleen, resulting in phlegm-dampness. Prolonged deficiency of stomach and the spleen rsulting in failure to control the transportation and transformation of water and food can lead to turbid phlegm. The phlegm-qi moves up-

饮食不节,或嗜食烟酒,熏灼肺胃;或过食辛辣肥甘炙煿,酿湿生痰;或过食生冷,损伤脾胃,痰湿内生;或脾胃素虚,运化失司,痰浊内生。痰气上干于肺,肺气上逆为咳。

ward to the lung which flows upward causing cough.

1.3 Disorder of the Mind and Spirit Causing Qi-fire Attacking the Lung

Depression and annoyance suppresses the lung qi which in turn transforms into fireand the fire attacks the lung causing cough.

1.3 情志失调，气火逆肺

抑郁恼怒，肝失条达，气郁化火犯肺为咳。

1.4 Lung Deficiency Due to Prolonged Diseases and Qi Flows Upward

Prolonged lung diseases hurt qi-yin. Asthenia-fire and cold phlegm grow inside and lung qi flows upward causing cough.

Cough mostly results from the lung but is also related to the liver and the spleen, the kidney as well if prolonged. Cough due to exogenous factors doesn't last long and it is sthenia, while cough due to endogenous factors lasts long and tends to relapse often. Phlegm and fire are the usual etiological factors and the co-existence of asthenia of healthy qi and sthenia of pathogenic factors is its etiological nature. Cough due to exogenous factors and cough due to endogenous factors can be inter-determined.

1.4 久病肺虚，气机上逆

肺病迁延，气阴耗伤，虚火寒痰内生，肺气上逆为咳。

咳嗽的主脏在肺，与肝、脾有关，久则及肾。外感咳嗽病程短属实，内伤咳嗽病程长，常反复发作，病理因素主要是痰与火，病理性质属邪实和正虚并见。外感咳嗽与内伤咳嗽又可互为因果。

2 Syndrome Differentiation and Treatment

2.1 Key Points of Syndrome Differentiation

Cough should be firstly identified as cough due to exogenous factors or due to endogenous factors by time and rhythmicity of the cough, aggravating factors, and the color, nature, quantity, smell of phlegm. Cough due to exogenous factors is mostly a new disease which comes and goes quickly with the exterior symptoms of lung defensive Qi such as cold and fever, headache, stuffy nose, which belong to sthenia of pathogenic factors. In contrast, cough due to endogenous factors starts gradually and last

2 辨证论治

2.1 辨治要点

咳嗽首辨外感与内伤。可从咳的时间、节律、加重因素及痰的色、质、量、味等特点来辨。外感咳嗽多是新病，起病急，病程短，初起多兼有寒热、头痛、鼻塞等肺卫表证，多属邪实。内伤咳嗽，起病慢，往往有较长的咳嗽病史，常兼他脏病证。由他脏及肺者，多因邪实导致正

long usually with a history of cough and diseases in other organs. If lung is affected by other organs, mostly it is that sthenia of pathogenic factors results in asthenia of healthy qi. If lung diseases already exist, it is mostly that asthenia results in sthenia.

虚;肺脏自病者,多因虚致实。

Cough due to exogenous factors of sthenia should be treated by eliminating pathogenic factors and restoring the lung's function. In light of the pathogenic nature, give treatment of dispelling wind, dispersing cold, clear awaying away heat and moisturizing dryness respectively. Cough due to endogenous factors of asthenia should be treated by eliminating pathogenic factors, stopping cough, strengthening healthy qi and replenishing deficiency to relieve both the secondary and the primary symptoms according to the relative predominance of sthenia or asthenia. Cough should be treated in a holistic way in which treatment of the spleen, the liver and the kidney should also be considered in addition to the lung. At the initial treatment, convergent herbs ought to be avoided to eliminate the pathogenic factors. Instead, make the best to improve the smoothness of lung qi to stop cough. For prolonged cough, eliminate the pathogenic factors to stop the cough, strengthen the healthy qi and replenish deficiency to relieve both the secondary and the primary symptoms.

外感咳嗽属实,治当祛邪利肺,按病邪性质分别予疏风、散寒、清热、润燥治法;内伤咳嗽多属于邪实正虚,治以祛邪止咳,扶正补虚,按虚实的主次标本兼顾。咳嗽的治疗,除直接治肺外,还应从整体出发,注意治脾、治肝、治肾等。咳嗽初期一般忌敛涩留邪,当因势利导,肺气宣畅则咳嗽自止;咳嗽日久,祛邪止咳,扶正补虚,标本兼顾。

2.2 Therapeutic Methods for Different Patterns

2.2 分型论治

2.2.1 Wind-cold Attacking the Lung

2.2.1 风寒袭肺证

Manifestations: bad cough with sound, short of breath, itching throat, thin and whitish phlegm, often with stuffy nose and clear away discharge, sore limb or severe aversion to cold and fever, no sweating; thin white tongue fur; floating tense

证候: 咳嗽声重,气急,咽痒,痰稀薄色白,常伴有鼻塞,流清涕,肢体酸楚,或见恶寒发热,无汗等表证。舌苔薄白,脉浮紧。

pulse.

Treatment: To dispel wind and disperse cold; disperse the lung and stop cough.

治法：疏风散寒，宣肺止咳。

Formulas and Herbs: *Rough and Ready Three Decoction* (San Ao Tang), usually usually composed of *Ephedrae Herba* (Ma Huang), *Armeniacae Semen Amaru* (Xing Ren) and *Glycyrrhizae Radix et Rhizoma* (Gan Cao) to disperse the lung and cold.

方药：三拗汤。常用麻黄、杏仁、甘草宣肺散寒。

Modification: For prolonged cough, use *Cough Stopping Power* (Zhi Ke San) to dispel wind and moisturize the lung; for cough complicated with phlegm-dampness with thick phlegm, chest suppression, grimy tongue fur, add *Pinelliae Rhizoma* (Ban Xia), *Magnoliae Officinalis Cortex* (Hou Po), *Poria* (Fu Ling) to moisturize dryness and resolve phlegm; for unrelieved exterior cold and suppressed interior heat, hoarse cough, thick phlegm, thirst, restlessness or fever, use *Ephedra, Apricot, Gypsum Fibrosum and Liquorice Decoction* (Ma Xing Shi Gan Tang) should be used to relieve the exterior and clear away heat.

加减：若咳嗽迁延不愈，用止嗽散疏风润肺；若夹痰湿，咳而痰黏、胸闷、苔腻者，加半夏、厚朴、茯苓以燥湿化痰；若表寒未解，里有郁热，咳而音哑，痰黏稠，口渴，心烦，或身热，用麻杏石甘汤解表清里。

2.2.2 Wind-heat Attacking the Lung

2.2.2 风热犯肺证

Manifestations: Frequent bad cough, ranting, sore throat, difficult expectoration, thick or yellow phlegm, sweating while coughing, often with yellow nasal discharge, thirst, headache, aversion to wind, fever; thin yellow tongue fur; rapid floating pulse.

证候：咳嗽频剧，气粗，咽痛，咯痰不爽，痰黏稠或稠黄，咳时汗出，常伴鼻流黄涕，口渴，头痛，肢楚，恶风，身热等表证。舌苔薄黄，脉浮数。

Treatment: To dispel wind and clear away heat; disperse the lung and resolve phlegm.

治法：疏风清热，宣肺化痰。

Formulas and Herbs: *Mulberry and Chrysanthemum Cool Decoction* (Sang Ju Yin), usually usually composed of *Chrysanthemi Flos* (Ju Hua), *Menthae Haplocalycis Herba* (Bo He) to disperse and clear a-

方药：桑菊饮。常用菊花、薄荷宣透风热；杏仁、桔梗、甘草轻宣肺气，祛痰止咳；连翘、芦根清热生津。

way wind-heat, *Armeniacae Semen Amaru* (Ku Xing Ren), *Platycodi Radix*(Jie Geng), *Glycyrrhizae Radix et Rhizoma* (Gan Cao) to disperse lightly lung qi and eliminate phlegm to stop cough, *Forsythiae Fructus* (Lian Qiao), *Phragmitis Rhiamoma* (Lu Gen) to clear away heat and generate body fluid.

Modification: For exuberant interior pathogenic heat, fever and thirst, add *Scutellariae Radix* (Huang Qin), *Anemarrhenae Rhizoma* (Zhi Mu) to clear away and purge lung-heat; for severe sore throat, add *Belamecandae Rhizoma* (She Gan), *Calyx Persistenes seu Fructus Physalis Franchetii* (Gua Jin Deng), *Paeoniae Radix Rubra* (Chi Shao) to clear away heat and relieve sore throat; for lung fluid injured by heat, dry throat and throat, add *Adenophorae Radix* (Nan Sha Shen), *Trichosanthis Radix*(Tian Hua Fen), *Phragmitis Rhiamoma* (Lu Gen) to clear away heat and generate body fluid.

加减：若热邪内盛，身热口渴明显者，加黄芩、知母清泄肺热；咽痛明显加射干、挂金灯、赤芍清热利咽；若热伤肺津，咽燥口干，加南沙参、天花粉、芦根清热生津。

2.2.3 Wind-dryness Attacking the Lung

Manifestations: Dry cough, choke after continued cough, itching throat, sore and dry throat, dry mouth and nose, no phlegm or little threadlike phlegm, difficult expectoration, or phlegm with blood, thirst, initially with stuffy nose, headache, slight aversion to cold, fever; thin white or thin yellow tongue fur, scarlet dry tongue; floating and rapid pulse or a little rapid.

Treatment: To disperse wind and clear away the lung; moisturize dryness to stop cough.

Formulas and Herbs: *Mori Folium and Armeniacae Semen Amaru Decoction* (Sang Xing Tang), usually with *Mori Folium* (Sang Ye) and *Sojae Semen Praeparatum* (Dou Chi) to relieve exterior with

2.2.3 风燥伤肺

证候：干咳，连声作呛，喉痒，咽喉干痛，唇鼻干燥，无痰或痰少而黏连成丝，不易咯出，或痰中带有血丝，口干，初起或伴鼻塞、头痛、微寒、身热等表证。舌苔薄白或薄黄，舌质红干而少津，脉浮数或小数。

治法：疏风清肺，润燥止咳。

方药：桑杏汤。常用：桑叶、豆豉辛凉解表、轻宣燥热之邪，配山栀清泄肺热；杏仁、川贝母宣肺化痰止咳；沙

pungent-cool herbs to lightly disperse pathogenic dry-heat along with *Gardeniae Fructus* (Zhi Zi) to clear away lung-heat; *Armeniacae Semen Amaru* (Ku Xing Ren), *Fritillariae Cirrhosae Bulbus* (Chuan Bei Mu) to disperse lung, resolve phlegm and stop cough; *Glehniae Radix(Bei Sha Shen)* and *Pear Peel* (Li Pi) to nourish yin, moisturize the lung and generate body fluid.

参、梨皮养阴润肺生津。

Modification: For evident dry-heat, add *Ophiopogonis Radix* (Mai Men Dong), *Anemarrhenae Rhizoma* (Zhi Mu), *Gypsum Fibrosum Fibrosum* (Shi Gao) to clear away the lung and purge heat; for phlegm with blood and epistaxis, add *Imperatae Rhizoma* (Bai Mao Gen), *Moutan Cortex* (Mu Dan Pi) and *Rehmannia Radix* (Sheng Di Huang) to clear away heat and stop blood; for coexistence of dry syndromes and wind-cold with dry cough, no or little phlegm, dry throat and nose along with aversion to cold, fever, headache, no sweating, thin white dry tongue fur, use *Apricot Kernel and Perilla Powder* (Xing Su San) to disperse lung, expel cold and stop cough in a warm and not dry way.

加减：燥热现象明显者，加麦门冬、知母、石膏清肺泄热；痰中夹血或鼻衄，加白茅根、牡丹皮、生地黄清热止血；燥证与风寒并见，表现为干咳、少痰或无痰、咽干鼻燥，兼有恶寒发热、头痛无汗、舌苔薄白而干，用杏苏散宣肺散寒止咳、温而不燥。

2.2.4 Phlegm-dampness Accumulated in the Lung

Manifestations: Frequent heavy cough with noise, plenty of phlegm which is sticky or thick or thin and aggravates particularly in the early morning, cough relieved after phlegm spit, suppressed chest, abdominal fullness, nausea and little in-take, loose stool, white and greasy tongue fur, soft and rolling pulse.

Treatment: To dry the dampness and resolve phlegm; regulate the flow of qi and stop cough.

Formulas and Herbs: *Er chen Decoction* (Er Chen Tang) and *Three-Seed Filial Devotion*

2.2.4 痰湿蕴肺

证候：反复咳嗽痰多，咳声重浊，痰白黏腻或稠厚或稀薄，每于晨间咳痰尤甚，因痰而嗽，痰出则咳缓，胸闷，脘痞腹胀，呕恶食少，大便时溏。舌苔白腻，脉濡滑。

治法：燥湿化痰，理气止咳。

方药：二陈汤合三子养亲汤。常用：半夏、茯苓燥湿

Decoction (San Zi Yang Qin Tang), usually usually composed of *Pinelliae Rhizoma* (Ban Xia), *Poria* (Fu Ling) to dry dampness and resolve phlegm; *Citri Reticulatae Pericarpium* (Chen Pi), *Glycyrrhizae Radix et Rhizoma* (Gan Cao) to regulate the flow of qi and harmonize zhong jiao, and *Sinapis Semen* (Jie Zi), *Perillae Fructus* (Su Zi), *Raphani Semen* (Lai Fu zi) to help qi descending, phlegm resolving and digestion.

化痰；陈皮、甘草理气和中；白芥子、苏子、莱菔子降气化痰消食。

Modification: For severe phlegm-dampness, cough with thick phlegm, abdominal fullness, greasy fur, add *Atractylodis Rhizoma* (Cang Zhu) and *Magnoliae Officinalis Cortex* (Hou Pu) to help to dry dampness and resolve phlegm; for severe phlegm-cold, sticky white foaming phlegm, aversion to cold, add *Zingiberis Rhizoma* (Gan Jiang) and *Asari Radix et Rhizoma* (Xi Xin) to warm the lung and resolve phlegm; for prolonged illness and spleen deficiency, tiredness, add moderately *Codonopsis Radix* (Dang Shen) and *Atractylodis Macrocephalae Rhizoma* (Bai Zhu) to strengthen qi and spleen and take *Six Nobles Pill* (Liu Jun Zi Wan) after symptoms are relieved.

加减：若痰湿较重，咳而痰多稠厚，胸闷，脘痞，苔腻，加苍术、厚朴以增强燥湿化痰之力；若寒痰较重，痰黏白如沫，怕冷者，加干姜、细辛温肺化痰；久病脾虚，神倦，酌加党参、白术益气健脾，症状平稳后可服六君子丸。

2. 2. 5 Phlegm-heat Accumulated in the Lung

2. 2. 5 痰热郁肺

Manifestations: Cough with hoarse and short breath, sound of phlegm in the throat, plenty of sticky and thick phlegm or thick yellow phlegm, difficult expectoration, hot stinking smell or blood expectoration, distention in the chest and pain in the chest while coughing, flushed face, fever, dry mouth and thirsty; red tongue; yellow thin greasy tongue fur; rapid rolling pulse.

证候：咳嗽气息粗促，或喉中有痰声，痰多质黏厚或稠黄，咯吐不爽，或有热腥味，或吐血痰，胸胁胀满，咳时引痛，面赤，或有身热，口干欲饮。舌质红，苔薄黄腻，脉滑数。

Treatment: To clear away heat and purify the lung; resolve phlegm and stop cough.

治法：清热肃肺，豁痰止咳。

Formulas and Herbs: *Metal-Clarifying and Phlegm-Resolving Decoction* (Qing Jin Hua Tan Tang), usually composed of *Mori Cortex* (Sang Bai Pi), *Scutellariae Radix* (Huang Qin), *Gardeniae Fructus* (Zhi Zi), *Anemarrhenae Rhizoma* (Zhi Mu) to purge the lung-heat; *Fritillariae Thunbergii Bulbus* (Zhe Bei Mu), *Trichosanthis Fructus* (Gua Lou), *Platycodi Radix* (Jie Geng), *Ophiopogonis Radix* (Mai Men Dong), *Poria* (Fu Ling) and *Glycyrrhizae Radix et Rhizoma* (Gan Cao) to resolve phlegm-heat.

方药: 清金化痰汤。常用:桑白皮、黄芩、山栀、知母清泄肺热;象贝母、瓜蒌、桔梗、麦门冬、茯苓、甘草化痰热。

Modification: For yellow pyoid or stinking phlegm, add moderately *Houttuyniae Herba* (Yu Xing Cao), *Rhizoma Fagopyri Cymosi* (Jin Qiao Mai Gen), *Coicis Semen* (Yi Yi Ren) and *Semen Benincasae* (Dong Gua Zi) to clear away heat, resolve phlegm and detoxify; for distention in the chest and severe cough and constipation, add *Descurainiae Semen Lepidii Semen* (Ting Li Zi) and *Rhei Radix et Rhizoma* (Da Huang) to purge the lung and dispel phlegm; for phlegm-heat injuring body fluid, add moderately *Adenophorae Radix* (Nan Sha Shen), *Asparagi Radix* (Tian Dong) and *Trichosanthis Radix* (Tian Hua Fen) to nourish yin and generate body fluid.

加减: 痰黄如脓或腥臭,酌加鱼腥草、金荞麦根、薏苡仁、冬瓜子清热化痰解毒;胸满咳逆,便秘,配葶苈子、大黄泻肺逐痰;痰热伤津,酌加南沙参、天门冬、天花粉养阴生津。

2.2.6 Liver-fire Invading the Lung

Manifestations: Paroxysmal cough with upward flow of qi, flushed face while coughing, dry throat and bitter mouth, feeling phlegm stuck in the throat, difficult expectoration, little phlegm but sticky, distending pain in the chest and hypochondria while coughing which aggravates and lessens with mood changes; red tongue; thin yellow tongue fur with little moisture; taut and rapid pulse.

2.2.6 肝火犯肺

证候: 上气咳逆阵作,咳时面红,咽干口苦,常感痰滞咽喉,咯之难出,量少质黏,胸胁胀痛,咳时引痛,症状可随情绪波动增减。舌质红,舌苔薄黄少津,脉弦数。

Treatment: To clear away the lung and purge the liver; regulate the flow of qi and subtract the pathogenic fire.

治法： 清肺泻肝，顺气降火。

Formulas and Herbs: *Clearing Away Lung Heat Powder* (Xie Bai San) combined with *Indigo Naturalis and Meretricis Concha Cyclinae ConchaPowder* (Dai Ha San), usually composed of *Mori Cortex* (Sang Bai Pi), *Lycii Cortex* (Di Gu Pi), *Scutellariae Radix* (Huang Qin) are often used to clear away the lung and purge the fire; *Indigo Naturalis* (Qing Dai) and *Meretricis Concha Cyclinae Concha* (Ha Ke) to purge the liver and resolve phlegm; *Glycyrrhizae Radix et Rhizoma* (Gan Cao) and *Semen Oryza Sativae* (Jing Mi) are used to resolve phlegm and stop cough.

方药： 泻白散合黛蛤散。常用：桑白皮、地骨皮、黄芩清肺泻火，青黛、蛤壳清肝化痰；甘草、粳米化痰止咳。

Modification: For predominate heat and flushed face and congested eyes, add *Gardeniae Fructus* (Zhi Zi), *Moutan Cortex* (Mu Dan Pi), *Scutellariae Radix* (Huang Qin) to clear away the lung and purge the liver; for sticky phlegm and difficult expectoration, add *Bryozoatum* (Hai Fu Shi), *Fritillariae Bulbus* (Bei Mu), *Trichosanthis Fructus* (Gua Lou) to clear away heat and resolve phlegm; for suppressed chest and upward flow of qi, add *Aurantii Fructus* (Zhi Qiao) and *Inulae Flos* (Xuan Fu Hua) to regulate the lung qi and reverse the upward movement of qi.

加减： 火热较盛，面赤目赤者，加山栀、牡丹皮、黄芩清肝泻火；痰黏难咯，加海浮石、贝母、瓜蒌清热化痰；胸闷气逆，加枳壳、旋覆花利肺降逆。

2.2.7 Deficiency and Exhaustion of Lung-yin

2.2.7 肺阴亏耗

Manifestations: Dry and short cough, phlegm with blood, or gradually hoarse throat, dry mouth and throat, feverish sensation in the afternoon, red cheeks, night sweating, emaciation, fatigue; red tongue with little tongue fur; thin and rapid pulse.

证候： 干咳，咳声短促，或痰中夹血丝，或声音逐渐嘶哑，口干咽燥，或午后潮热、颧红，盗汗，日渐消瘦，神疲。舌质红，少苔，脉细数。

Treatment: To nourish yin and moisturize the

治法： 滋阴润肺，化痰止

lung; resolve phlegm and stop cough.

Formulas and Herbs: *Glehnia and Ophiopogonis Radix Decoction* (Sha Shen Mai Dong Tang), usually composed of *Glehniae Radix (Bei Sha Shen)*, *Ophiopogonis Radix* (Mai Dong), *Trichosanthis Radix* (Tian Hua Fen) and *Polygonati Odorati Rhizoma* (Yu Zhu) to nourish lung-yin; *Mori Folium* (Sang Ye) to clear away and dispel lung-heat, *Lablab Semen Album* (Bian Dou) and *Glycyrrhizae Radix et Rhizoma* (Gan Cao) to slowly harmonize zhong jiao.

Modification: For dry cough with little phlegm, add *Fritillariae Cirrhosae Bulbus* (Chuan Bei Mu) and *Prunus Amygdalus Dulcis* (Tian Xing Ren) to moisturize the lung and resolve phlegm; for phlegm with blood, add *Moutan Cortex* (Mu Dan Pi), *Gardeniae Fructus* (Zhi Zi) and *Nelumbinis Rhizomatis Nodus* (Ou Jie) to clear away heat and stop bleeding; for feverish sensation and night sweating, add *Folium Mahoniae* (Gong Lao Ye), *Stellariae Radix* (Yin Chai Hu), *Ostreae Concha* (Sheng Mu Li) and *Fructus Tritici Levis* (Fu Xiao Mai) to clear away asthenia-heat and stop sweating.

2.2.8 Asthenia-cold of Lung Qi

Manifestations: Weak coughing, clear away and thin phlegm, aversion to wind and sweating, tired and lazy to talk, little intake; pale tongue and white tongue fur; thin weak pulse.

Treatment: To replenish qi and warm the lung; resolve phlegm and stop cough.

Formulas and Herbs: *Lung Warming Decoction* (Wen Fei Tang), usually composed of *Ginseng Radix et Rhizoma* (Ren Shen), *Cinnamomi Cortex* (Rou Gui) to warm and replenish the lung and the

咳。

方药：沙参麦冬汤。常用：沙参、麦门冬、天花粉、玉竹滋养肺阴，润肺止咳；桑叶清散肺热；扁豆、甘草甘缓和中。

加减：干咳少痰，可加川贝母、甜杏仁润肺化痰；痰中带血，加牡丹皮、栀子、藕节清热止血；潮热盗汗，加功劳叶、银柴胡、生牡蛎、浮小麦清虚热、收敛止汗。

2.2.8 肺气虚寒

证候：咳声低微无力，咳痰清稀，畏风自汗，神疲懒言，食少。舌淡苔白，脉细弱。

治法：补气温肺，止咳化痰。

方药：温肺汤。常用：人参、肉桂温补肺肾；钟乳石重镇纳气；半夏、橘红、干姜、木香、甘草温脾化痰；理气止

kidney; *Stalactitum* (Zhong Ru Shi) to help the reception of qi; *Pinelliae Rhizoma* (Ban Xia), *Citri Exocarpium Rubrum* (Ju Hong), *Zingiberis Rhizoma* (Gan Jiang), *Aucklandiae Radix* (Mu Xiang) and *Glycyrrhizae Radix et Rhizoma* (Gan Cao) to warm the kidney, resolve phlegm, regulate qi and stop cough.

咳。

Modification: For plenty of clear away and thin phlegm, add *Sinapis Semen* (Jie Zi) and *Asari Radix et Rhizoma* (Xi Xin) to warm the lung, disperse cold and resolve fluid retention; for aversion to cold and cold limbs, add *Aconm Lateralis Radix Praeparata* (Fu Zi) to warm the kidney-yang; for severe cough and short breath which aggravates in action, add *Psoraleae Fructus* (Bu Gu Zhi) and *Aquilariae Lignum Resinatum* (Chen Xiang) to invigorate the kidney to absorb qi.

加减：痰多清稀，加白芥子、细辛温肺散寒化饮；畏寒肢冷加附子温肾阳；咳逆气短，动则更甚，加补骨脂、沉香补肾纳气。

Asthma

哮 病

Retained phlegm in the lung, triggered by exogenous pathogenic factors, improper diet, emotional disturbance and over strain, leads to the obstruction of qi and phlegm and the lung's failure to disperse and descend, which results in asthma, a dyspnea disease with wheezing. During attack, there is wheezing in the throat and respiratory dyspnea, even difficult to lie down when it is severe.

哮病是由于宿痰伏肺，遇外邪侵袭、饮食不当、情志失调、劳倦等诱因触发引起痰气交阻，肺失宣降而形成的一种发作性的痰鸣气喘疾患。发时喉中有哮鸣声，呼吸气促困难，甚则喘息不能平卧。

1 Etiology and Pathogenesis

1 病因病机

Retained phlegm in the lung is the etiological origin which is triggered by exogenous pathogenic factors, improper diet, emotional disturbance and overstrain, resulting in phlegm obstructing the airway and

哮病的病理基础为宿痰伏肺，每因外邪侵袭、饮食不当、情志失调、劳倦等诱因引动而触发，以致痰壅气道，肺

the failure of dispersion and descending of lung-qi.

气宣降功能失常。

1.1 Exogenous Pathogenic Factors Attacks and Lung-qi is Obstructed

Exogenous wind-cold or pathogenic wind-heathidden in the lung or inhalation of smoke, dust, pollen, animal scarf and odorous gas lead to the obstruction of lung-qi which fails to transform fluid which when retained fluid turns into phlegm, causing asthma.

1.1 外邪侵袭,壅阻肺气

外感风寒或风热之邪,邪蕴于肺;或因吸入烟尘、花粉、动物毛屑、异味气体等,壅阻肺气,气不布津,聚液生痰而致哮。

1.2 Improper Diet Leads to Retention of Dampness and Phlegm

Over intake of cold food, or favor for sour, salty, sweet and greasy food, or intake of seafood, leads to the dysfunction of the spleen and then turbid phlegm is generated which moves upwards and stays in the lung and obstructs the airway resulting in asthma.

1.2 饮食不当,聚湿生痰

过食生冷,或嗜食酸咸甘肥,或进食海腥发物,以致脾失健运,痰浊内生,上干于肺,壅塞气道,诱发哮病。

1.3 Weak Constitution When Attacked by Pathogenic Factors Triggers Asthma

Congenital defect, kidney-deficiency and imbalance between zang organs and fu organs contribute to turbid phlegm retained in the lung. Weak constitution after diseases, such as measles and whooping cough, or recurrence of cold and prolonged cough will lead to lung-deficiency. Due to yang-asthenia and weak qi, the lung fails to transform body fluid resulting in phlegm and remaining fluid in the lung. While, in case of yin-asthenia and yang-excess, heat exuberates and fluid gathers, which leads to phlegm-heat retains in the lung. When triggered by exogenous pathogenic factors, improper diet, emotional disturbance and overstrain, phlegm retaining in the lung provokes asthma.

1.3 体虚病后,遇感触发

先天禀赋不足,肾虚脏腑失调,痰浊内伏。或病后体弱,罹患麻疹、顿咳;或反复感冒、咳嗽日久等导致肺虚。阳虚气弱,肺不化津,痰饮内伏;阴虚阳盛,热蒸液聚,则痰热伏肺。当遇外邪、饮食、情志、劳倦等诱因,则触动伏痰,发生哮病。

Lung is the pathological position of asthma, but is related to the spleen, the kidney and the heart.

哮病的病位在肺,与脾、肾、心有关。病理因素以痰

Phlegm retaining in the lung is the pathological factor and "obstinate root". Improper diet, emotional disturbance, overstrains and particularly climate change are the triggers. The pathological change is that phlegm long retaining in the lung when triggered, ascend with qi while phlegm was obstructed, struggles with phlegm and together they congest the airway and narrow lung pipes which affects the dispersion and descending of lung-qi. When asthma attacks, pathogenic sthenia is the predominant pathological change. Repeated attacks of asthma for long periods can injure the healthy-qi and give rise to syndromes of weakened lung, spleen and kidney in remission stage. A severe attack in which symptoms cannot be relieved, pathogenic sthenia and healthy-asthenia co-exist might lead to respiratory failure.

为主，痰伏于肺，则成为发病的“夙根”。气候失常、饮食不当、情志失调、劳累等为本病的诱发因素，其中尤以气候变化为主。发作时的基本病理变化为“伏痰”遇感引触，痰随气升，气因痰阻，相互搏结，壅塞气道，肺管狭窄，通畅不利，肺气宣降失常。发作期病变以邪实为主。若长期反复发作，正气耗伤，在缓解期可出现肺、脾、肾虚弱之候。大发作时病情持续不解，邪实与正虚错综并见，甚至发生喘脱危候。

2 Syndrome Differentiation and Treatment

2 辨证论治

2.1 Key Points of Syndrome Differentiation

2.1 辨治要点

Doctors should first identify theacute episodes and remission stage according to asthmatic wheezing. In acute episades, doctors shoud differentiate cold-asthma, heat-asthma, heat-asthma trapped by cold or phlegm-asthma, according to phlegm, cold-heat features along with the tongue and pulse. In remission stage, doctors shoud differentiate which zang-fu organs are weakened and injured.

依据哮喘痰鸣情况辨发作期与缓解期，发作期依据痰液及寒热特点结合舌脉辨寒哮、热哮、寒包热哮及痰哮。缓解期辨脏腑虚损所在。

The treatment principle is relieving the secondary symptoms inacute episodes and treating the primary symptoms in remission stage. To relieve the secondary symptoms and overcome the pathogenic factors in attack stage, doctors should give treatments of warming to disperse the lung, clear awaying to purify the lung, warming and clear awaying at the same time, dispel-

治疗时当以“发时治标，平时治本”为基本原则。发作期攻邪治标，可予温化宣肺、清化肃肺、温清并施、祛痰利气等法，并兼顾正虚；若寒郁化热，药随证变，当改投清化痰热，肃肺利气之品；因

ling phlegm to regulate qi without ignoring asthenia and sthenia. If depressed cold transforms into heat, prescription should change as pattern changes and doctors should give treatments of purifying to disseminate phlegm-heat and purging the lung to regulate qi. For asthma triggered by exogenous pathogenic factors, treatments should be focused on dispelling wind, purging and dispersing. In remission stage, treatment should be focused on strengthening healthy qi and dealing with the primary symptoms by means of invigorating the lung, strengthening the spleen and tonifying the kidney. For severe attacks, doctors should take quick action in case it is too late.

2.2 Therapeutic Methods of Different Types of Asthma

2.2.1 Acute Episades

2.2.1.1 Cold-asthma

Manifestations: Wheezing in the throat that sounds like frogs, short breath, distention and oppression in the chest and diaphragm, slight cough, little white foamy phlegm but difficult to expectorate, no thirsty or thirsty but favorable for hot drinks, aversion to cold, likely to have attacks in cold weather or after cold attacks; dark and bluish complexion; pale tongue with white smooth tongue fur; taut tense pulse or floating tense pulse.

Treatment: To disperse the lung and dispel cold; resolve phlegm and relieve asthma.

Formulas and Herbs: *Belamecandae Rhizoma* and *Ephedrae Herba Decoction* (She Gan Ma Huang Tang), usually composed of *Belamecandae Rhizoma* (She Gan) and *Ephedrae Herba* (Ma Huang) to disperse the lung and stop dyspnea; *Zingiberis Rhizoma*, (Gan Jiang), *Asari Radix et Rhizoma* (Xi Xin) and

外感风邪触发者，重视祛风宣泄。缓解期扶正治本，分别采取补肺、健脾、益肾等法。哮病大发作，应积极救治，以免贻误病情。

2.2 分型论治

2.2.1 发作期

2.2.1.1 冷哮

证候：喉中哮鸣如水鸡声，呼吸急促，胸膈满闷如塞，咳不甚，痰少咯吐不爽，色白而多泡沫，口不渴或渴喜热饮，形寒怕冷，天冷或受寒易发，面色青晦。舌苔白滑，脉弦紧或浮紧。

治法：宣肺散寒，化痰平喘。

方药：射干麻黄汤。常用：射干、麻黄宣肺平喘；干姜、细辛、半夏温肺化饮降逆；紫菀、款冬花化痰止咳；五味子收敛肺气；大枣、甘草和中。

Pinelliae Rhizoma (Ban Xia) to warm the lung, transform retained fluid and suppress the upward flow of qi; *Asteris Radix et Rhizoma* (Zi Yuan) and *Farfarae Fols* (Kuan Dong Hua) to resolve phlegm and stop cough, *Jujubae Fructus* (Da Zao) and *Glycyrrhizae Radix et Rhizoma* (Gan Cao) to harmonize zhong jiao.

Modification: For exterior cold and fluid retention inside, and severe cold manifestations, use modified *Small Blue Dragon Decoction* (Xiao Qing Long Tang); for up-surging phlegm and upward flow of qi so much as not able to lie down, add *Descurainiae Semen Lepidii Semen* (Ting Li Zi) and *Perillae Fructus* (Zi Su Zi) to purge the lung and suppress the upward flow of qi; *Armeniacae Semen Amaru* (Ku Xing Ren), *Mori Cortex* (Sang Bai Pi) and *Citri Reticulatae Pericarpium* (Chen Pi) to resolve phlegm and regulate qi.

加减：若表寒里饮、寒象较重者，可用小青龙汤加减；若痰涌气逆不得平卧，加葶苈子、苏子泻肺降逆，杏仁、白前、橘皮等化痰利气。

2.2.1.2 Heat-asthma

Manifestations: Wheezing in the throat that sound like roaring, gasping and hoarse breath, over-inflated chest and distension in the hypochondria, frequent irritable cough, white and thick phlegm, difficult expectoration, bitter mouth, favorable for hot drinks, sweating, flushed face, fever, prone to attack in summer; red tongue with yellow and greasy tongue fur; rolling rapid pulse or taut rolling pulse.

Treatment: To clear away heat and disperse the lung; resolve phlegm and relieve asthma.

Formulas and Herbs: *Asthma-Relieving Decoction* (Ding Chuan Tang), usually composed up of *Ephedrae Herba* (Ma Huang) to relieve asthmatic dyspnea; *Scutellariae Radix* (Huang Qin) and *Mori Cortex* (Sang Bai Pi) to clear away heat and disperse the

2.2.1.2 热哮

证候：喉中痰鸣如吼，喘而气粗息涌，胸高胁胀，咳呛阵作，咯痰色黄，黏浊稠厚，咯吐不利，口苦，口渴喜饮，汗出，面赤，或有身热，或好发于夏季。舌苔黄腻、质红，脉滑数或弦滑。

治法：清热宣肺，化痰定喘。

方药：定喘汤。常用：麻黄宣肺平喘；黄芩、桑白皮清热肃肺；杏仁、半夏、款冬花、苏子化痰降逆；白果敛肺，防麻黄过于耗散；甘草调

lung; *Armeniacae Semen Amaru* (Ku Xing Ren), *Pinelliae Rhizoma* (Ban Xia), *Farfarae Flos* (Kuan Dong Hua) and *Perillae Fructus* (Zi Su Zi) to resolve phlegm and suppress the upward flow of qi; *Ginkgo Semen* (Bai Guo) to accumulate the lung-qi against the possible effect of over-dispelling by *Ephedrae Herba* (Ma Huang); *Glycyrrhizae Radix et Rhizoma* (Gan Cao) to harmonize all the ingredients.

和诸药。

Modification: For obstructed lung-qi, wheezing and hoarse breath too much to lie down, add *Descurainiae Semen Lepidii Semen* (Ting Li Zi) and *Pheretima* (Di Long) to purge the lung and relieve cough; for lung-heat, severe obstruction, yellow thick phlegm, add *Meretricis Concha Cyclinae Concha* (Hai Ha ke), *Belamecandae Rhizoma* (She Gan), *Anemarrhenae Rhizoma* (Zhi Mu) and *Houttuyniae Herba* (Yu Xing Cao) to clear away heat and resolve phlegm; for constipation, add *Major Purgative Decoction* (Da Cheng Qi Tang).

加减:若肺气壅实,痰鸣息涌不得卧,加葶苈子、地龙泻肺平喘;肺热壅盛,痰吐稠黄,加海蛤壳、射干、知母、鱼腥草清热化痰;大便秘结,加大承气汤。

2.2.1.3 Heat-asthma Trapped by Cold

2.2.1.3 寒包热哮

Manifestations: Wheezing in the throat, restlessness and suppression in the chest and diaphragm, short breath, difficult expectoration, yellow sticky phlegm or white-yellow phlegm, irritable, fever, aversion to cold, no sweating, body sores, dry mouth and thirsty, dry stool; white-yellowish greasy tongue fur; red on the edge and tip of the tongue; taut tight pulse.

证候:喉中鸣息有声,胸膈烦闷,呼吸急促,喘咳气逆,咯痰不爽,痰黏色黄,或黄白相兼,烦躁,发热,恶寒,无汗,身痛,口干欲饮,大便偏干。舌苔白腻罩黄,舌边尖红,脉弦紧。

Treatment: To relieve exterior and dispel cold; clear away to resolve phlegm-heat.

治法:解表散寒,清化痰热。

Formulas and Herbs: *Small Blue Dragon Decoction* (Xiao Qing Long Tang) and *Gypsum Fibrosum Decoction* (Shi Gao Tang), usually composed of *Ephedrae Herba* (Ma Huang) and *Cinnamomi Ramulus*

方药:小青龙加石膏汤。常用:麻黄、桂枝散寒解表,宣肺平喘;细辛、干姜、半夏温化痰饮;石膏清泄肺热,

(Gui Zhi) to dispel cold and relieve exterior, disperse the lung and relieve asthma; *Asari Radix et Rhizoma* (Xi Xin), *Zingiberis Rhizoma* (Gan Jiang) and *Pinelliae Rhizoma* (Ban Xia) to warm to resolve retained phlegm and fluid; *Gypsum Fibrosum* (Shi Gao) to purge lung-heat; *Glycyrrhizae Radix et Rhizoma* (Gan Cao) and *Jujubae Fructus* (Da Zao) to harmonize all the ingredients.

甘草、大枣调和诸药。

Modification: For severe wheezing and short breath, add *Descurainiae Semen Lepidii Semen* (Ting Li Zi) and *Perillae Fructus* (Zi Su Zi) to eliminate phlegm and relieve asthma; for yellow sticky phlegm, add *Scutellariae Radix* (Huang Qin), *Fritillariae Thunbergii Bulbus* (Zhe Bei Mu) and *Trichosanthis Fructus* (Gua Lou) to clear away phlegm-heat.

加减: 若痰鸣气急较甚,加葶苈子、苏子祛痰降气平喘;若痰吐稠黄较黏,加黄芩、象贝母、瓜蒌皮清化痰热。

2.2.1.4 Wind-phlegm Asthma

2.2.1.4 风痰哮

Manifestations: Wheezing in the throat that sounds like sawing, acute dyspnea and chest distention, sticky greasy phlegm and difficult expectoration, or white foaming phlegm, no manifestation of heat or cold, dark and bluish complexion; thick turbid tongue fur; rolling replete pulse.

证候: 喉中痰鸣声如曳锯,喘急胸满,咯痰黏腻难出,或为白色泡沫痰液,无明显寒热倾向,面色青暗。舌苔厚浊,脉滑实。

Treatment: To cleanse phlegm and disinhibit orifices; suppress qi and relieve asthma.

治法: 涤痰利窍,降气平喘。

Formulas and Herbs: *Three-Seed Filial Devotion Decoction* (San Zi Yang Qin Tang), usually composed of *Sinapis Semen* (Jie Zi) to warm the lung, regulate qi and cleanse phlegm; *Perillae Fructus* (Zi Su Zi) to suppress the upward flow of qi and resolve phlegm; *Raphani Semen* (Lai Fu zi) to help qi flow and dispel phlegm.

方药: 三子养亲汤。常用:白芥子温肺利气涤痰;苏子降气化痰,止咳平喘;莱菔子行气祛痰。

Modification: For phlegm obstruction and acute dyspnea too much to lie down, add *Descurainiae Semen Lepidii Semen* (Ting Li Zi) and *Pheretima* (Di

加减: 若痰壅喘急,不能平卧,加葶苈子、地龙泻肺涤痰,必要时可暂予控涎丹

Long) to purge the lung and cleanse phlegm and use if necessary for time being, Saliva-Control Pills to purse the lung and dispel phlegm; for asthma triggered by pathogenic wind, add *Perillae Folium* (Zi Su Ye), *Cicada Periostracum* (Chan Tui) and *fructus xanthii* (Cang Er Zi) to dispel wind and resolve phlegm.

泻肺祛痰;若感受风邪而发作者,加苏叶、蝉蜕、苍耳子祛风化痰。

2. 2. 2　Remission Stage

2. 2. 2　缓解期

2. 2. 2. 1　Lung-qi Deficiency and Spleen-qi Deficiency

2. 2. 2.1　肺脾气虚

Manifestations: Short breath and low voice, or light wheezing in the throat, white clear away thin phlegm, spontaneous sweating, aversion to wind, prone to get cold, fatigue, little intake, loose stool; pale tongue with white tongue fur; fine weak pulse.

证候: 气短而声低,或喉中时有轻度哮鸣,痰白清稀,自汗,怕风,常易感冒,倦怠无力,食少便溏。舌质淡,苔白,脉细弱。

Treatment: To strengthen the spleen and invigorate qi; strengthen the earth and generate the metal.

治法: 健脾益气,补土生金。

Formulas and Herbs: *Six Nobles Decoction* (Liu Jun Zi Tang), usually composed of *Codonopsis Radix* (Dang Shen), *Atractylodis Macrocephalae Rhizoma* (Bai Zhu) to strengthen the spleen and invigorate qi; *Poria* (Fu Ling) to transform the dampness and strengthen the spleen; *Pinelliae Rhizoma* (Ban Xia) and *Citri Reticulatae Pericarpium* (Chen Pi) to dry the dampness and resolve phlegm; *Glycyrrhizae Radix et Rhizoma* (Gan Cao) to strengthen qi and harmonize zhong jiao.

方药: 六君子汤。常用:党参、白术健脾益气;茯苓化湿健脾;半夏、橘皮燥湿化痰;甘草补气调中。

Modification: For exterior deficiency and spontaneous sweating and proneness to cold attack, add *Jade screen Powder* (Yu Ping Feng San) to strengthen qi and consolidate exterior; for aversion to wind and cold, add *Cinnamon-Twig Decoction* (Gui Zhi Tang) to harmonize nourishing blood (ying xue) and defensive qi (Wei (Defensive) Qi); for plenty of phlegm, add *Puerariae Lobatae Radix* (Qian Hu) and

加减: 表虚自汗,易感冒,加玉屏风散补气固表;怕冷、恶风,加桂枝汤调和营卫;痰多者加前胡、杏仁。

Armeniacae Semen Amaru (Ku Xing Ren).

2.2.2.2 Lung Deficiency and Spleen Deficiency

Manifestations: Short breath which worsens with actions, sticky expectoration, dizzy and tinnitus, sore in the waist and knees, palpitation, easy to get tired, or feverish sensation over the five centers, flushed cheek, dry mouth; red tongue with little tongue fur, thin and rapid pulse; or aversion to cold, pale complexion, enlarged tongue with pale white tongue fur, fine deep pulse.

Treatment: To strengthen the lung and invigorate the kidney.

Formulas and Herbs: *Pulse-Engendering and Rehmannia Decoction* (Sheng Mai Di Huang Tang) and *Metal-Water and Six Nobles Brew* (Jin Shui Liu Jun Jian), usually composed of *Rehmanniae Radix Praeparata* (Shu Di Huang), *Corni Fructus* (Shan Yu Rou) and *Juglandis Semwn* (He Tao Rou) to invigorate the kidney and gather qi; *Ginseng Radix et Rhizoma* (Ren Shen), *Ophiopogonis Radix* (Mai Dong) and *Schisandrae Chinensis Fructus* (Wu Wei Zi) to strengthen lung-qi and lung-yin; *Poria* (Fu Ling) and *Glycyrrhizae Radix et Rhizoma* (Gan Cao) to invigorate qi and strengthen the spleen; *Pinelliae Rhizoma* (Ban Xia) and *Citri Reticulatae Pericarpium* (Chen Pi) to regulate qi and resolve phlegm.

Modification: For kidney-yang deficiency, apply *Golden Chamber Kidney Qi Pills* (Jin Kui Shen Qi Wan); for notable lung-qi deficiency, add *Astragali Radix* (Huang Qi), *Atractylodis Macrocephalae Rhizoma* (Bai Zhu) and *Lilii Bulbus* (Bai He); take regularly Dried Human Placenta Powder, *Ginseng and Gecko Powder* (Shen Ge San) or Canterpiller Fungus Powder to strengthen the lung and kidney to promote

2.2.2.2 肺肾两虚

证候：短气息促，动则为甚，咯痰质黏，头晕耳鸣，腰膝酸软，心慌，不耐劳累；或五心烦热，颧红，口干，舌质红少苔，脉细数；或畏寒肢冷，面色苍白，舌苔淡白、质胖，脉沉细。

治法：补肺益肾。

方药：生脉地黄汤合金水六君煎。常用：熟地、山萸肉、胡桃肉补肾纳气；人参、麦冬、五味子补益肺之气阴；茯苓、甘草益气健脾；半夏、陈皮理气化痰。

加减：若肾阳亏虚者可用金匮肾气丸；肺气虚明显者加黄芪、白术、百合；可常服紫河车粉、参蛤散或冬虫夏草粉补肺益肾纳气。

qi absorption.

Dyspnea

Dyspneais is caused by lung's failure to disperse and kidney's failure to gather and accumulate due to six exogenous pathogenic factors, improper diet, emotional disturbance, overstrain and prolonged illness, which has the symptoms of difficult breath, even by opening mouth, raising shoulders, quivering nostrils, and difficult in lying down. When it turns serious, patients will present symptoms such as prolonged dyspnea, restlessness, bluish lips, cold limbs, heavy sweating, and floating rootless pulse.

1 Etiology and Pathogenesis

Etiologically, the causes of dyspnea can be categorized into two types: exogenous and endogenous. The former refer to six exogenous pathogenic factors attacking the lung while the latter means upward flow of lung qi leading to lung's failure to disperse or qi lacking in controlance leading to kidney's failure to gather due to improper diet, emotional disturbance, overstrain and prolong illness.

1.1 Lung's Failure to Disperse Due to Attacks by Exogenous Pathogenic Factors

When wind-cold attacks the lung, the sweat pores on skins will close, and therefore lung-qi is suppressed inside. Or before the exterior is relieved, the wind-cold in the interior has transformed into heat which cannot be dispersed. Or, pathogenic cold depresses constant lung-heat. Or, frequent exuberante of pulmony pathogenic cold. Or lung qi is obstructed and blocked due to wind-heat attack. Or phlegm-heat ob-

喘　证

喘证是因六淫外邪、饮食不当、情志失调、久病劳欲等病因导致肺失宣降，肾失摄纳，出现呼吸困难，甚至张口抬肩，鼻翼翕动，不能平卧为特征的病证。严重者喘促持续不解，烦躁不安，面唇青紫，肢冷，汗出如珠，脉浮大无根，发为喘脱。

1 病因病机

喘证的病因有外感、内伤两大类。外感为六淫外邪侵袭肺系；内伤为饮食不当、情志失调、久病劳欲等病因致使肺气上逆，宣降失职，或肾失摄纳，气无所主而成。

1.1 外邪侵袭，肺失宣肃

风寒袭肺，外闭皮毛，内遏肺气，或表邪未解，内已化热，热不得泄；或肺热素盛，寒邪外束，热为寒郁；或风热犯肺，肺气壅实；或痰热壅肺，均可致肺失宣肃，升降失常，气机壅阻，上逆作喘。

structs the lung. Under such circumstances, the lung fails to disperse and purge and lose control of the ascending and descending of qi which will bring about the blockage of qi and the upward flow of qi leading to dyspnea.

1.2 Phlegm Obstructing the Lung Due to Improper Diet

Too much intake of cold and raw, greasy and sweatfood or heavy drinking will injure zhong jiao which leads to the dysfunction of the spleen and phlegm generated due to accumulated dampness and the phlegm will obstruct the lung. Or phlegm-fire blocks the lung and the lung-qi cannot flow downward. Or damp phlegm transforms into cold which gathers in the lung and when triggered by exogenous pathogenic factors, the cold will obstruct the airway. All these will lead to dyspnea.

1.2 饮食不当，生痰阻肺

过食生冷、肥甘，或嗜酒伤中，脾运失健，聚湿生痰，壅阻肺气；或痰火阻肺，肺气不降；或湿痰寒化，寒饮伏肺，常因外邪引动伏饮，壅阻气道，均可发为喘促。

1.3 Disturbed Emotions leading to the Liver-qi's Upward Flow to the Lung

Emotional dissatisfaction, worries andanxiety lead to qi stagnation which results in abstruction of lung-qi, or anger damage the liver which results in the liver-qi flows upward to injure the lung. Both will bring about the unsmooth flow of qi and when qi flows upward, dyspnea attacks.

1.3 情志所伤，肝气逆肺

情志不遂，忧思气结，肺气痹阻；或郁怒伤肝，肝气上逆于肺，均可致气机不利，气逆而喘。

1.4 Overstrain and Prolonged Illness Leading to Deficiency of the Lung and Kidney

Prolong illness will result in lung-deficiency, consumption of qi-yin and loss of controlance of qi while overstrain injures the kidney, damages primordial qi of the kidney and qi cannot be gathered and accumulated. Or water diffusion due to kidney-deficiency attacks the lung and heart, resulting in the upward flow of lung-qi. Or zhong jiao qi weakness leads to malnu-

1.4 劳欲久病，肺肾亏虚

久病肺虚，气阴亏耗，气失所主；或劳欲伤肾，肾元亏损，气失摄纳；或肾虚水泛，干肺凌心，心阳不振，肺气上逆；或中气虚弱，肺气失养，均可因虚致喘。

trition. All these cause dyspnea due to deficiency.

The lung and the kidney are the pathological basis of dyspnea. The liver and the spleen are affected as well. Pathologically, dyspnea differs in deficiency and excess. Dyspnea of excess type lies in the lung while dyspnea of deficiency type, in the lung as well as the kidney. When it turns severe, not only the lung and the kidney become deficient but the heart is affected when solitary yang tends to escape and even breath failure will occur due to yin depletion and yang depletion.

喘证的发病部位主要在肺和肾，涉及肝脾。病理性质有虚实之分，实喘在肺，虚喘责之肺肾两脏。喘证的严重阶段，不但肺肾俱虚，在孤阳欲脱之时，每多影响到心，甚至出现亡阴、亡阳的喘脱危证。

2 Syndrome Differentiation and Treatment

2.1 Key Points of Syndrome Differentiation

As for dyspnea, it is critically important to differentiate deficiency and excess. Dyspnea of excess type has features like deep hoarse breath but short exhalation. Dyspnea of deficiency type has features like short breath and low voice which worsens over strain. Dyspnea of excess type should be identified as exogenous or endogenous. Exogenous dyspnea of excess type usually start quickly but doesn't last long which is trigged by exogenous pathogenic factors often with exterior symptoms. In contrast, endogenous dyspnea of excess type lasts long and tends to relapse withont exterior symptoms, which is usually triggered by turbid phlegm or liver-qi attacking the lung. Dyspnea of deficiency type should be identified according to the pathological zang-fu organs.

In terms of the treatment principles, treatment in dyspnea of excess type should be focused on dispelling pathogenic factor to regulate qi while dyspnea of deficiency type be focuses on nurturing, replenishing and gathering qi. As for dyspnea of excess type, doc-

2 辨证论治

2.1 辨治要点

喘证辨证，首先注意分清虚实。实喘者，呼吸深长气粗，呼出为快；虚喘者，呼吸短促声低，遇劳加重。实喘又当辨外感内伤，外感者起病急，病程短，常因外感所致，多伴有表证；内伤病程较长，或反复发作，无表证，常因痰浊或肝气犯肺。虚喘者还应辨病变脏腑所属。

喘证治疗原则，实喘以祛邪利气为主，虚喘以培补摄纳为主。实喘治肺，选用温宣、清肃、化痰、降气诸法祛邪利气；虚喘分脏腑，别阴

tors should give treatments on the lung with methods like warming and dispersing, clear awaying and purging, resolving phlegm and qi descending to dispel the pathogenic factors and regulate qi. Dyspnea of deficiency type differs in different zang-fu organs, yin and yang which could be treated with strengthening the lung and the spleen, invigorating the kidney and nurturing the heart, replenishing and gathering qi. If there is complication of both dyspnea of excess type and deficiency type, cold and heat, doctors should first identity the major conflict and the minor conflict, the primary symptoms and the secondary symptoms. Moreover, treatment of the original diseases should not be overlooked as dyspnea is often triggered by those chronic diseases.

阳,可用补肺、健脾、补肾、养心等法培补摄纳。若虚实夹杂、寒热并见者,应分清主次,权衡标本。此外,由于喘证多继发于各种急慢性疾病中,应当注意积极治疗原发病。

2.2 Therapeutic Methods of Different Types of Dyspnea

2.2 分型论治

2.2.1 Wind-cold Attacking the Lung

Manifestations: Short breath, distention and suppression in the chest, cough with white thin foamy phlegm in great amounts, often with headache, aversion to cold or fever, no thirst, no sweating; thin and white and slippery tongue fur; floating tight pulse.

Treatment: To disperse the lung and dispel cold.

Formulas and Herbs: *Ephedrae Herba Decoction* (Ma Huang Tang) and *Canopy Powder* (Hua Gai San), usually composed of *Ephedrae Herba* (Ma Huang) and *Cinnamomi Ramulus* (Gui Zhi) to warm the lung and dispel cold; *Perillae Fructus* (Su Zi) and *Mori Cortex* (Sang Bai Pi) to disperse the lung and stop dyspnea; *Citri Reticulatae Pericarpium* (Chen Pi), *Armeniacae Semen Amaru* (Ku Xing Ren), *Poria* (Fu Ling) and *Glycyrrhizae Radix et Rhizoma* (Gan Cao) to resolve phlegm and lower qi.

2.2.1 风寒袭肺

证候:呼吸急促,胸部胀闷,咳嗽,痰白,量多稀薄带泡沫,常伴有头痛,恶寒,或有发热,口不渴,无汗。苔薄白而滑,脉浮紧。

治法:宣肺散寒。

方药:麻黄汤合华盖散。常用:麻黄、桂枝温肺散寒,苏子、桑白皮宣肺定喘;陈皮、杏仁、茯苓、甘草化痰降气。

Modification: For heavy cold-phlegm, use *Small Blue Dragon Decoction* (Xiao Qing Long Tang) to warm the lung, resolve phlegm and relieve dyspnea; for heavy cough and gasping, add *Belamecandae Rhizoma* (She Gan), *Puerariae Lobatae Radix* (Qian Hu) and *Magnoliae Officinalis Cortex* (Hou Po) to disperse the lung, lower qi and resolve phlegm.

加减: 若寒痰较重,用小青龙汤温肺化痰平喘;若咳喘重,加射干、前胡、厚朴宣肺降气化痰。

2.2.2 Exterior-cold and Lung-Heat

2.2.2 表寒肺热

Manifestations: Gasping, distention or pain in the chest, cough with thick sticky phlegm which is difficult to expectorate, physical cold, fever, irritation, sore body, sweating or no sweating, thirst; white thin tongue fur with yellow covering, red tongue edge; floating rapid or rolling pulse.

证候: 气喘,胸胀或痛,咳嗽,痰稠黏而不爽,伴形寒,身热,烦闷,身痛,有汗或无汗,口渴。苔薄白或罩黄,舌边红,脉浮数或滑。

Treatment: To relieve the exterior and clear away the interior, resolve phlegm and relieve dyspnea.

治法: 解表清里,化痰平喘。

Formulas and Herbs: *Ephedra, Apricot, Gypsum Fibrosum and Liquorice Decoction* (Ma Xing Shi Gan Tang), usually composed of *Ephedrae Herba* (Ma Huang) to disperse the lung and relieve the exterior; *Gypsum Fibrosum Fibrosum* (Shi Gao) to clear away the interior heat; *Armeniacae Semen Amaru* (Ku Xing Ren) and *Glycyrrhizae Radix et Rhizoma* (Gan Cao) to resolve phlegm and lower qi.

方药: 麻杏石甘汤。常用:麻黄宣肺解表;石膏清泄里热;杏仁、甘草化痰降气。

Modification: For severe aversion to exterior cold, add *Cinnamomi Ramulus* (Gui Zhi) to disperse cold and relieve the exterior; for phlegm-heat, add *Trichosanthis Pericarpium* (Gua Lou Pi) and *Fritillariae Thunbergii Bulbus* (Zhe Bei Mu) to clear away phlegm-heat; for short and heavy breath, add *Descurainiae Semen Lepidii Semen* (Ting Li Zi), and *Belamecandae Rhizoma* (She Gan) to purge the lung and relieve dyspnea.

加减: 表寒重加桂枝解表散寒;痰热重加瓜蒌皮、象贝母清化痰热;气急重加葶苈子、射干泻肺平喘。

2.2.3 Phlegm-heat Depresses the Lung

Manifestations: Gasping and cough, distention and pain in the chest, sticky phlegm in great amounts in color of yellow or blood-stained, fever, sweating, thirst and favor for cold drink, flushed face, dry throat, dark and painful urine, dry stool; red tongue with thin yellowish or greasy tongue fur; rapid rolling pulse.

Treatment: To clear away heat and resolve phlegm, disperse the lung and relieve dyspnea.

Formulas and Herbs: *Mori Cortex Decoction* (Sang Bai Pi Tang), usually composed of *Mori Cortex* (Sang Bai Pi), *Pinelliae Rhizoma* (Ban Xia), *Perillae Fructus* (Su Zi), *Armeniacae Semen Amaru* (Ku Xing Ren) and *Fritillariae Cirrhosae Bulbus* (Bei Mu) to resolve phlegm and relieve dyspnea; *Scutellariae Radix* (Huang Qin), *Forsythiae Fructus* (Lian Qiao) and *Gardeniae Fructus* (Zhi Zi) to clear away the lung and purge heat.

Modification: For high fever, add *Gypsum Fibrosum Fibrosum* (Shi Gao) and *Anemarrhenae Rhizoma* (Zhi Mu) to purge heat; for dyspnea with plenty of phlegm, add *Descurainiae Semen Lepidii Semen* (Ting Li Zi) *Meretricis Concha Cyclinae Concha* (Hai Ha ke), *Houttuyniae Herba* (Yu Xing Cao) and *Benincasa Hispida Congniaux* (Dong Gua Ren) to clear away the lung and resolve phlegm; for unsmooth flow of zang-qi, add *Trichosanthis Semen* (Gua Lou Zi), *Rhei Radix et Rhizoma* (Da Huang) and *Mirabilite Efflorescence* (Feng Hua Xiao) to purge fu-organs and eliminate heat.

2.2.3 痰热郁肺

证候：气喘咳嗽，胸部胀痛，痰多质黏，痰色黄或夹有血色，伴身热，汗出，口渴而喜冷饮，面赤，咽干，小便赤涩，大便或秘。舌质红，舌苔薄黄或腻，脉滑数。

治法：清热化痰，宣肺平喘。

方药：桑白皮汤。常用：桑白皮、半夏、苏子、杏仁、川贝母化痰定喘；黄芩、黄连、栀子清肺泄热。

加减：身热重，加石膏、知母清泄里热；喘甚痰多，加葶苈子、海蛤壳、鱼腥草、冬瓜仁清肺化痰；腑气不通，加瓜蒌仁、大黄或风化硝通腑泄肺。

2.2.4 Turbid Phlegm Obstructing the Lung

Manifestations: Gasping and suppression in the chest, cough with plenty of white sticky phlegm as

2.2.4 痰浊阻肺

证候：喘而胸闷，咳嗽痰多质黏色白，兼有呕恶，食

well as nausea, little intake, sticky in the mouth but not thirsty; white greasy tongue fur; rolling or soft pulse.

少,口黏不渴。舌苔白腻,脉象滑或濡。

Treatment: To eliminate phlegm and lower the reverse flow; disperse the lung and relieve dyspean.

治法: 祛痰降逆,宣肺平喘。

Formulas and Herbs: *Erchen Decoction* (Er Chen Tang) and *Three-Seed Filial Devotion Decoction* (San Zi Yang Qin Tang), usually composed *Pinelliae Rhizoma* (Ban Xia) and *Poria* (Fu Ling) to dry dampness and resolve phlegm; *Citri Reticulatae Pericarpium* (Chen Pi) and *Glycyrrhizae Radix et Rhizoma* (Gan Cao) to regulate qi and harmonize zhong jiao; *Sinapis Semen* (Jie Zi), *Perillae Fructus* (Su Zi) and *Raphani Semen* (Lai Fu Zi) to lower qi and resolve phlegm.

方药: 二陈汤合三子养亲汤。常用:半夏、茯苓燥湿化痰;陈皮、甘草理气和中;白芥子、苏子、莱菔子降气化痰。

Modification: For serious phlegm-dampness and thick greasy tongue fur, add *Atractylodis Rhizoma* (Cang Zhu) and *Magnoliae Officinalis Cortex* (Hou Po) to dry dampness, regulate qi and eliminate phlegm; for evident spleen-deficiency, lassitude, little intake, loose stool, add *Codonopsis Radix* (Dang Shen) and *Atractylodis Macrocephalae Rhizoma* (Bai Zhu) to invigorate the spleen and strengthen qi; for severe accumulation of phlegm and fluid, white thin clear away phlegm, and aversion to cold, add *Zingiberis Rhizoma* (Gan Jiang) and *Asari Radix et Rhizoma* (Xi Xin).

加减: 痰湿较重,舌苔厚腻,加苍术、厚朴燥湿理气化痰;脾虚明显,神疲、纳少便溏,加党参、白术健脾益气;痰饮较甚,痰色白清稀,畏寒,加干姜、细辛。

2.2.5 Suppression of Lung-qi

2.2.5 肺气郁痹

Manifestations: Dyspnea triggered by emotional stimulation, sudden occurrence of short breath in attack, distention and pain in the chest, suffocating in the throat, no wheezing or expectoration, much anxiety and depression in ordinary times, insomnia, palpitation; thin tongue fur; taut pulse.

证候: 每遇情志刺激而诱发气急,发时突然呼吸短促,胸闷胁胀,咽中如窒,无哮鸣咳痰,平素多忧思抑郁,不寐,心悸。苔薄,脉弦。

Treatment: To break depression, lower qi and relieve dyspnea.

治法: 开郁降气平喘。

Formulas and Herbs: *Five Milled Ingredients Decoction* (Wu Mo Yin Zi), usually composed of *Linderae Radix* (Wu Yao), *Aucklandiae Radix* (Mu Xiang) and *Aurantii Fructus*(Zhi Qiao) to regulate qi and resolve depression; *Aquilariae Lignum Resinatum* (Chen Xiang) and *Arecae Semen* (Bing Lang) to regulate qi and lower reverse flow of qi; *Perillae Fructus* (Su Zi), *Haematitum* (Zhe Shi) to lower reverse flow of qi and relieve dyspnea.

方药: 五磨饮子。常用:乌药、木香、枳壳行气解郁;沉香、槟榔行气降逆;苏子、金沸草、代赭石降逆平喘。

Modification: For serious distention and oppression in the chest, add *Bupleuri Radix* (Chai Hu), *Curcumae Radix* (Yu Jin), *Citri Reticulatae Pericarpium Viride* (Qing Pi) to disperse the liver and regulate qi; for palpitation and insomnia, add *Lilii Bulbus* (Bai He), *Alibiziae Cortex* (He Huan Pi) and *Ziziphi Spinosae Semen* (Suan Zao Ren) to tranquilize the heart and mind; for distention in abdomen and constipation, add *Rhei Radix et Rhizoma* (Da Huang) to purge fu-organs and lower qi.

加减: 胸胁满闷较重者,加柴胡、郁金、青皮疏肝理气;心悸、不寐者,加百合、合欢皮、酸枣仁宁心安神;腹胀便秘,加大黄通腑降气。

2.2.6 Lung Deficiency

2.2.6 肺脏虚损

Manifestations: Gasping and short breath, low voice, snoring sound in the throat, weak and low coughing sound, thin expectoration, spontaneous sweating, aversion to wind, or cough and choke with little but sticky phlegm, feverish sensation, discomfort in the throat and pharynx, flushed cheeks; pink tongue with peeling tongue fur; soft weak pulse or fine rapid pulse.

证候: 喘促短气,声低,喉有鼾声,咳声低弱,痰吐稀薄,自汗畏风,或见咳呛痰少质黏,烦热而渴,咽喉不利,面颧潮红。舌质淡红或有苔剥,脉软弱或细数。

Treatment: To invigorate the lung, strengthen qi and nurturing yin.

治法: 补肺益气养阴。

Formulas and Herbs: *Pulse-Engendering Powder* (Sheng Mai San) and *Lung-Invigorating Decoction*

方药: 生脉散合补肺汤。常用:人参、麦门冬、五

(Bu Fei Tang), usually composed of *Ginseng Radix et Rhizoma* (Ren Shen), *Ophiopogonis Radix* (Mai Men Dong), *Schisandrae Chinensis Fructus* (Wu Wei Zi), *Astragali Radix* (Huang Qi) and *Rehmanniae Radix Praeparata* (Shu Di Huang) to invigorate the lung and strengthen qi; *Aster Radix et Rhizoma* (Zi Yuan) and *Mori Cortex* (Sang Bai Pi) to resolve phlegm and relieve dyspnea.

味子、黄芪、熟地黄补肺益肾;紫菀、桑白皮化痰止喘。

Modification: For coughing and gasping with thin and little expectoration, add *Pinellinae Rhizoma Praeparatum* (Fa Ban Xia), *Farfarae Flos* (Kuan Dong Hua) and *Perillae Fructus* (Zi Su Zi) to warm the lung, stop coughing and relieve dyspnea; for coughing and gasping with sticky expectoration, add *Fritillariae Cirrhosae Bulbus* (Chuan Bei Mu), *Stemonae Radix* (Bai Bu), *Trichosanthis Pericarpium* (Gua Lou Pi) to resolve phlegm and purge the lung; for little intake and loose stool, and middle-qi drop in the abdomen, use *Center-Supplementing qi-Boosting Decoction* (Bu Zhong Yi Qi Tang) to invigorate the spleen, nourish the lung, boost qi and reverse the drop.

加减: 咳喘咯痰稀薄者,加法半夏、款冬花、苏子温肺止咳定喘;咳喘咯痰稠黏,加川贝母、百部、瓜蒌皮化痰肃肺;食少便溏,腹中气坠者,可配合补中益气汤补脾养肺、益气升陷。

2.2.7 Kidney Deficiency and Failure to Receive Qi

2.2.7 肾虚不纳

Manifestations: Prolonged dyspnea which gets worse in movement, difficulty in catching breath, emaciation and lassitude, swollen instep, sweating and cold limbs, bluish lips and complexion, white pale tongue fur or dark moist slippery tongue fur; fine faint pulse or deep weak pulse.

证候: 喘促日久,动则喘甚,气不得续,形瘦神惫,足背浮肿,汗出肢冷,面唇青紫。舌苔淡白或黑而润滑,脉微细或沉弱。

Treatment: To invigorate the spleen to receive qi.

治法: 补肾纳气。

Formulas and Herbs: *Golden Chamber Kidney Qi Pills* (Jin Kui Shen Qi Wan) and *Ginseng and Gecko Powder* (Shen Ge San), usually composed of *Aconm Lateralis Radix Praeparata* (Fu Zi), *Cinnamomi*

方药: 金匮肾气丸合参蛤散。常用:附子、肉桂、地黄、山茱萸、山药、牡丹皮、茯苓、泽泻温补肾阳;人参、蛤

Cortex (Rou Gui), *Rehmannia Radix* (Di Huang), *Corni Fructus* (Shan Zhu Yu), *Dioscoreae Rhizoma* (Shan Yao), *Moutan Cortex* (Mu Dan Pi), *Poria* (Fu Ling) and *Alismatis Rhizoma* (Ze Xie) to warm and invigorate kidney-yang; *Ginseng Radix et Rhizoma* (Ren Shen) and *Gecko* (Ge Jie) to invigorate qi and enable the kidney to receive qi.

蚧补气纳肾。

Modification: For kidney-yin with signs like gasping and coughing, flushed face, irritation, dry throat and mouth, cold feet, oily sweating, red tongue with little fluid and fine rapid pulse, use *Seven-Ingredients Boosting* Qi Pills (Qi Wei Du Qi Wan) and *Pulse-Engendering Powder* (Sheng Mai San) to nourish the kidney and receive qi; for Biao (secondary symptoms)-sthenia with symptoms of upper excess and lower deficiency, turbid phlegm blocking the lung, gasping with much phlegm, short breath, distention in the chest and greasy tongue fur, use *Fructus-Perillae-Lowering-Qi Decoction* (Su Zi Jiang Qi Tang) to resolve phlegm and lower the upward flow of qi, warm the kidney and receive qi.

加减：肾阴虚者，证见喘咳，面红烦躁，口咽干燥，足冷，汗出如油，舌红少津，脉细数，用七味都气丸合生脉散以滋肾纳气；若兼有标实，上盛下虚，痰浊壅肺，喘咳痰多，气急，胸闷，苔腻，可用苏子降气汤化痰降逆、温肾纳气。

2.2.8 Health-qi Deficiency and Breath Failure

Manifestations: Severe dyspnea with reverse flow of qi even when patients open mouth and raise shoulders, short of breath with flapping nostrils, heavy beady sweating, cold limbs; rootless floating pulse or sometimes with pauses and difficult to be caught.

2.2.8 正虚喘脱

证候：喘逆剧甚，张口抬肩，鼻翕气促，端坐不能平卧，稍动则咳喘欲绝，或有痰鸣，心慌动悸，烦躁不安，面青唇紫，汗出如珠，肢冷。脉浮大无根，或见歇止，或模糊不清。

Treatment: To boost yang to prevent breath failure, settle and gather kidney-qi.

治法：扶阳固脱，镇摄肾气。

Formulas and Herbs: *Black Tin Pills* (Hei Xi Dan) and *Gecko Powder* (Ge Jie Fen) taken with *Ginseng and Aconite Decoction* (Shen Fu Tang), in

方药：参附汤送服黑锡丹、蛤蚧粉。人参、附子扶阳固脱，黑锡丹镇摄肾气，蛤蚧

which *Ginseng Radix et Rhizoma* (Ren Shen) and *Aconm Lateralis Radix Praeparata* (Fu Zi) can boost yang to prevent breath failure while *Black Tin Pills* (Hei Xi Dan) and Gecko (Ge Jie) help to strengthen the lung and invigorate qi as well as gather qi and reliever dyspnea.

补肺益肾、纳气定喘。

Modification: For yang-deficiency with symptoms of weak breath, sweating, cold limbs, pale tongue and deep fine pulse, add *Cinnamomi Cortex* (Rou Gui), *Zingiberis Rhizoma* (Gan Jiang), *Os Draconis* (Long Gu), *Ostreae Concha* (Mu Li); for yin-deficiency, short breath, irritation, interior heat, sweating palms, thirst, red tongue and deep fine pulse, add *Ophiopogonis Radix* (Mai Men Dong), *Asparagi Radix* (Tian Dong), *Corni Fructus* (Shan Zhu Yu), *Panacis Quinquefolii Radix* (Xi Yang Shen) instead of *Ginseng Radix et Rhizoma* (Ren Shen); for unconsciousness, add *Polygalae Radix* (Yuan Zhi) and *Acori Tatarinowii Rhizoma* (Shi Chang Pu) to calm the mind, eliminate phlegm and promote resuscitation; for edema and little urine, add *Poria* (Fu Ling) and *Radix Rohdea japonica* (Wan Nian Qing Gen) to warm yang and regulate fluid.

加减：阳虚甚，气息微弱，汗出肢冷，舌淡，脉沉细，加肉桂、干姜、龙骨、牡蛎；阴虚甚，气息急促，心烦内热，汗出黏手，口干舌红，脉沉细数，加麦门冬、天门冬、山茱萸，人参改西洋参；神昧不清，加远志、石菖蒲安神祛痰开窍；浮肿少尿，加茯苓、万年青根温阳利水。

Hemoptysis

咳　血

Hemoptysis is usually caused by exogenous pathogenic factors attacks, emotional and spiritual excess, overstrain, prolonged illness or fever diseases, in which the burning heat forces the blood to move frenetically off the regular way and the blood breaks the constrain of the lung and airway, coughed out via mouth. Therefore, hematemesis is often manifested as blood-stained phlegm or blood-mixed phlegm or

咳血是因感受外邪、情志过极、劳倦过度、久病或热病后导致火热熏灼，迫血妄行，血液不循常道，由肺及气管外溢，经口而咳出，表现为痰中带血，或痰血相兼，或纯血鲜红的病证。

blood expectoration only.

1 Etiology and Pathogenesis

Hemoptysis is caused by both exogenous and endogenous pathogenic factors in which lung-qi is being attacked, resulting in the lung's failure to clear away and purge, and lung collaterals injured, causing blood overflowing vessels.

1 病因病机

咳血是因内外之邪,干及肺气,肺失清肃,损伤肺络,血溢脉外所致。

1.1 Attacks by Exogenous Pathogenic Factors Injuring Blood Vessels

Wind-heat, wind-dryness, wind-warm attack the lung and the heat damages pulmonary small vessels for which the lung fails to clear away and purge, which, in turn leads to hematemesis.

1.1 感受外邪,损伤血络

风热、风燥、风温之邪袭肺,热伤肺络,肺失清肃,引起咳血。

1.2 Depressive Emotions Leading to Liver Depression Transforming into Fire

Excess of worries and anger depresses liver-qi which transforms into fire and the liver-fire attacks the lung and damages pulmonary small vessels, leading to hematemesis.

1.2 情志郁结,肝郁化火

忧思恼怒过度,肝气郁结化火,肝火犯肺,肺络损伤,引起咳血。

1.3 Fluid consumption and blood-heat due to Weak Constitution after Illness

Asthenia-fire burns inside, injuring pulmonary small vessels, leading to hematemesis due to lack of moisturizing and nourishing of the lung after fever diseases or lung and kidney yin-deficiency after prolonged illness.

1.3 体虚病后,津亏血热

热病之后,或久病肺肾阴虚,肺失濡养,虚火内灼,损伤肺络,以致咳血。

The cause of hematemesis can be exogenous or endogenous. The pathogenesis is burning heat forcing the blood to move frenetically. By pathology, some are due to deficiency while some are due to excess. During pathological development, it can be often seen that excess turns into deficiency. Yin-deficiency and fire-excess is pathological factor as well as the result.

咳血的病因有外感和内伤;病机特点为火热熏灼,迫血妄行;病理性质有虚有实,火热之中分虚实,疾病发展过程中常由实转虚。阴虚火旺既是导致出血的病理因素,又是出血所导致的后果。

2　Syndrome Differentiation and Treatment

2.1　Key Points of Syndrome Differentiation

Hemoptysis should be distinguished from nasal bleeding, dental bleeding and vomiting blood according to clinical history and clinic symptoms. Deficiency and excess should be identified by pathogenic features and the color of blood. By excess heat, it is acute bleeding for short in scarlet, usually with symptoms of excess like wind-heat, phlegm-heat and liver-fire while deficiency heat is prolonged process with dark red blood which goes on and off with symptoms of yin-deficiency.

The treatment of hematemesis should be focused on clearing away heat and moisturize the lung, cleansing the liver and purgeing the lung, nourishing yin and moisturizing the lung, and tranquilize small vessels and stoping bleeding.

2.2　Therapeutic Methods on Different Patterns

2.2.1　Dry-heat Attacks the Lung

Manifestations: Cough with itchy throat, scarlet-blooded stained phlegm, dry mouth and nose, possibilities of fever; red tongue with little fluid; thin yellow tongue fur; rapid pulse.

Treatment: To clear away heat and moisturize the lung, calm small vessels and stop bleeding.

Formulas and Herbs: *Mori Folium and Armeniacae Semen Amaru Decoction* (Sang Xing Tang), usually composed of *Mori Folium* (Sang Ye), *Gardeniae Fructus* (Zhi Zi) and *Sojae Semen Praeparatum* (Dan Dou Chi) to clear away and disperse lung-heat, *Glehniae Radix(Bei Sha Shen)* and *Pear Peel* (Li Pi) to nourish yin and moisturize dryness; *Fritillariae Cirrhosae Bulbus* (Chui Bei Mu) and *Armeniacae Semen*

2　辨证论治

2.1　辨治要点

咳血应根据病史及临床表现与鼻衄、齿衄及呕血相鉴别。从发病特点及出血颜色以辨清虚实。出血急骤，病程较短，血色鲜红，常伴有风热、痰热、肝火等实证的证候，多为热证实证；病程较久，血色暗红，时发时止，伴有阴虚证候的多为虚热证。

咳血的治疗以清热润肺、清肝泻肺和滋阴润肺、宁络止血为主。

2.2　分型论治

2.2.1　燥热伤肺

证候：咳嗽咽痒，痰中带血，血色鲜红，口干鼻燥，或有身热。舌质红少津，苔薄黄，脉数。

治法：清热润肺，宁络止血。

方药：桑杏汤。常用：桑叶、栀子、淡豆豉清宣肺热；沙参、梨皮养阴润燥；贝母、杏仁润肺化痰止咳。

Amaru (Ku Xing Ren) to moisturize the lung, resolve phlegm and stop coughing.

Modification: For relatively heavy bleeding, add *Imperatae Rhizoma* (Bai Mao Gen), *Rubiae Radix et Rhizoma* (Qian Cao), *Nelumbinis Rhizomatis Nodus* (Ou Jie) and *Platycladi Cacumen Preparata* (Ce Bai Ye) to cool blood and stop bleeding; for with further symptoms such as fever, headache, cough, sore throat and floating rapid pulse, add *Lonicerae Japonicae Flos* (Jin Yin Hua), *Forsythiae Fructus* (Lian Qiao), *Amomi Fructus* (Niu Bang Zi) to cool and reliever exterior, and clear away heat and relieve sore throat; for severe damage to body fluid, cough without phlegm, add *Ophiopogonis Radix* (Mai Men Dong), *Asparagi Radix* (Tian Dong), *Scrophulariae Radix*(Xuan Shen), *Trichosanthis Radix* (Tian Hua Fen) to nourish yin and moisturize dryness.

加减：出血较多者，加白茅根、茜草、藕节、侧柏叶凉血止血；兼见发热、头痛、咳嗽、咽痛、脉浮数，加金银花、连翘、牛蒡子辛凉解表，清热利咽；若津伤较甚，干咳无痰，加麦门冬、天门冬、玄参、天花粉等养阴润燥。

2.2.2 Liver-fire Attacks the Lung

2.2.2 肝火犯肺

Manifestations: Paroxysmal coughing with scarlet-blooded stained phlegm or cough with scarlet blood, distention and pain in the chest and hypochondria, irritation, bitter mouth; red tongue with thin yellow tongue fur; taut rapid pulse.

证候：咳嗽阵作，痰中带血或纯血鲜红，胸胁胀痛，烦躁易怒，口苦。舌质红，苔薄黄，脉弦数。

Treatment: To cleanse the liver and purge the lung, cool blood and stop bleeding.

治法：清肝泻肺，凉血止血。

Formulas and Herbs: *Lung-Heat Expelling Power* (Xie Bai San) and *Meretricis Concha Cyclinae Concha* and *Indigo Naturalis* Powder (Ha Dai San), in which *Mori Cortex* (Sang Bai Pi) and *Lycii Cortex* (Di Gu Pi) can clear away and purge lung-heat, *Indigo Naturalis* (Qing Dai), *Meretricis Concha Cyclinae Concha*(Hai Ha ke) and *Glycyrrhizae Radix et Rhizoma* Praeparata (Zhi Gan Cao) to clear away the lung and resolve phlegm.

方药：泻白散合黛蛤散。常用：桑白皮、地骨皮清泻肺热；青黛清肝凉血；海蛤壳、甘草清肺化痰。

Modification: For severe live-fire, dizziness, bloodshot eyes and irritation, add *Gardeniae Fructus* (Zhi Zi) and *Scutellariae Radix* (Huang Qin) to purge the liver and dispel fire; for excess heat forcing blood to move frenetically with symptoms of coughing scarlet blood in amounts, use *Rhinoceros Horn and Rehmannia Decoction* (Xi Jiao Di Huang Tang) and *Notoginseng Radix et Rhizoma Powder* (San Qi Fen) to clear away heat and purge fire, cool blood and stop bleeding.

加减: 若肝火较甚,头晕目赤,心烦易怒,加栀子、黄芩清肝泻火;热甚迫血妄行,咳血量较多,纯血鲜红者,可用犀角地黄汤加三七粉冲服以清热泻火、凉血止血。

2.2.3 Lung-heat Due to Yin-deficiency

2.2.3 阴虚肺热

Manifestations: Cough with little phlegm, blood-stained phlegm, continual coughing scarlet blood, dry mouth and throat, flushed cheeks, feverish sensations and night-sweating; red tongue; fine rapid pulse.

证候: 咳嗽痰少,痰中带血,或反复咳血,血色鲜红,口干咽燥,颧红,潮热盗汗。舌质红,脉细数。

Treatment: To nourish yin and moisturize the lung, calm small vessels and stop bleeding.

治法: 滋阴润肺,宁络止血。

Formulas and Herbs: *Lily Metal-Consolidating Decoction* (Bai He Gu Jin Tang), usually composed of *Lilii Bulbus* (Bai He), *Ophiopogonis Radix* (Mai Men Dong), *Scrophulariae Radix* (Xuan Shen), *Rehmannia Radix* (Sheng Di Huang), *Rehmanniae Radix Praeparata* (Shu Di Huang) to nourish yin and clear away heat, and nourish the lung and generate fluid; *Angelicae Sinensis Radix* (Dang Gui) and *Paeoniae Radix Alba* (Bai Shao) to soften, moisturize and nourish blood, *Fritillariae Cirrhosae Bulbus* (Chuan Bei Mu) and *Glycyrrhizae Radix et Rhizoma* (Gan Cao) to purge the lung, resolve phlegm and stop coughing.

方药: 百合固金汤。常用:百合、麦门冬、玄参、生地黄、熟地黄滋阴清热,养肺生津;当归、白芍药柔润养血;贝母、甘草肃肺化痰止咳。

Modification: For heavy coughing blood, add *Ten-Ashes Powder* (Shi Hui San) to cool blood and stop bleeding; for continual coughing blood, add *Asini Corii Colla* (E Jiao) and *Notoginseng Radix et*

加减: 咳血量多者,兼服十灰散凉血止血;反复咳血加阿胶、三七养血止血;潮热颧红者,加青蒿、鳖甲、地

Rhizoma (San Qi) to nourish blood and stop bleeding; for flushed cheeks, add *Artemisiae Annuae Herba* (Qing Hao), *Trionycis Carapax* (Bie Jia) and *Lycii Cortex* (Di Gu Pi) to clear away and subtract deficiency-heat.

骨皮等清退虚热。

Chapter 2 Heart System Diseases

第2章 心系病证

Palpitation

心 悸

Palpitation is a disease of perturbing and upsetting heart and mind, caused by many factors. Patients with palpitation feel uneasiness and alertness inside and sometimes out of control. Light palpitation is called palpitation which is usually triggered by exogenous factors and takes an acute onset, off and on but the whole body conditions are quite well. Severe palpitation is triggered by pathological changes in the heart or other zang-fu organs, which starts gradually without particular periods of time and the whole body conditions are quite bad.

心悸是由多种因素引起心神不安，临床以患者自觉心中悸动，惊惕不安，甚则不能自主的一种病证。病情较轻者为惊悸，常因外来刺激所引起，起病迅速，时作时止，全身情况较好；病情较重者为怔忡，常由心或其他脏腑病变所引起，起病缓慢，发作无时，全身情况较差。

1 Etiology and Pathogenesis

1 病因病机

The main causes of palpitation can be weak constitution, overstrain, injury of seven emotions, attacks by exogenous pathogenic factors and improper herbstion and diet. The pathogenesis is deficiency of qi, blood, yin and yang. The heart fails to be nourished or pathogenic factors interfere with the heart and mind, leading to perturbation.

心悸的致病原因主要有体虚劳倦、七情所伤、感受外邪、药食不当。心悸的基本病机是气血阴阳亏虚，心失所养，或邪扰心神，心神不宁。

1.1 Lack of Nourish of the Heart due to Weak Constitution and Prolonged Illness

1.1.1 The heart failing to be nourishd due to deficiency of qi and blood

Congenital defects or lack of proper care after birth leads to the deficiency of qi and blood and the heart and mind are not well nourishd, which results in palpitation.

1.1.2 Heart-Fire interfereing upwards due to kidney-yin deficiency

Ageing and prolonged illness, overstrain or excess desire exhaust and damage kidney-essence, which cannot nourish heart-yin, leading to heart-yin deficiency. Then hear-fire interferes upward with the heart and mind, resulting in heart palpitation.

1.1.3 Heart meridian failing to be warmed and nourishd due to weak heart-yang

Weak constitution after prolonged illness injuries heart-yang and as the heart fails to be warmed andnourishd, palpitation is resulted.

1.2 Emotional and Spiritual Stimulations Injurying the Heart and the Spleen

Excess of worry strains the heart and the spleen, gradually leading to deficiency of qi and blood thatnourish the heart. As the heart fails to be nourishd, palpitation attacks. Or imbalance of emotions and minds, leading to the stagnation of liver-qi, which along with accumulation of fluid turns into phlegm. As depressive phlegm transforms into fire, it interferes upward with the heart and mind, causing palpitation.

In a word, palpitation pathologically not only lies with the heart but also closely related to other organs like liver, spleen, kidney and lung. It comes

1.1 体虚久病,心失所养

1.1.1 气血不足,心失所养

先天禀赋不足或后天失调,造成气血不足,心神失养,而致心悸。

1.1.2 肾阴不足,心火上扰

年老久病或劳欲过度,耗伤肾精,肾精不能滋养心阴,心阴亏虚,心火上扰心神,故而心悸。

1.1.3 心阳虚弱,不能温养心脉

久病体虚,心阳受损,心失温养,导致心悸。

1.2 情志刺激,损伤心脾

忧思过度,劳伤心脾,渐致气血亏虚,心失所养,而成心悸;或情志失调,肝气郁结,气结津聚为痰,痰郁化火,上扰心神,则成心悸。

综上所述,心悸的病位在心,与肝、脾、肾、肺四脏密切相关。病理性质主要有虚

into two types: deficiency and excess. By palpitation of deficiency type, it is deficiency of qi, blood, yin and yang that lead to the failure of the heart being nourishd, resulting in palpitation while by palpitation of excess type, it is phlegm-fire interference with the heart and fluid invasion upward or stasis of heart blood that cause the unsmooth circulation of qi and blood resulting in palpitation. These two types interfere and interchange. Pathological factors include qi stagnation, blood stasis, turbid phlegm and retention of fluid in the body.

实两方面，虚者为气、血、阴、阳亏损，使心失滋养，而致心悸；实者多由痰火扰心，水饮上凌或心血瘀阻，气血运行不畅而引起；虚实之间可以相互夹杂或转化。心悸的病理因素包括气滞、血瘀、痰浊、水饮。

2　Syndrome Differentiation and Treatment

2.1　Key Points of Syndrome Differentiation

Doctors should first identify the types ofpalpitation. For palpitation of deficiency type, identify which is deficiency, qi, blood, yin or yang of zang-fu organs. For palpitation of excess type, identify which is the primary pathogenic factor, phlegm, fluid retention, stasis or fire. Palpitation with short breath, tiredness and weakness, spontaneous sweating is qi-deficiency. Palpitation with dizziness, pale face indicates blood deficiency. Feverish sensation and dry mouth is yin-deficiency and palpitation with cold limbs, aversion to cold, gasping is yang-deficiency. Palpitation with facial edema, little urine belongs to fluid retention. Palpitation with heartache, dark lips and purple tongue is due to blood stasis. Palpitation with irritation, bitter mouth and dry stool is due to phlegm-fire. In term of co-occurrence of two types, doctors should distinguish what is due to deficiency and what is due to excess. Also, doctors should identify the pulse changes. Palpitation often goes along with irregular

2　辨证论治

2.1　辨治要点

心悸的辨证首先应辨虚实，虚证者要辨别脏腑气、血、阴、阳何者偏虚，实证者须分清痰、饮、瘀、火何邪为主。常见虚证：心悸气短，神疲乏力，自汗者属气虚；心悸头晕，面色不华者属血虚；心悸盗汗，潮热口干者属阴虚；心悸肢冷，畏寒气喘者属阳虚。常见实证：心悸面浮，尿少肢肿者为水饮；心悸心痛，唇暗舌紫者为瘀血；心悸烦躁，口苦便秘者为痰火。虚实夹杂者还要分清孰虚孰实。其二还需辨脉象之变化。心悸常伴有脉律失常，临证应仔细体会结、代、促、数、缓、迟等脉。一息六至为数脉，一息四至为缓脉，一息三至为迟脉；脉象见数时一

heartbeat. Therefore, doctors ought to feel carefully different types of pulse such as knotted pulse, slow pulse, quick pulse, rapid pulse, gentle pulse and retarded pulse. Six beats for a breath is known as rapid pulse while four beats for a breath is gentle pulse. Three beats is retarded pulse. Rapid beats with irregular intervals is called quick pulse while slow regular intermittent beats is called knotted pulse. Slow and weak beats with regular intervals is called slow pulse. Quick pulse often indicates yang-excess. Rapid pulse and quick pulse are usually signs of heat. Nevertheless, rapid or quick pulse but deep fine or weak fine with facial edema and swollen limb, short breath in action, physical cold and cold limbs, pale tongue is usually indication of deficiency cold. Knotted pulse is usually due to yin-excess. Retarded pulse, knotted pulse and slow regular intermittent pulse are likely to be deficiency cold. Knotted pulse means qi stagnation and blood stasis; slow regular intermittent pulse relates to deficiency and weakness of primordial qi and slight weakness of zang-qi. However, if retarded pulse, knotted pulse and slow regular intermittent pulse turn to be energetic when pressed, along with dry mouth and red tongue, it means injured yang affecting yin leading to deficiency of both yin and yang.

止，止无定数为促脉，脉象见缓时一止，止无定数为结脉；脉来更代，几至一止，止有定数为代脉。阴盛则促，数脉、促脉多为热象，但若脉虽数、促却沉细、微细，伴有面浮肢肿，动则气短，形寒肢冷，舌淡等症，为虚寒之证。阴盛则结，脉象迟、结、代者，一般多属虚寒。其中：结脉表示气血凝滞；代脉常为元气虚衰，脏气衰微。但若脉象呈迟、结、代而按之有力，伴有口干舌红者为阳损及阴所致阴阳两虚。

The treatment should follow the principles of deficiency and excess. Forpalpitation of deficiency type, treat by invigorating qi, nurturing blood, nourishing yin and warming yang; for excess type, dispel phlegm, resolve fluid retention, clear away fire and remove stasis. However, palpitation is often a complication of deficiency and excess with differences in predominance and acuteness. There-

心悸的治疗应分虚实。虚证分别治以补气、养血、滋阴、温阳；实证则应祛痰、化饮、清火、行瘀。但本病以虚实错杂为多见，且虚实的主次、缓急各有不同，故治当相应兼顾。同时，由于心悸以心神不宁为其病理特点，故

fore, both should be taken into consideration. At the same time, since palpitation has the pathologic features of uneasiness and perturbation of the heart and mind, add into formula, herbs of calming the mind and tranquilizing the mind.

应酌情配入镇心安神之法。

2.2 Thereuptic Methods for Different Patterns

2.2 分型论治

2.2.1 Heart-deficiency and Timidity

2.2.1 心虚胆怯

Manifestations: Palpitation and uneasiness, proneness to frightened and terrified, fidget, sleeplessness with plenty of dreams, fear for noises, little intakes and poor appetite; thin white tongue fur; rapid fine pulse or fine taut pulse.

证候: 心悸不宁,善惊易恐,坐卧不安,不寐多梦而易惊醒,恶闻声响,食少纳呆。苔薄白,脉细略数或细弦。

Treatment: To tranquilize the heart and mind, nourish the heart and calm the mind.

治法: 镇惊定志,养心安神。

Formulas and Herbs: *Spirit-calming and Mind-tranquilizing Pills* (An Shen Ding Zhi Wan), usually composed of *Codonopsis Radix* (Dang Shen), *Poria* (Fu Ling) and *Glycyrrhizae Radix et Rhizoma* (Gan Cao) to invigorate qi; *Polygalae Radix* (Yuan Zhi), *Acori Tatarinowii Rhizoma* (Shi Chang Pu) and *Dens Draconis* (Long Chi) to calm the spirits and relieve fright; *Chuanxiong Rhizoma* (Chuan Xiong) and *Ziziphi Spinosae Semen* (Suan Zao Ren) to regulate bold and nourish the heart; *Anemarrhenae Rhizoma* (Zhi Mu) to clear away heat and relieve irritation.

方药: 安神定志丸。常用:党参、茯苓、甘草益气;远志、石菖蒲、龙齿安神定惊;川芎、酸枣仁调血养心;知母清热除烦。

Modification: For insufficiency of heart-yang, distention in the chest, short breath, physical cold and cold limbs, change *Cinnamomi Cortex* (Rou Gui) for *Cinnamomi Ramulus* (Gui Zhi) and add *Aconm Lateralis Radix Praeparata* (Fu Zi) to warm and invigorate heart-yang; for further symptoms such as deficiency of qi and blood, dizziness, vertigo and pale complexion, add *Asini Corii Colla* (E

加减: 若见心阳不振,胸闷气短,形寒肢冷,用肉桂易桂枝,加附子以温通心阳;兼心血不足,头晕目眩,面色无华,加阿胶、首乌、龙眼肉以滋养心血;兼心气郁结,夜寐不安,情志抑郁,加柴胡、郁金、合欢皮、绿萼梅以疏肝解

Jiao), *Polygoni Multiflori Radix* (He Shou Wu) and *Longan Arillus* (Long Yan Rou) to nourish and nourish heart-blood; for further symptoms such as depressive heart-qi, restless sleep, depressive emotions and mind, add *Bupleuri Radix* (Chai Hu), *Curcumae Radix* (Yu Jin), *Alibiziae Cortex* (He Huan Pi) and *Prunus mume var. viridicalyx* (Lü E Mei) to disperse the liver and relieve depression.

郁。

2.2.2 Deficiency of Qi and Blood

Manifestations: Palpitation, short breath, dizziness, vertigo, insomnia, amnesia, pale complexion, tiredness and weakness, poor appetite, little intake; pink tongue; fine weak pulse.

Treatment: To supplement blood and nourish the heart, invigorate qi and calm the mind.

Formulas and Herbs: *Angelica Splenic Decoction* (Gui Pi Tang), usually composed of *Codonopsis Radix* (Dang Shen), *Astragali Radix* (Huang Qi) and *Atractylodis Macrocephalae Rhizoma* (Bai Zhu) to invigorate qi and strengthen the spleen; *Angelicae Sinensis Radix* (Dang Gui) to supplement blood, *Polygalae Radix* (Yuan Zhi), *Ziziphi Spinosae Semen* (Suan Zao Ren) and *Longan Arillus* (Long Yan Rou) to nourish the heart, calm the spirits and minds; *Aucklandiae Radix* (Mu Xiang) and *Citri Reticulatae Pericarpium* (Chen Pi) to regulate qi and invigorate spleen.

Modification: For feverish sensations in the five centers, spontaneous sweating, night sweating, distention in the chest, irritation, red tongue with little tongue fur, fine rapid pulse or knotted slow pulse, deficiency of both yin and yang, use modified *Honeyed Liquorice Decoction* (Zhi Gan Cao Tang) to invigorate qi and nourish blood, and nourish yin

2.2.2 心血不足

证候: 心悸气短,头晕目眩,失眠健忘,面色无华,倦怠乏力,纳呆食少。舌淡红,脉细弱。

治法: 补血养心,益气安神。

方药: 归脾汤。常用:党参、黄芪、白术益气健脾;当归补血;远志、酸枣仁、龙眼肉养心安神定志;木香、陈皮理气健脾。

加减: 若五心烦热,自汗盗汗,胸闷心烦,舌红少苔,脉细数或结代,为气阴两虚,治以益气养血,滋阴安神,用炙甘草汤加减;失眠多梦,加合欢皮、夜交藤、五味子、柏子仁、莲子心等养心安神;若

and calm the spirits; for insomnia with plenty of dreams, add *Alibiziae Cortex* (He Huan Pi), *Polygoni Multiflori Caulis* (Shou Wu Teng), *Schisandrae Chinensis Fructus* (Wu Wei Zi), *Platycladi Semen* (Bai Zi Ren) and *Nelumbinis Semen* (Lian Zi) to nourish the heart and calm the spirits; for palpitation due to heart-yin damage after fever disease, use modified *Pulse-Engendering Powder* (Sheng Mai San) to invigorate qi, nourish yin and invigorate the heart.

热病后期损及心阴而心悸者,以生脉散加减,有益气养阴补心之功。

2.2.3 Insufficiency of Heart-yang

Manifestations: Palpitation, anxiety, distension in the chest, short breath which gets worse in action, pale complexion; pale tongue with white tongue fur; weak pulse or deep fine weak pulse.

Treatment: To warm and invigorate heart-yang, calm the spirits and relieve palpitation.

Formulas and Herbs: *Cinnamon-Twig, Glycyrrhizae, Os Draconis and Ostreae Concha Decoction* (Gui Zhi Gan Cao Long Gu Mu Li Tang) and *Ginseng and Aconite Decoction* (Shen Fu Tang), usually composed of *Cinnamomi Ramulus* (Gui Zhi) and *Glycyrrhizae Radix et Rhizoma* (Gan Cao) to warm and invigorate heart-yang; *Os Draconis* (Long Gu) and *Ostreae Concha* (Mu Li) to calm the spirits and relieve palpitation; *Ginseng Radix et Rhizoma* (Ren Shen) and *Aconm Lateralis Radix Praeparata* (Fu Zi) to invigorate qi and warm yang.

Modification: For physical cold and cold limbs, increase the amount of *Ginseng Radix et Rhizoma* (Ren Shen), *Astragali Radix* (Huang Qi), *Aconm Lateralis Radix Praeparata* (Fu Zi) and *Cinnamomi Cortex* (Rou Gui) to warm yang and dispel cold; for water-fluid retention, add *Descurainiae Semen*

2.2.3 心阳不振

证候:心悸不安,胸闷气短,动则尤甚,面色苍白,形寒肢冷。舌淡苔白,脉象虚弱或沉细无力。

治法:温补心阳,安神定悸。

方药:桂枝甘草龙骨牡蛎汤合参附汤。常用:桂枝、甘草温补心阳;龙骨、牡蛎安神定悸;人参、附子益气温阳。

加减:若形寒肢冷者,重用人参、黄芪、附子、肉桂温阳散寒;兼见水饮内停者,加葶苈子、五加皮、车前子、泽泻等利水化饮;若心阳不振,以致心动过缓者,酌加炙麻

Lepidii Semen (Ting Li Zi), *Acanthopanacis Cortex* (Wu Jia Pi), *Plantaginis Semen* (Che Qian Zi) and *Alismatis Rhizoma* (Ze Xie) to regulate water and fluid and resolve retention; for bradycardia due to insufficiency of heart-yang, add moderately *Ephedrae Herba* Praeparata (Zhi Ma Huang), *Psoraleae Fructus* (Bu Gu Zhi) and increase the amount of *Cinnamomi Ramulus* (Gui Zhi) to warm and invigorate heart-yang.

黄、补骨脂，重用桂枝以温通心阳。

2.2.4 Water and Fluid Retention Attacks the Heart

Manifestations: Palpitation, vertigo, short breath, distention in the chest and fullness in abdomen, thirst without desire for drink, short and little urine, or edema of lower limbs, physical cold and cold limbs, along with nausea, likeliness to vomit and drooping; pale enlarged pulse with white slippery tongue fur; taut rolling pulse or deep fine rolling pulse.

Treatment: To boost heart-yang, transform qi and regulate water, calm the heart and the spirits.

Formulas and Herbs: *Poria, Cinnamomi, Atractylodes and Glycyrrhizae Decoction* (Ling Gui Zhu Gan Tang), usually composed of *Cinnamomi Ramulus* (Gui Zhi) and *Poria* (Fu Ling) to warm yang, regulate water and resolve retention; *Atractylodis Macrocephalae Rhizoma* (Bai Zhu) and *Glycyrrhizae Radix et Rhizoma* (Gan Cao) to invigorate spleen and dispel dampness.

Modification: For further symtoms such as lung's failure to disperse, phlegm-dampness in the lung, gasping, distention in the chest, add *Armeniacae Semen Amaru* (Ku Xing Ren), *Puerariae Lobatae Radix* (Qian Hu) and *Platycodi Radix* (Jie Geng) to disperse the lung; *Descurainiae Semen*

2.2.4 水饮凌心

证候：心悸眩晕气急，胸闷痞满，渴不欲饮，小便短少，或下肢浮肿，形寒肢冷，伴恶心、欲吐、流涎。舌淡胖，苔白滑，脉象弦滑或沉细而滑。

治法：振奋心阳，化气行水，宁心安神。

方药：苓桂术甘汤。常用：桂枝、茯苓温阳利水化饮；白术、甘草健脾除湿。

加减：兼见肺气不宣，肺有痰湿，出现咳喘、胸闷者，加杏仁、前胡、桔梗以宣肺，葶苈子、五加皮、防己以泻肺利水；兼见瘀血，有舌紫暗，脉涩者，加当归、川芎、刘寄

Lepidii Semen (Ting Li Zi), *Acanthopanacis Cortex* (Wu Jia Pi) and *Stephaniae Tetrandrae Radix* (Fang Ji) to purge the lung and regulate water; for further symptoms such as blood stasis, dark purple tongue, uneven pulse, add *Angelicae Sinensis Radix* (Dang Gui), *Chuanxiong Rhizoma* (Chuan Xiong), *Artemisiae Annuae Herba* Anomalae (Liu Ji Nu), *Lycopi Herba* (Ze Lan) and *Leonuri Herba* (Yi Mu Cao); for edema, little urine, paroxysmal cough at night or sitting-breathing due to incomplete heart function, increase the amounts of such herbsl herbs that can warm yang and regulate water as *True Warrior Decoction* (Zhen Wu Tang).

奴、泽兰叶、益母草；若见因心功能不全而致浮肿、尿少、阵发性夜间咳喘或端坐呼吸者，当重用温阳利水之品，如真武汤。

2. 2. 5　Yin-deficiency and Fire-excess

Manifestations: Palpitation, easy to be frightened, irritation, insomnia, feverish sensation in five centers, thirst, night sweating, worsened with worries and concerns, tinnitus, pain in the back, dizziness, vertigo, easy to fly into a rage; red tongue with little fluid or no tongue fur; find rapid pulse.

Treatment: To nourish yin and clear away fire, nourish the heart and calm the spirits

Formulas and Herbs: *Celestial Emperor Heart-Supplementing Elixir* (Tian Wang Bu Xin Dan) and *Cinnabar and Spirit-Calming Pills* (Zhu Sha An Shen Wan). The former usually is composed of *Rehmannia Radix* (Sheng Di Huang), *Scrophulariae Radix* (Xuan Shen) and *Ophiopogonis Radix* (Mai Men Dong) to nourish yin and clear away heat; *Ginseng Radix et Rhizoma* (Ren Shen) to supplement and invigorate heart-qi; *Cinnabaris* (Zhu Sha), *Poria* (Fu Ling), *Polygalae Radix* (Yuan Zhi), *Ziziphi Spinosae Semen* (Suan Zao Ren),

2. 2. 5　阴虚火旺

证候: 心悸易惊，心烦失眠，五心烦热，口干，盗汗，思虑劳心则症状加重，伴耳鸣腰酸、头晕目眩、急躁易怒。舌红少津，苔少或无，脉象细数。

治法: 滋阴清火，养心安神。

方药: 天王补心丹合朱砂安神丸。前方用：生地黄、玄参、麦门冬滋阴清热；当归、丹参补血养心；人参补益心气；朱砂、茯苓、远志、酸枣仁、柏子仁、五味子养心安神。后方用：朱砂安神；当归、生地黄养血滋阴；黄连泻心火。

Platycladi Semen (Bai Zi Ren) and *Rehmannia Radix* (Sheng Di Huang) to nourish the heart and calm the spirits. The latter formula usually is composed of *Cinnabaris* (Zhu Sha) to calm spirits; *Angelicae Sinensis Radix* (Dang Gui) and *Rehmannia Radix* (Sheng Di Huang) to nourish blood and nourish yin; *Coptidis Rhizoma* (Huang Lian) to clear away heart-fire.

Modification: For deficiency of kidney-ying, frenetical movement of deficiency-fire, spermatorrhea and pain in the back, add *Testudinis Carapax et Plastrum* (Gui Jia), *Rehmanniae Radix Praeparata* (Shu Di Huang), *Anemarrhenae Rhizoma* (Zhi Mu), *Phellodendri Chinensis Cortex* (Huang Bo) or *Anemarrhena, Phellodendron, and Rehmannia Pills* (Zhi Bai Di Huang Wan); for yin-deficiency without evident symptoms of fire-heat, use only *Celestial Emperor Heart-Supplementing Elixir* (Tian Wang Bu Xin Dan); for yin-deficiency and stasis-heat, add *Paeoniae Radix Rubra* (Chi Shao), *Moutan Cortex* (Mu Dan Pi), *Persicae Semen* (Tao Ren), *Carthami Flos* (Hong Hua) and *Curcumae Radix* (Yu Jin) to clear away heat and cool blood, and promote blood circulation and eliminate stasis.

加减：若肾阴亏虚，虚火妄动，遗精腰酸者，加龟甲、熟地黄、知母、黄柏，或加服知柏地黄丸；若阴虚而火热不明显者，可单用天王补心丹；若阴虚兼有瘀热者，加赤芍药、牡丹皮、桃仁、红花、郁金等清热凉血、活血化瘀。

2.2.6 Stasis Blocking the Heart

2.2.6 瘀阻心脉

Manifestations: Palpitation, anxiety, distention and discomfort in the chest, occasional needling-like heartache, bluish lips and nails; dark purple tongue or sometimes with stasis spots; uneven pulse or knotted pulse or slow regular intermittent pulse.

证候：心悸不安，胸闷不舒，心痛时作，痛如针刺，唇甲青紫。舌质紫暗或有瘀斑，脉涩或结或代。

Treatment: To promote blood circulation and removing blood stasis, regulate qi and dredge collaterals.

治法：活血化瘀，理气通络。

Formulas and Herbs: *Peach Seed and Carthami*

方药：桃仁红花煎合桂

Decoction (Tao Ren Hong Hua Jian) and *Cinnamon, Glycyrrhizae, Os Draconis and Ostreae Concha Decoction* (Gui Zhi Gan Cao Long Gu Mu Li Tang). The former is composed of *Persicae Semen* (Tao Ren), *Carthami Flos* (Hong Hua), *Salviae Miltiorrhizae Radix et Rhizoma Radix* (Dan Shen), *Paeoniae Radix Rubra* (Chi Shao) and *Chuanxiong Rhizoma* (Chuan Xiong) to promote blood circulation and remove blood stasis; *Corydalis Rhizoma* (Yan Hu Suo), *Cyperi Rhizoma* (Xiang Fu) and *Citri Reticulatae Pericarpium Viride* (Qing Pi) to regulate qi and stop pain; *Rehmannia Radix* (Sheng Di Huang) and *Angelicae Sinensis Radix* (Dang Gui) to nourish and harmonize blood. The latter is composed of *Cinnamomi Ramulus* (Gui Zhi) and *Glycyrrhizae Radix et Rhizoma* (Gan Cao) to warm and supplement heart-yang, *Os Draconis* (Long Gu) and *Ostreae Concha* (Mu Li) to calm the spirits and stop fright.

枝甘草龙骨牡蛎汤。前方用：桃仁、红花、丹参、赤芍药、川芎活血化瘀；延胡索、香附、青皮理气止痛；生地黄、当归养血和血。后方用：桂枝、甘草温补心阳；龙骨、牡蛎安神定悸。

Modification: For stasis due to deficiency, delete herbs for regulating qi, add *Astragali Radix* (Huang Qi), *Codonopsis Radix* (Dang Shen) and *Polygonati Rhizoma* (Huang Jing); for turbid phlegm, distention and oppressive pain in the chest, turbid greasy tongue fur, add *Trichosanthis Pericarpium* (Gua Lou Pi), *Allii Macrostemonis Bulbus* (Xie Bai) and *Citri Reticulatae Pericarpium* (Chen Pi); for severe chest pain, add *Olibanum* (Ru Xiang), *Myrrha* (Mo Yao), *Faeces Trogopterorum* (Wu Ling Zhi), *Typhae Pollen* (Pu Huang) and *Notoginseng Radix et Rhizoma Powder* (San Qi Fen).

加减：若因虚致瘀者去理气之品，气虚加黄芪、党参、黄精；夹痰浊，胸满闷痛，苔浊腻，加瓜蒌、薤白、半夏、广陈皮；胸痛甚，加乳香、没药、五灵脂、蒲黄、三七粉等。

2.2.7 Phlegm-fire Interfering With the heart

2.2.7 痰火扰心

Manifestations: Palpitation off and on, easiness to be frightened, distention in the chest, irritation,

证候：心悸时发时止，受惊易作，胸闷烦躁，失眠多

insomnia, plenty of dreams, dry and bitter mouth, dry stool, short dark urine; red tongue with yellow greasy tongue fur; taut rolling pulse.

梦，口干苦，大便秘结，小便短赤。舌红，苔黄腻，脉弦滑。

Treatment: To clear away heat and reslove phlegm, tranquilize the heat and calm the spirits.

治法： 清热化痰，宁心安神。

Formulas and Herbs: *Coptis-Warming-Gallbladder Decoction* (Huang Lian Wen Dan Tang), usually composed of *Coptidis Rhizoma* (Huang Lian) to cleanse the heart and remove irritation; *Pinelliae Rhizoma* (Ban Xia), *Citri Exocarpium Rubrum* (Ju Hong), *Poria* (Fu Ling), *Aurantii Fructus Immaturus* (Zhi Shi) and *Bambusae Caulis in Taenias* (Zhu Ru) to dry dampness and resolve phlegm.

方药： 黄连温胆汤。常用：黄连清心除烦；半夏、橘红、茯苓、枳实、竹茹燥湿化痰。

Modification: For intangled phlegm and heat, and dry stool, add *Rhei Radix et Rhizoma* (Sheng Da Huang); for severe palpitation, add *Margaritifera Concha* (Zhen Zhu Mu), *Haliotidis Concha* (Shi Jue Ming) and *Magnetitum* (Ci Shi) to oppress and calm the spirits; for yin injury by depressive fire, add *Ophiopogonis Radix* (Mai Men Dong), *Polygonati Odorati Rhizoma* (Yu Zhu), *Asparagi Radix* (Tian Dong) and *Rehmannia Radix* (Sheng Di Huang) to nourish yin and clear away heat.

加减： 若痰热互结，大便秘结者，加生大黄；心悸重者，加珍珠母、石决明、磁石重镇安神；火郁伤阴者，加麦门冬、玉竹、天门冬、生地黄养阴清热。

Chest Discomfort

胸　痹

Chest discomfort is caused by blockade of heart vessel due to many factors, which has main clinical symptoms such as oppressional pain in the chest that can even reaches the back, dyspnea as severe as not able to lie down. Patients of light chest discomfort feels suffocating oppression in the chest and difficult breath while patients of severe chest discomfort feel

胸痹是由多种因素引起心脉痹阻，临床以胸部闷痛，甚则胸痛彻背，喘息不得卧为主症的一种疾病，轻者仅感胸闷如窒，呼吸欠畅，重者则有胸痛，严重者心痛彻背，背痛彻心。

heartache reaching the back and pain in the back reaching the heart.

1 Etiology and Pathogenesis

Chest discomfort can be caused mainly by cold pathogenic factors invading inside, improper diet, emotional disturbance, overstrain, internal injuries, weak constitution due to old age, leading to the dysfunction ofthe liver, spleen, kidney and the blockade of heart vessel.

1 病因病机

胸痹的致病原因主要有寒邪内侵、饮食不节、情志失调、劳倦内伤、年迈体虚，导致心肝脾肾功能失调，心脉痹阻而产生本病。

1.1 Weak Constitution Due to Old Age and Heart-yin Deficiency

As one gets old, kidney-qi gets weak. The weakness and deficiency of kidney-yang results in insufficiency of heart-yang or heart-qi, because of which blood cannot circulate well and heart vessel are blocked, leading to chest discomfort. In another case, insufficiency of heart-yin due to kidney-yin deficiency, and heart vessel lacks in moisturizing and nourishing due to yin-blood deficiency, cause chest discomfort.

1.1 年老体虚，心肾亏虚

年老之人，肾气渐衰，肾阳虚衰导致心阳不振或心气不足，血脉运行不利，心脉痹阻则成胸痹。若肾阴亏虚导致心阴不足，阴血亏虚心脉失于濡养，而成胸痹。

1.2 Cold Pathogenic Factors Invading Inside and Blocking Chest-yang

Cold pathogenic factors attacks and blocks chest-yang, which hinders the circulation of qi and blood, which leads to the blockade ofheart vessel. Therefore, chest discomfort is caused.

1.2 寒邪内侵，痹阻胸阳

寒邪内侵，胸阳被遏，气血运行不畅导致心脉痹阻发为胸痹。

1.3 Improper Diet and Spleen and Stomach Injuries

Over intake of sweet, fat food and over-drinking will damage the tranferring and transforming functions of the spleen and stomach. Dampness gathers and turns into phlegm, which finally blocks the heart vessel. Or when the spleen and the stom-

1.3 饮食不节，脾胃损伤

过食甘肥、饮酒过度，脾胃受损运化失司，湿聚为痰，痹阻心脉；或脾胃受损，气血生化乏源，心脉失养，而成胸痹。

ach get injured, qi and blood cannot be generated and tranformed. And the heart vessel lacks in nurturing, leading to chest discomfort.

1.4 Emotional Disturbance Injures the Liver and the Spleen

Depressive anger injures the liver. When liver fails to disperse and purge, functional activities of qi will be affected. Or when the spleen injured by worries fails to transfer, then turbid phlegm appears. Both qi-stagnation and phlegm-blockade can lead to unsmooth circulation of blood which brings about chest discomfort.

In a word, pathologically, chest discomfort is the blockade ofheart vessel that lies in the heart but is related to the liver, the lung, the spleen and the kidney. Its nature is primary deficiency and secondary excess. The former includes qi deficiency, qi-yin deficiency and deficiency and weakness of yang-qi while the latter includes blood stasis, cold clots, turbid phlegm and qi stagnation which can co-occur.

2 Syndrome Differentiation and Treatment

2.1 Key Points of Syndrome Differentiation

Doctors firstly should identify the severity of the disease. Pain that lasts for a short period of time and disappear shortly after is usually of light condition while pain that lasts long and attacks continually are of serious condition. And pain that last for hours or days without likeliness to end is of life-threatening condition. Pain attacks after strain but is relieved after rest or herbstion is known as normal development while pain that cannot be relieved after herbstion is known as of dangerous situation. Secondly, doctors should distinguish deficiency from

1.4 情志失调,损伤肝脾

郁怒伤肝,肝失疏泄,气机阻滞;或忧思伤脾,脾失健运,痰浊内生。气滞或痰阻均可导致血行不畅,心脉痹阻成为胸痹。

综上所述,胸痹的基本病机为心脉痹阻,病位在心,涉及肝、肺、脾、肾等脏。其病性为本虚标实,虚实夹杂。本虚有气虚、气阴两虚及阳气虚衰;标实有血瘀、寒凝、痰浊、气滞,且可相兼为病。

2 辨证论治

2.1 辨治要点

首先辨病情轻重,其次辨标本虚实。疼痛持续时间短暂,瞬息即逝者多轻;持续时间长,反复发作者多重;若持续数小时甚至数日不休者常为重症或危候。疼痛遇劳发作,休息或服药后能缓解者为顺症;服药后难以缓解者常为危候。其次需辨别虚实,分清标本。标实者:闷重而痛轻,兼见胸胁胀满,喜太

excess, the primary symptoms from the secondary symptoms. Excess of the primary symptoms is such that severe oppresion and light pain along with distention and fullness in the chest, deep sigh, suffocation, thin white tongue fur, taut pulse are due to qi stagnation; suffocation and pain in the chest with drooping and phlegm expectoration, pale tongue with whilte tongue fur, taut rolling pulse or taut pulse are due to turbid phlegm; twisting pain in the chest which attacks or aggravates because of cold, aversion to cold, cold limbs, pale tongue with white tongue fur, fine pulse are due to cold freezing the heart vessel; unstable stabbing pain but a fixed pain spot, attacks in nights, purple dark tongue or with stasis spots, knotted slow pulse or uneven pulse are due to stagnation and stasis of the heart vessel. Primary deficiency are like such. Dull pain and oppression in the chest over strain, palpitation, short breath, tiredness, pale and enlarged tender tongue with teeth marks on its edge, deep fine pulse or knotted slow pulse are due to insufficiency of heart-qi; twisting pain, distention in the chest, short breath, cold limbs, spirtual tiredness, spontaneous sweating, deep fine pulse are due to insuffciency of heart-yang; endless dull pain off and on that attacks in movement, thirst, pale red tongue with little tongue fur, deep fine rapid pulse are due to deficiency of both qi and yin.

息，憋气，苔薄白，脉弦者，多属气滞；胸部窒闷而痛，伴唾吐痰涎，苔腻，脉弦滑或弦数者，多属痰浊；胸痛如绞，遇寒则发，或得冷加剧，伴畏寒肢冷，舌淡苔白，脉细，为寒凝心脉所致；刺痛固定不移，痛有定处，夜间多发，舌紫暗或有瘀斑，脉结代或涩，由心脉瘀滞所致。本虚者：心胸隐痛而闷，因劳累而发，伴心慌，气短、乏力，舌淡胖嫩，边有齿痕，脉沉细或结代者，多属心气不足；若绞痛兼见胸闷气短，四肢厥冷，神倦自汗，脉沉细，则为心阳不振；隐痛时作时止，缠绵不休，动则多发，伴口干，舌淡红而少苔，脉沉细而数，则属气阴两虚表现。

The principle of treatment should be treating the secondary symptoms first and the primary symptoms next. Doctors should start from dispelling the pathogenic factors to strengthening the healthy factors or treat both according to predominance of excess, deficiency, the primary symptoms, the sec-

本病的治疗原则应先治其标，后治其本，先从祛邪入手，然后再予扶正，必要时可根据虚实标本的主次，兼顾同治。治标尤重活血通脉，治本尤重补益心气。

ondary symptoms. When treating the secondary symptoms, focus on promoting blood circulation and dredging collaterals. When treating the primary symptoms, focus on supplementing and invigorating heart-qi.

2.2 Therapeutic Methods of Different Types of Chest Pain

2.2.1 Heart-blood Stasis Blocks

Manifestations: Stabbing or twisting pain in the chest, fixed pain, pain aggravating in night, pain in the heart reaching the back and pain in the back reaching the heart or pain stretching out to shoulders and back, prolonged oppression in the chest that aggravates over strain; purple dark tongue with stasis spots; thin tongue fur; taut uneven pulse.

Treatment: To promote blood circulation and remove blood stasis, dredge vessels and stop pain.

Formulas and Herbs: *Sanguine Mansion Stasis-Expelling Decoction* (Xue Fu Zhu Yu Tang), usually composed of *Persicae Semen* (Tao Ren), *Carthami Flos* (Hong Hua), *Angelicae Sinensis Radix* (Dang Gui), *Paeoniae Radix Rubra* (Chi Shao) and *Chuanxiong Rhizoma* (Chuan Xiong) to promote blood circulation and remove stasis; *Bupleuri Radix* (Chai Hu) and *Aurantii Fructus*(Zhi Qiao) to regulate qi.

Modification: For severe blood stasis and chest pain, add *Olibanum* (Ru Xiang), *Myrrha* (Mo Yao), *Curcumae Radix* (Yu Jin), *Dalbergiae Odoriferae Lignum* (Jiang Xiang), *Salviae Miltiorrhizae Radix et Rhizoma Radix* (Dan Shen); for severe blood-stasis and qi-stagnation, severe pain in the chest, add *Aquilariae Lignum Resinatum* (Chen Xiang), *Santali Albi Lignum* (Tan Xiang) and *Piperis Longi Fructus* (Bi Bo) to regualate qi and stop

2.2 分型论治

2.2.1 心血瘀阻

证候：心胸疼痛，如刺如绞，痛有定处，入夜为甚，甚则心痛彻背，背痛彻心，或痛引肩背，伴有胸闷，日久不愈，可因暴怒、劳累而加重。舌质紫暗，有瘀斑，苔薄，脉弦涩。

治法：活血化瘀，通脉止痛。

方药：血府逐瘀汤。常用：桃仁、红花、当归、赤芍药、川芎活血化瘀；柴胡、枳壳调整气机。

加减：瘀血痹阻重证，胸痛剧烈，可加乳香、没药、郁金、降香、丹参等；血瘀气滞并重，胸闷痛甚者，可加沉香、檀香、荜茇等辛香理气止痛之药；若卒然心痛发作，可含化复方丹参滴丸、速效救心丸等活血化瘀、芳香止痛之品。

pain; for sudden heart pain attacks, use *Compound Salviae Miltiorrhizae Droplets* (Fu Fang Dan Shen Di Ji) and *Heart Disease Relieve & Cure Pills* (Su Xiao Jiu Xin Wan) to promote blood circulation and remove blood stasis and stop pain.

2.2.2 Qi stagnating in the Heart and Chest

Manifestations: Distention and fullness in the chest, recurring dull pain, fixed pain, deep breath for times, triggered or worsened by emotional and spiritual disturbance, or distention and fullness in the abdomen which is relieved after burping or flatus; thin or greasy tongue fur; fine taut pulse.

Treatment: To disperse the liver and regulate qi, promote blood circulation and dredge collaterals.

Formulas and Herbs: *Bupleurum-Dispersing-Liver Powder* (Chai Hu Shu Gan San), usually composed of *Bupleuri Radix* (Chai Hu), *Cyperi Rhizoma* (Xiang Fu) and *Aurantii Fructus* (Zhi Qiao) to disperse the liver, regulate qi and stop pain; *Chuanxiong Rhizoma* (Chuan Xiong) to promote blood circulation and stop pain, *Paeoniae Radix Alba* (Bai Shao) and *Glycyrrhizae Radix et Rhizoma* (Gan Cao) to relieve and stop pain.

Modification: For evident oppression in the chest and heartache that is a sign of qi-stagnation and blood-stasis, add *Great Guffaw Powder* (Shi Xiao San); for depressive qi transforming into heat, irritation, thirst, constipation, red tongue with yellow tongue fur, taut rapid pulse, use *Moutan Cortex and Gardeniae- Free Wanderer Pills* (Dan Zhi Xiao Yao Wan); for severe constipation, add *Angelicae Sinensis and Aloe Pills* (Dang Gui Lu Hui Wan) to purge depressive fire.

2.2.2 气滞心胸

证候：心胸满闷，隐痛阵发，痛有定处，时欲太息，遇情志不遂时容易诱发或加重，或兼有脘腹胀闷，得嗳气或矢气则舒。苔薄或薄腻，脉细弦。

治法：疏肝理气，活血通络。

方药：柴胡疏肝散。常用：柴胡、香附、枳壳疏肝理气止痛；川芎活血止痛；芍药、甘草缓急止痛。

加减：胸闷心痛明显，为气滞血瘀之象，可合用失笑散；气郁化热，心烦易怒，口干便秘，舌红苔黄，脉弦数者，用丹栀逍遥散；便秘严重者，加当归芦荟丸以泻郁火。

2.2.3 Turbid Phlegm Blocks the Chest

Manifestations: Severe oppression in the chest, slight heartache, plenty of phlegm, short breath, heavy limbs, obesity, attacks or aggravation on overcast or raining days, fatigue, weakness, poor appetite, loose stool, phlegm expectoration and drooping; enlarged tongue with teeth marks on the edge; turbid greasy or white slippery pulse; rolling pulse.

Treatment: To activate yang and purge turbidity, remove phlegem and eliminate blockade.

Formulas and Herbs: *Trichosanthis, Allii Macrostemonis Bulbus and Pinelliae Decoction* (Gua Lou Xie Bai Ban Xia Tang) and *Phlegm-Cleansing Decoction* (Di Tan Tang), usually composed of *Trichosanthis Fructus* (Gua Lou), *Pinelliae Rhizoma* (Ban Xia), *Arisaematis Rhizoma* (Tian Nan Xing) and *Bambusae Caulis in Taenias* (Zhu Ru) to resolve phlegm and disperse clots; *Allii Macrostemonis Bulbus* (Xie Bai) to activate yang and resolve phlegm; *Acori Tatarinowii Rhizoma* (Shi Chang Pu) to resolve phlegm and induce resuscitation; *Citri Reticulatae Pericarpium* (Chen Pi) and *Aurantii Fructus Immaturus* (Zhi Shi) to regulate qi and stop pain; *Ginseng Radix et Rhizoma* (Ren Shen), *Poria* (Fu Ling) and *Glycyrrhizae Radix et Rhizoma* (Gan Cao) to supplement and invigorate heart-qi.

Modification: For depressive turbid phlegm transforming into heart with signs such as thick yellow phlegm, constipation, yellow greasy tongue fur, use *Coptis-Warming-Gallbladder Decoction* (Huang Lian Wen Dan Tang) and *Curcumae Radix* (Yu Jin); for phlegm and blood stasis blocking each other with signs such as suffocating oppression in

2.2.3 痰浊闭胸

证候: 胸闷重而心痛微,痰多气短,肢体沉重,形体肥胖,遇阴雨天而易发作或加重,伴有倦怠乏力,纳呆便溏,咯吐痰涎。舌体胖大且边有齿痕,苔浊腻或白滑,脉滑。

治法: 通阳泄浊,豁痰宣痹。

方药: 栝蒌薤白半夏汤合涤痰汤。常用:瓜蒌、半夏、天南星、竹茹化痰散结;薤白通阳化痰;石菖蒲化痰开窍;陈皮、枳实理气止痛;人参、茯苓、甘草补益心气。

加减: 若患者痰黄稠,便秘,苔黄腻,为痰浊郁而化热者,用黄连温胆汤加郁金;若痰瘀交阻,症见胸闷如窒,心胸隐痛或绞痛阵作,舌紫暗,苔白腻,可加桃仁、红花。

the chest, dull pain in the heart and chest or paroxysmal twisting pain, purple dark tongue, greasy white tongue fur, add *Persicae Semen* (Tao Ren) and *Carthami Flos* (Hong Hua).

2.2.4 Cold Freezing Heart Vessel

Manifestations: Sudden twisting pain in the heart reaching the back, gasping too much to lie down, attacks or aggravation due to sudden attacks by wind-cold or temperature drop, physical cold even with cold limbs, spontaneous cold sweating, oppression in the chest, short breath, palpitation, pale complexion; thin white tongue fur; deep tense pulse or deep fine pulse.

Treatment: To dispel cold with pungent and warming herbs.

Formulas and Herbs: *Aurantii Immaturus, Allii Macrostemonis Bulbus and Cinnamomi Decoction* (Zhi Shi Xie Bai Gui Zhi Tang) and *Angelicae Sinensis-Four Disorder Decoction* (Dang Gui Si Ni Tang), usually composed of *Allii Macrostemonis Bulbus* (Xie Bai), *Cinnamomi Ramulus* (Gui Zhi) and *Asari Radix et Rhizoma* (Xi Xin) to connect yang and disperse cold; *Angelicae Sinensis Radix* (Dang Gui) and *Paeoniae Radix Rubra* (Chi Shao) to promote blood circulation and remove blood stasis; *Aurantii Fructus Immaturus* (Zhi Shi) and *Tetrapanacis Medulla* (Tong Cao) to regulate activities of qi.

Modification: For severe chest pain due to extreme of yin-cold with signs like endless sharp pain in the chest, physical cold and cold limbs, short breath and gasp, deep tense pulse or deep weak pulse, use *Aconite Main Tuber and Halloysite Pill* (Wu Tou Chi Shi Zhi Wan) and *Piperis Longi*

2.2.4 寒凝心脉

证候：卒然心痛如绞，心痛彻背，喘不得卧，多因气候骤冷或骤感风寒而发病或加重，伴形寒，甚则手足不温，冷汗自出，胸闷气短，心悸，面色苍白。苔薄白，脉沉紧或沉细。

治法：辛温散寒，宣通心阳。

方药：枳实薤白桂枝汤合当归四逆汤。常用：薤白、桂枝、细辛通阳散寒；当归、芍药活血化瘀；枳实、通草调畅气机。

加减：阴寒极盛之胸痹重症，表现胸痛剧烈，痛无休止，伴身寒肢冷，气短喘息，脉沉紧或沉微者，用乌头赤石脂丸加荜茇、高良姜、细辛等；若心痛剧而四肢不温，冷

Fructus (Bi Bo), *Alpiniae Officinarum Rhizoma* (Gao Liang Jiang) and *Asari Radix et Rhizoma* (Xi Xin); for sharp pain in the heart and cold limbs, cold-sweating, take immediately beneath the tongue *Styrax Pills* (Su He Xiang Wan) or *Moschus-Heart-Securing Pills* (She Xiang Bao Xin Wan) to regulate qi, warmly activate yang and induce resusciation.

汗自出，即刻舌下含苏合香丸或麝香保心丸，以芳香化浊，理气温通开窍。

2.2.5 Deficiency of Yin and Qi

Manifestations: Dull pain in the heart and chest from time to time, palpitation, short breath, aggravation in movements, tiredness and fatigue, low voice and weak breath, pale complexion, sweating; pale red enlarged tongue with teeth marks on the edge; thin white tongue fur; weak fine gentle or knotted slow pulse.

Treatment: To invigorate qi and nourish yin, promote blood circulation and dredge collaterals.

Formulas and Herbs: *Pulse-Engendering Powder* (Sheng Mai San) and *Ginseng Tonic Decoction* (Ren Shen Yang Rong Tang), usually composed of *Ginseng Radix et Rhizoma* (Ren Shen), *Astragali Radix* (Huang Qi), *Atractylodis Macrocephalae Rhizoma* (Bai Zhu), *Poria* (Fu Ling) and *Glycyrrhizae Radix et Rhizoma* (Gan Cao) to invigorate qi and strengthen the spleen; *Ophiopogonis Radix* (Mai Men Dong), *Rehmannia Radix* (Di Huang), *Angelicae Sinensis Radix* (Dang Gui) and *Paeoniae Radix Alba* (Bai Shao Yao) to nourish yin and nourish blood; *Polygalae Radix* (Yuan Zhi) and *Schisandrae Chinensis Fructus* (Wu Wei Zi) to nourish the heart and calm the spirits.

Modification: For dry mouth, dry stool, add *Rehmannia Radix* (Sheng Di Huang), *Polygoni Multiflori Radix* (He Shou Wu), *Polygonati Odorati*

2.2.5 气阴两虚

证候：心胸隐痛，时作时休，心悸气短，动则益甚。伴倦怠乏力，声息低微，面色㿠白，易汗出。舌质淡红，舌体胖且边有齿痕，苔薄白，脉虚细缓或结代。

治法：益气养阴，活血通脉。

方药：生脉散合人参养荣汤。常用：人参、黄芪、白术、茯苓、甘草益气健脾；麦门冬、地黄、当归、白芍药滋阴养血；远志、五味子养心安神。

加减：口干舌燥，大便干结，可加生地黄、何首乌、玉竹、石斛；自汗，纳呆，便溏，

Rhizoma (Yu Zhu) and *Dendrobii Caulis* (Shi Hu); for spontaneous sweating, poor appetite and loose stool, delete *Rehmannia Radix* (Di Huang), *Angelicae Sinensis Radix* (Dang Gui) and *Ophiopogonis Radix* (Mai Men Dong) and add *Dioscoreae Rhizoma* (Shan Yao), *Amomi Fructus* (Sha Ren) and *Saposhnikoviae Radix*(Fang Feng).

去地黄、当归、麦门冬，加山药、砂仁、防风。

2. 2. 6　Deficiency of Heart-yin and Kidney-yin

Manifestations: Oppression and pain in the heart, palpitation, night-sweating, pseudo-irritation, sleeplessness, soreness of the waist and weakness of knees, dizziness, tinnitus, dry mouth, constipation, red tongue with little fluid; thin tongue fur or peeling tongue fur; fine weak pulse or quick pulse.

Treatment: To nourish yin and clear away fire, nourish the heart and harmonize collaterals.

Formulas and Herbs: *Celestial Emperor Heart-Supplementing Elixir* (Tian Wang Bu Xin Dan) and *Honeyed Liquorice Decoction* (Zhi Gan Cao Tang), usually composed of *Glycyrrhizae Radix et Rhizoma Praeparata* (Zhi Gan Cao), *Ginseng Radix et Rhizoma* (Ren Shen) and *Poria* (Fu Ling) to invigorate and supplement heart-qi; *Rehmannia Radix* (Sheng Di Huang), *Ophiopogonis Radix* (Mai Men Dong), *Asparagi Radix* (Tian Dong), *Scrophulariae Radix* (Xuan Shen) and *Asini Corii Colla* (E Jiao) to nourish yin and clear away fire; *Schisandrae Chinensis Fructus* (Wu Wei Zi), *Polygalae Radix* (Yuan Zhi), *Ziziphi Spinosae Semen* (Suan Zao Ren) and *Platycladi Semen* (Bai Zi Ren) to nourish the heart and calm the spirits.

Modification: For pseudo-irritation and sleeplessness, red tongue-lip with little fluid, use Wild

2. 2. 6　心肾阴虚

证候：心痛憋闷，心悸盗汗，虚烦不寐，腰酸膝软，头晕耳鸣，口干便秘，舌红少津。苔薄或剥，脉细数或促代。

治法：滋阴清火，养心和络。

方药：天王补心丹合炙甘草汤。常用：炙甘草、人参、茯苓补益心气；生地黄、麦门冬、天门冬、玄参、阿胶养阴清火；五味子、远志、酸枣仁、柏子仁养心安神。

加减：若见虚烦不寐，舌尖红少津者，可用酸枣仁汤；

Jujube Seed Decoction (Suan Zao Ren Tang); for dizziness and vertigo, dumb limbs and trembling hands, add *Margaritifera Concha* (Zhen Zhu Mu), *Magnetitum* (Ci Shi), *Haliotidis Concha* (Shi Jue Ming) and *Succinum* (Hu Po) to restrain yang; for dizziness and vertigo, spermatorrhea, night-sweating, palpitation, restlessness, dry mouth and throat, applp *Kidney Yin-Reinforcing Drink* (Zuo Gui Yin).

若见头晕目眩,肢麻手抖,加用珍珠母、灵磁石、石决明、琥珀等重镇潜阳之品;若见头晕目眩,遗精盗汗,心悸不宁,口燥咽干,用左归饮。

2.2.7 Yang-deficiency of the Heart and the Kidney

Manifestations: Palpitation and heartache, oppression in the chest and short breath which aggravates in movements, spontaneous sweating, pale complexion, lassitude, fear of cold, cold limbs or edema, pale and enlarged tongue with white or greasy tongue fur; deep retarded fine pulse.

Treatment: To warm and supplement yang qi and boost heart-yang.

Formulas and Herbs: *Ginseng and Aconite Decoction* (Shen Fu Tang) and *Kidney Yin-Reinforcing Drink* (Zuo Gui Yin), usually composed of *Ginseng Radix et Rhizoma* (Ren Shen) to reinforce vital energy; *Aconm Lateralis Radix Praeparata* (Fu Zi) and *Cinnamomi Cortex* (Rou Gui) to warmly activate heart yang and kidney yang; *Rehmanniae Radix Praeparata* (Shu Di Huang) and *Corni Fructus* (Shan Zhu Yu), *Dioscoreae Rhizoma* (Shan Yao), *Lycii Fructus* (Gou Qi Zi), *Eucommiae Cortex* (Du Zhong) and *Cuscutae Semen* (Tu Si Zi) to nourish and strengthen kidney-essence; *Angelicae Sinensis Radix* (Dang Gui) to promote blood circulation and dredge the collaterals.

Modification: For edema, dyspnea, palpitation, use *True Warrior Decoction* (Zhen Wu Tang)

2.2.7 心肾阳虚

证候: 心悸而痛,胸闷气短,动则更甚,自汗,面色㿠白,神倦怯寒,四肢欠温或肿胀。舌质淡胖,边有齿痕,苔白或腻,脉沉细迟。

治法: 温补阳气,振奋心阳。

方药: 参附汤合右归饮。常用:人参大补元气;附子、肉桂温通心肾之阳;熟地黄、山茱萸、山药、枸杞子、杜仲、菟丝子补益肾精;当归活血通络。

加减: 若见水肿、喘促、心悸,用真武汤加黄芪、汉防

with *Astragali Radix* (Huang Qi), *Stephaniae Tetrandrae Radix* Tetrandrae (Han Fang Ji), *Polyporus* (Zhu Ling), *Plantaginis Semen* (Che Qian Zi) to warm kidney-yang and resolve water and fluid retention; for yang-deficiency and coma due to frenetic activities of qi with signs like pale complexion, cold limbs, heavy cold sweating, weak and barely perceptible pulse, use *Four Disorders Decoction* (Si Ni Tang) and *Ginseng Decoction* (Ren Shen Tang) to warm yang and invigorate qi, resuscitate and stop disorder.

己、猪苓、车前子温肾阳而化水饮；若阳虚欲脱厥逆者，症见面色苍白，四肢厥冷，冷汗淋漓，脉微欲绝，用四逆加人参汤，温阳益气，回阳救逆。

Insomnia

不　寐

Insomnia is a sleep disorder in which there is an inability to attain normal sleep often due to yang's not going into yin, characterized by inadequate time and depth of sleep. Patients with light insomnia can be difficult to fall into sleep, light sleep, waking up at times or awake as long as one desires. Serious insomnia can be sleepless overnight.

不寐是因为阳不入阴所引起的经常不能获得正常睡眠为特征的一类病证。主要表现为睡眠时间、深度的不足。轻者入睡困难，或寐而不酣，时寐时醒，或醒后不能再睡，重则彻夜不眠。

1　Etiology and Pathogenesis

1　病因病机

Emotional and spiritual dissatisfaction, excess diet, unbalance between work and rest, weak constitution with constant illness are the main causes of insomnia. And the pathogenesis is yang-excess and yin-deficiency and the imbalance between yin and yang.

本病病因主要有情志不遂、饮食不节、劳逸失调、体弱多病。基本病机为阳盛阴衰，阴阳失衡。

1.1　Emotional and Spiritual Dissatisfaction and Restlessness

1.1　情志失调，心神不安

Excess of the seven emotions such as the liver hurt by rage, the spleen injured by worry, the heart injured by overjoy, will lead to restlessness or the

七情过极，如怒伤肝、思伤脾、喜伤心等均可导致心神不安或心神失养，造成不

heart and spirits lacks in nourish, resulting in insomnia.

寐。

1.2 Excess Diet Damaging the Harmony between the Spleen and the Stomach

1.2 饮食不节,脾胃不和

Gluttony injures the spleen and the stomach, which leads to the disharmony between the spleen and the stomach. Therefore, yang roams outside which results in restlessness.

暴饮暴食,损伤脾胃,胃气失和,阳浮越于外,以致睡卧不安。

1.3 Depressive Heat in the Liver and the Gallbladder, Phlegm-fire Interfering Upward

1.3 肝胆郁热,痰火上扰

The meridians of the liver and the gallbladder are depressed inside by phlegm heat, and phlegm-fire interferes upward the heart and spirits, leading to insomnia.

肝胆之经痰热内郁,痰火上扰心神,而成不寐。

1.4 Timidness due to Heart-deficiency and Mental Derangement

1.4 心虚胆怯,神不守舍

Habitual qi-deficiency in the heart and gallbladder leads to the lack of nurturing of the heart and spirits due to heart-qi deficiency and restlessness due to gallbladder-qi deficiency respectively, which finally causes pseudo-irritation and sleeplessness, dreaminess and easiness to wake up.

平素心胆气虚,心气不足则心神失养,胆气亏虚而心神不宁,终成虚烦不眠,多梦易醒。

1.5 Weak Constitution Due to Prolonged Illness Leading to Deficiency of Essence and Blood

1.5 久病体虚,精血亏虚

Congenital defects and too much intercourse will cause the deficiency of kidney-yin, lack of nourish of the heart and spirits. Then the heart-yang is so excited that cannot settle down into yin, which leads to insomnia. Or deficiency of qi and blood due to weak constitution after prolonged illness will lead to insufficiency of qi and blood which are unable to nourish the heart and the spirits, resulting in insomnia.

先天禀赋不足、房劳过度以致肾阴亏虚,心神失养,心阳亢于上,阳不入阴而为不寐;或久病体虚,气血亏虚而致心血不足,心神失养遂成不寐。

In a word, pathologically, insomnia lies in the

综上所述,不寐其病位

heart, but is closely related to the liver, the spleen and the kidney. By pathogenesis, insomnia differs in deficiency and excess. Insomnia of excess type is caused by liver depression turning into fire and phlegm interferes inside. And yang-excess cannot settle into yin that leads to insomnia. Insomnia of deficiency type is caused by deficiency in both the heart and the spleen. Timidness due to heart-deficiency will stop the connection between the heart and the kidney, prevent water and fire from coordinating each other, which will leads to the lack of nourish of the heart and the spirits, and yin-deficiency is not able to take in yang. Insomnia is therefore resulted in. Prolonged insomnia will have symptoms of both two types.

在心，与肝、脾、肾密切相关。不寐的病机有虚实之分，实证由肝郁化火，痰热内扰，阳盛不得入于阴而致，虚证多由心脾两虚，心虚胆怯，心肾不交，水火不济，心神失养，阴虚不能纳阳而发。失眠久病亦可出现虚实夹杂之证。

2 Syndrome Differentiation and Treatment

2.1 Key Points of Syndrome Differentiation

To treat insomnia, doctors first should distinguish the types, the excess or the deficiency. Insomnia of deficiency typeare mainly due to insufficient yin-blood, and the heart and the spirits lack in nourish, which has clinical characteristics of emaciation, lusterless complexion, lassitude and unwillingness to talk, palpitation and forgetfulness. On the other hand, insomnia of excess type is due to pathogenic heat interfering with the heart and has symptoms of uneasiness, irritation, bitter mouth and dry throat, constipation and dark urine. Secondly, doctors should identify the pathological location. Heart is the primary location. Because of the lack of heart and spirits nourish or uneasiness, the spirits are not well guarded, which leads to insomnia. Besides, the liver, the gallbladder, the spleen,

2 辨证论治

2.1 辨治要点

本病辨证首分虚实。虚证，多属阴血不足，心失所养，临床特点为体质瘦弱，面色无华，神疲懒言，心悸健忘；实证为邪热扰心，临床特点为心烦易怒，口苦咽干，便秘溲赤。次辨病位，病位主要在心。由于心神的失养或不安，神不守舍而不寐，且与肝、胆、脾、胃、肾相关。如：急躁易怒而不寐，多为肝火内扰；脘闷苔腻而不寐，多为胃腑宿食，痰热内盛；心烦心悸，头晕健忘而不寐，多为阴虚火旺，心肾不交；面色少华，肢倦神疲而不寐，多属脾

the stomach and the kidney are closely related to the disease. For instance, insomnia due to irritation is very much likely to be caused by liver-fire interfering inside. Insomnia due to distention in the abdomen and greasy tongue fur is more likely to be caused by undigested food in the stomach and exuberance of phlegm-heat. Insomnia due to irritation and palpitation, dizziness, forgetfulness is likely to be caused by yin-deficiency and fire-excess, discordance between heart and spleen. Insomnia due to weakness and lassitude is mostly caused by dysfunction of the spleen and spleen-deficiency, the lack of nourish of the heart and spirits. Insomnia due to restlessness, easiness to be frightened is more likely to be caused by qi-deficiency of the heart and gallbladder.

虚不运，心神失养；心烦不寐，触事易惊，多属心胆气虚等。

Insomnia should be treated through supplementing deficiency and purging excess to restore the balance of yin and yang in zang-fu organs. For insomnia of excess type, eliminate surplus, for example, between dispersing the liver and purge fire, clear awaying and transforming phlegm-heat, promoting digestion and harmonizing the middle-Jiao. For insomnia of deficiency type, supplement what is short by invigorating qi and nourishing blood, strengthening the spleen, the liver and the kidney. Moreover, doctors should also pay attention to using such methods as calming spirits and tranquilizing the minds, nourishing blood and calm the spirits, suppressing and calming the spirits, cleansing the heart and calming the spirits. For disharmony of the emotions and the minds, along with herbstion, patients need psychological treatment to calm down, which can help the whole treatment.

不寐的治疗当以补虚泻实，调整脏腑阴阳为原则。实证泻其有余，如疏肝泻火、清化痰热、消导和中；虚证补其不足，如益气养血、健脾补肝益肾。在此基础上予安神定志、养血安神、镇惊安神、清心安神。对于情志失调者除药物外，辅以心理治疗稳定情绪增加疗效。

2.2 Therapeutic Methods for Different Patterns

2.2.1 Liver-fire Interferes with the Heart

Manifestations: Insomnia with many dreams, even sleeplessness overnight, irritation and impatience, dizziness and feeling fullness in the head, reddish eyes, tinnitus, bitter and dry mouth, no desire for food or drink, constipation, dark urine; red tongue with yellow tongue fur; taut and rapid pulse.

Therapeutic: To disperse the liver and purge fire to calm the heart and spirits.

Formulas and Herbs: *Gentian Liver-Draining Decoction* (Long Dan Xie Gan Tang), usually composed of *Cinnabaris* (Zhu Sha) to suppress and calm the spirits; *Coptidis Rhizoma* (Huang Lian) to clear away the heart and eliminate fire; *Rehmannia Radix* (Sheng Di Huang) and *Angelicae Sinensis Radix* (Dang Gui) to nourish yin and nourish blood.

Modification: For distention in the chest and fullness in the hypochondria with deep sighs, add *Cyperi Rhizoma* (Xiang Fu), *Curcumae Radix* (Yu Jin), *Citri Saroodactylis Fructus* (Fo Shou) and *Prunus mume var. viridicalyx* (Lü E Mei) to disperse the liver and resolve depression; for dizziness and vertigo, severe headache, sleeplessness and irritation, constipation, use *Angelicae Sinensis, Gentianae and Aleo Pills* (Dang Gui Long Hui Wan).

2.2.2 Phlegm-heatInterferes with the Heart

Manifestation: Restlessness and sleeplessness, distention in the chest and fullness in the abdomen, nausea and belch, bitter mouth, feeling heavy in the head, vertigo; reddish tongue with yellow greasy tongue fur; rapid rolling pulse.

Therapeutic: To clear away and transform phlegm-heat, harmonize zhong jiao and calm the

2.2 分型论治

2.2.1 肝火扰心

证候: 不寐多梦,甚则彻夜不眠,急躁易怒,伴头晕头胀,目赤耳鸣,口干而苦,不思饮食,便秘溲赤。舌红苔黄,脉弦而数。

治法: 疏肝泻火,镇心安神。

方药: 龙胆泻肝汤。常用:朱砂重镇安神;黄连清心泻火;生地黄、当归滋阴养血。

加减: 胸闷胁胀,善太息者,加香附、郁金、佛手、绿萼梅以疏肝解郁;若头晕目眩,头痛欲裂,不寐躁怒,大便秘结者,可用当归龙荟丸。

2.2.2 痰热扰心

证候: 心烦不寐,胸闷脘痞,泛恶嗳气,伴口苦,头重,目眩。舌偏红,苔黄腻,脉滑数。

治法: 清化痰热,和中安神。

spirits.

Formulas and Herbs: *Coptis-Warming-Gallbladder Decoction* (Huang Lian Wen Dan Tang), usually composed of *Gentianae Radix et Rhizoma* (Long Dan), *Scutellariae Radix* (Huang Qin) and *Gardeniae Fructus* (Zhi Zi) to clear away the liver and purge fire; *Alismatis Rhizoma* (Ze Xie), *Akebiae Caulis* (Mu Tong) and *Plantaginis Semen* (Che Qian Zi) to clear away heat and promote diuresis; *Rehmannia Radix* (Sheng Di Huang) and *Angelicae Sinensis Radix* (Dang Gui) to nourish yin and soften the liver; *Bupleuri Radix* (Chai Hu) to disperse the liver and regulate qi.

方药：黄连温胆汤。常用：龙胆草、黄芩、栀子清肝泻火；泽泻、木通、车前子清热利湿；生地黄、当归滋阴柔肝；柴胡疏肝理气。

Modification: For insomnia with distention in the chest and belch, fullness in the abdomen, sticky stool, greasy tongue fur, rolling pulse, add *Pinelliae and Setariae Decoction* (Ban Xia Shu Mi Tang); for palpitation and uneasiness, add *Margaritifera Concha* (Zhen Zhu Mu), *Succinum* (Hu Po) and *Cinnabaris* (Zhu Sha) to suppress fright and calm the spirits; for sleeplessness overnight, constipation, use *Chlorite-Expelling-Phlegm Pills* (Meng Shi Gun Tan Wan).

加减：不寐伴胸闷嗳气，脘腹胀满，大便不爽，苔腻脉滑，加用半夏秫米汤；若心悸不安，加珍珠母、琥珀、朱砂以镇惊安神；如彻夜不眠，大便秘结不通者，用礞石滚痰丸。

2.2.3 Disharmony of Stomach-qi

2.2.3 胃气不和

Manifestation: Restless sleep, discomfort in the stomach, belch and acid regurgitation, distention in the abdomen, stick stool or constipation; yellow greasy tongue fur; deep rolling pulse.

证候：睡卧不安，胃脘不适，嗳腐吞酸，腹胀，大便不爽或便秘。苔黄腻，脉沉滑。

Treatment: To promote digestion to eliminate food retention, harmonize the stomach and calm the spirits.

治法：消食化滞，和胃安神。

Formulas and Herbs: *Pachyma Compound Digestive Tonic Pills* (Bao He Wan), usually composed of *Crataegi Fructus* (Shan Zha), *Massa Fermentata*

方药：保和丸。常用：山楂、神曲、莱菔子消食导滞；苍术、半夏、茯苓、陈皮和胃

Medicinalis (Shen Qu) and *Raphani Semen* (Lai Fu Zi) to promote digestion and eliminate food retention; *Atractylodis Rhizoma* (Cang Zhu), *Pinelliae Rhizoma* (Ban Xia), *Poria* (Fu Ling) and *Citri Reticulatae Pericarpium* (Chen Pi) to harmonize the stomach and remove distention. *Alibiziae Cortex* (He Huan Pi) and *Polygoni Multiflori Caulis* (Ye Jiao Teng) can be added to calm the mind and spirits.

除满。本方可加合欢皮、夜交藤宁心安神。

Modification: For distention and fullness in the abdomen, add *Magnoliae Officinalis Cortex* (Hou Po) and *Arecae Semen* (Bing Lang); for evident signs of heat, add *Coptidis Rhizoma* (Huang Lian) and *Gardeniae Fructus* (Zhi Zi); for distention in the abdomen and constipation, use *Aurantii Immaturus-Promoting-Digestion Pills* (Zhi Shi Dao Zhi Wan).

加减: 脘腹胀满者,加厚朴、槟榔;若热象明显,可加黄连、山栀;腹胀便秘者,用枳实导滞丸。

2.2.4 Deficiency of the Heart and the Spleen

2.2.4 心脾两虚

Manifestation: Difficulty to fall asleep, dreaminess and easiness to wake up, palpitation, forgetfulness, lassitude, little intake, dizziness, vertigo, physical fatigue, distention in the abdomen, loose stool, lusterless face; pale tongue with thin tongue fur; thin weak pulse.

证候: 不易入睡,多梦易醒,心悸健忘,神疲食少,伴头晕目眩,四肢倦怠,腹胀便溏,面色少华。舌淡苔薄,脉细无力。

Treatment: To invigorate the heart and the spleen, nourish blood and calm the spirits.

治法: 补益心脾,养血安神。

Formulas and Herbs: *Angelica Spl enic Decoction* (Gui Pi Tang), usually composed of *Codonopsis Radix* (Dang Shen), *Astragali Radix* (Huang Qi) and *Atractylodis Macrocephalae Rhizoma* (Bai Zhu) to invigorate qi and strengthen the spleen; *Angelicae Sinensis Radix* (Dang Gui) to supplement blood; *Polygalae Radix* (Yuan Zhi), *Ziziphi Spinosae Semen* (Suan Zao Ren) and *Longan Arillus* (Long

方药: 归脾汤。常用:党参、黄芪、白术益气健脾;当归补血;远志、酸枣仁、龙眼肉养心安神;木香、陈皮理气健脾。

Yan Rou) to nourish the heart and calm the spirits; *Aucklandiae Radix* (Mu Xiang) and *Citri Reticulatae Pericarpium* (Chen Pi) to regulate qi and strengthen the spleen.

Modification: For insufficiency of heart-blood with symptoms such as pale complexion, palpitation and vertigo, add *Rehmanniae Radix Praeparata* (Shu Di Huang), *Paeoniae Radix Alba* (Bai Shao) and *Asini Corii Colla* (E Jiao) to nourish heart-blood; for severe insomnia, add *Schisandrae Chinensis Fructus* (Wu Wei Zi), *Polygoni Multiflori Caulis* (Ye Jiao Teng), *Alibiziae Cortex* (He Huan Pi) and *Platycladi Semen* (Bai Zi Ren) to nourish the heart and calm the spirits; for oppression in the abdomen, poor appetite, greasy tongue fur, use *Atractylodis Macrocephalae Rhizoma* (Bai Zhu) in great amount and add *Atractylodis Rhizoma* (Cang Zhu), *Pinelliae Rhizoma* (Ban Xia), *Citri Reticulatae Pericarpium* (Chen Pi), *Poria* (Fu Ling) and *Magnoliae Officinalis Cortex* (Hou Po) to regulate qi and resolve phlegm.

加减: 心血不足较甚者,症见面色苍白,心悸眩晕者,加熟地、芍药、阿胶以养心血;不寐较重者,加五味子、夜交藤、合欢皮、柏子仁养心安神;兼见脘闷纳呆,苔腻,重用白术,加苍术、半夏、陈皮、茯苓、厚朴以健脾燥湿、理气化痰。

2.2.5 Disharmony between the Heart and the Kideny

Manifestation: Restlessness and sleeplessness, difficulty to fall asleep, palpitation, dreaminess, dizziness, vertigo, soreness in the waist and weakness in the knees, feverish sensations, night-sweating, feverish dysphoria of the five centers, dry throat with little fluid, spermatorrhea, irregular menstruation; red tongue with little tongue fur; deep rapid pulse.

Treatment: To nourish yin and subtract fire, restore harmony between the heart and the kidney.

Formulas and Herbs: *Rehmannia Pills with Six Ingredients* (Liu Wei Di Huang Wan) and *Coordination*

2.2.5 心肾不交

证候: 心烦不寐,入睡困难,心悸多梦,伴头晕耳鸣,腰膝酸软,潮热盗汗,五心烦热,咽干少津,男子遗精,女子月经不调。舌红少苔,脉细数。

治法: 滋阴降火,交通心肾。

方药: 六味地黄丸合交泰丸。前方滋阴补肾;后方

Restoring Pills (Jiao Tai Wan). The first formula is to nourish yin and invigorate kidney and the second is to coordinate between the heart and the kidney and guide fire back to its origin.

交通心肾,引火归原。

Modification: For restlessness and sleeplessness, sleeplessness overnight, add *Cinnabaris* (Zhu Sha), *Magnetitum* (Ci Shi), *Os Draconis* (Long Gu) and *Dens Draconis* (Long Chi) to suppress and calm the spirits; for restlessness, bitter mouth, red tongue with little tongue fur mainly due to insufficiency of heart-yin, use *Celestial Emperor Heart-Supplementing Elixir* (Tian Wang Bu Xin Dan) to nourish yin and nourish blood, and strengthen the heart and calm the spirits.

加减: 心烦不寐,彻夜不眠者,加朱砂、磁石、龙骨、龙齿重镇安神;心阴不足为主者,见心烦口干,舌红少苔,可用天王补心丹以滋阴养血、补心安神。

2.2.6 Qi-deficiency in the Heart and the Gallbladder

2.2.6 心胆气虚

Manifestations: Restlessness and sleeplessness, easiness to be frightened, timidity and palpitation, short breath, spontaneous sweating; pale tongue; taut thin pulse.

证候: 心烦不寐,触事易惊,胆怯心悸,伴气短自汗,倦怠乏力。舌淡,脉弦细。

Treatment: To invigorate qi and suppress fright, calm the spirits and settle down the minds.

治法: 益气镇惊,安神定志。

Formulas and Herbs: *Spirit-calming and Mind-tranquilizing Pills* (An Shen Ding Zhi Wan), usually composed of *Codonopsis Radix* (Dang Shen), *Poria* (Fu Ling) and *Glycyrrhizae Radix et Rhizoma* (Gan Cao) to invigorate qi; *Polygalae Radix* (Yuan Zhi), *Acori Tatarinowii Rhizoma* (Shi Chang Pu) and *Dens Draconis* (Long Chi) to calm the spirits; *Chuanxiong Rhizoma* (Chuan Xiong) and *Ziziphi Spinosae Semen* (Suan Zao Ren) to regulate blood and nourish the heart; *Anemarrhenae Rhizoma* (Zhi Mu) to clear away heat and eliminate irritation.

方药: 安神定志丸。常用:党参、茯苓、甘草益气;远志、石菖蒲、龙齿安神;川芎、酸枣仁调血养心;知母清热除烦。

Modification: For severe palpitation, uneasiness, likeliness to be frightened, add *Os Draconis*

加减: 心悸甚,惊惕不安者,加生龙骨、生牡蛎、朱砂

Crudus (Sheng Long Gu), *Ostreae Concha* Crudus (Sheng Mu Li) and *Cinnabaris* (Zhu Sha) to suppress fright and calm the spirits; for frequent deep sighs, poor appetite and distention in the abdomen, add *Bupleuri Radix* (Chai Hu), *Citri Reticulatae Pericarpium* (Chen Pi), *Dioscoreae Rhizoma* (Shan Yao) and *Atractylodis Macrocephalae Rhizoma* (Bai Zhu) to disperse the liver and strengthen the spleen; for deficiency of the heart, liver and blood, palpitation, sweating, use *Ginseng Radix et Rhizoma* (Ren Shen) in great amounts, and add *Paeoniae Radix Alba* (Bai Shao), *Angelicae Sinensis Radix* (Dang Gui) and *Astragali Radix* (Huang Qi) to strengthen and nourish the liver-blood.

以重镇安神;喜太息,纳呆腹胀者,加柴胡、陈皮、山药、白术以疏肝健脾;心肝血虚,惊悸汗出者,重用人参,加白芍药、当归、黄芪以补养肝血。

Epilepsy

Epilepsy is a disease of periodic sudden loss of control of the mind which is caused by imbalance of zang-fu organs, turbid phlegm blockade, frenetic qi activities, wind-phlegm interferes inside and blockage of upper orifices, which can be resulted in by many factors. It has clinical manifestations like sudden loss of consciousness, even falling to the ground unconscious, violent convulsion, drooping with foam at the mouth, eyes staring upward, strange shrieks. When consciousness is regained after a period of time, patients are no more different than a normal people. Before epilepsy attacks, there can be some pre-symptoms such as vertigo, oppression in the chest and after the attacks, patients usually feel fatigue.

痫　病

痫病是一种由多种原因造成脏腑失调,痰浊阻滞,气机逆乱,风痰内动,蒙蔽清窍所致的发作性神志异常的病证。临床以突然意识丧失,甚则仆倒,不省人事,强直抽搐,口吐涎沫,两目上视或口中怪叫为特征,移时苏醒,一如常人为特征。发作前可伴眩晕、胸闷等先兆,发作后常有疲倦乏力等症状。

1 Etiology and Pathogenesis

Epilepsy is mainly caused by congenital factors, lost balance of seven emotions, uncontrolled diet andhead damage. And the pathogenesis are the imbalance of zang-fu organs, turbid phlegm blockade, frenetic qi activities, wind-phlegm interference inside and blockage of upper orifices.

1.1 Disorder of Zang-qi due to Congenital Defects

Children will be born with congenital defocts if their parents have epilepsy. Or fright during pregnancy will lead to disorder of zang-fu organs and frenetic qi activity, resulting in epilepsy.

1.2 Injured Liver, Spleen and Kidney due to Emotional Disturbance

Frequent fright and frenetic qi activity make damages to the zang-fu organs. When the liver and the kidney are injured, yin is unable to restrain yang andthen the yang transform into heat and wind. When the spleen is injured, turbid phlegm is generated and can block orifices of the heart, leading to epilepsy.

1.3 Spleen and Stomach Injury due to Uncontrolled Diet

Over intake of sweat and greasy food, and overdrinking damages the spleen and stomach which lose the controlance of transportation and transference. Damp gathers into phlegm blocking the orifices of the heart, leading to epilepsy.

1.4 Blockade of Blood Stasis due to Head Damage

Brain damage due to external injury, partum injury or stroke will cause blood stasis to remain in-

1 病因病机

痫证的致病原因主要有先天因素、七情失调、饮食不节、脑部受损。基本病机是脏腑失调，痰浊阻滞，气机逆乱，风痰内动，蒙蔽清窍。

1.1 先天不足，脏气不平

父母有痫证，造成小儿先天禀赋不足，或母亲怀孕期间受惊吓，导致脏腑失调，气机逆乱，成为本病。

1.2 七情失调，肝脾肾受损

屡受惊恐，气机逆乱，脏腑受损。若肝肾受损，阴不敛阳，化热生风。或脾气受损，痰浊内生，蒙蔽心窍，而致痫病。

1.3 饮食不节，脾胃损伤

过食甘肥、饮酒过度，脾胃受损，运化失司，湿聚为痰，蒙蔽心窍，而成痫病。

1.4 脑部受损，瘀血阻滞

外伤、产伤、中风造成颅脑损伤，瘀血内留，阻滞经

side, which blocks the meridians and collaterals. The head and spirits lacks nourish, leading to epilepsy.

络,脑神失养,遂为本病。

In a word, epilepsy lies in the head but is related to the liver, spleen, heart and kidney, among which, the damage of the liver is the main pathological basis for epilepsy attacks. Among the pathological factors of wind, fire, phlegm and stasis, phlegm is the most important one. The pathological nature is primary deficiency and secondary excess. The former refers to zang-fu organs' damage and the latter refers to wind, fire, phlegm and stasis, which interact to cause epilepsy.

综上所述,本病的病位在脑,涉及肝、脾、心、肾诸脏。其中肝脾肾的损伤是痫病发生的主要病理基础。病理因素主要有风、火、痰、瘀,又以痰为重要。病理性质属于本虚标实,本虚为脏腑受损,标实为风、火、痰、瘀,四者并非孤立致病,多是互相结合,互相影响而发病。

2 Syndrome Differentiation and Treatment

2 辨证论治

2.1 Key Points of Syndrome Differentiation

2.1 辨治要点

Doctors should first identify the seriousness of the disease and distinguish the deficiency type from excess type according to the manifestations. Then, doctors should judge the pathological nature of wind, phlegm, heat or stasis. Generallyspeaking, severe epilepsy lasts long at short intervals while light epilepsy doesn't last long and at long intervals. At the attack stage, it is usually epilepsy of excess type due to wind-phlegm obstruction, or phlegm-fire, or stasis-heat interference with the spirits. At the intermittent stage, it is usually epilepsy of deficiency type or deficiency mixed with excess, often due to deficiency of the heart and spleen, yin-deficiency of the liver and kidney intermingled with wind, phlegm and stasis. Sudden attack, faint and falling to the ground, losing consciousness, clenched jaws and teeth, stiffened neck and nape, limb convulsion are symptoms of wind-type epilepsy. Droo-

痫病的辨证首先要辨病情轻重,其次辨证候的虚实;再确定病理性质,即风、痰、热、瘀。一般而言,本病发作持续时间长,发作间隔时间短者,为病重;发作持续时间短,发作间隔时间长者,为病轻。痫病发作期多实,多由风痰闭阻,痰火或瘀热扰动神明;间歇期多虚,或虚中夹实,常由心脾两虚,肝肾阴虚,夹风夹痰夹瘀所致。来势急骤,神昏猝倒,不省人事,口噤牙紧,颈项强直,四肢抽搐者,病性属风;发作时口吐涎沫,气粗痰鸣,呆木无知,发作后或有情志错乱,幻听,错觉,或有梦游者,病情

ping with foam at the mouth, hoarse breath, wheezing, dumbness and unconsciousness during attack, and emotional and spiritual disturbance, phonism, illusion, or sleepwalking after attack, are symptoms of phlegm-type epilepsy. Sudden fall, crowing, red face, fever, blood-stained foam at the mouth, constipation at usully times or after attack, stinky mouth with yellow tongue fur are symptoms of heat-type epilepsy. Complexion changing from red, purple red or bluish during attack, bluish lips with clinical history of internal head damages or partum injuries are symptoms of stasis-type epilepsy.

属痰；有猝倒啼叫，面赤身热，口流血沫，平素或发作后有大便秘结，口臭苔黄者，病性属热；发作时面色潮红、紫红，继则青紫，口唇紫绀，或有颅脑外伤、产伤等病史者，病性属瘀。

The reatment principle of epilepsyshould be treating the secondary symptoms in case of frequent attacks by clear awaying and purging liver-fire, resolving phlegm and stopping wind, opening orifices and settling epilepsy. For prolonged epilepsy, treat the primary symptoms with supplementing deficiency by invigorating qi and nurturing blood, strengthening the spleen and resolving phlegm, nourishing and invigorating the liver and kidney, calming the mind and tranquilizing the spirits.

痫病的治疗原则：频繁发作，以治标为主，着重清泻肝火、豁痰息风、开窍定痫；平时病缓，则补虚以治其本，宜益气养血、健脾化痰、滋补肝肾、宁心安神。

2.2 Therapeutic Methods of Different Types of Epilepsy

2.2 分型论治

2.2.1 Epilepsy Due to Wind-phlegm Obstruction

2.2.1 风痰闭阻

Manifestation: Frequent vertigo, dizziness, oppression in the chest, fatigue, plenty of phlegm and unhappiness before attacks, diversity at the attack stage such as sudden fall, loss of consciousness, convulsion, drooping, or screaming and fecal incontinence, or temporal unconsciousness, glassy eyes, blank look, conversation stopped, objects falling from hand, or trance without convulsion; red

证候：发病前常有眩晕，头昏，胸闷，乏力，痰多，心情不悦。发作呈多样性，或见突然跌倒，神志不清，抽搐吐涎，或伴尖叫与二便失禁，或短暂神志不清，双目发呆，茫然所失，谈话中断，持物落地，或精神恍惚而无抽搐。

tongue with white greasy tongue fur; taut rolling powerful pulse.

舌质红，苔白腻，脉弦滑有力。

Treatment: To cleanse phlegm and stop wind, open orifices and settle epilepsy.

治法：涤痰息风，开窍定痫。

Formulas and Herbs: *Modified Epilepsy-Settling Pills* (Ding Xian Wan), usually composed of *Succus Bambosae* (Zhu Li), *Fritillariae Thumbergii Bulbus* (Zhe Bei Mu), *Citri Reticulatae Pericarpium* (Chen Pi), *Acori Tatarinowii Rhizoma* (Shi Chang Pu), *Arisaema cum Bile* (Dan Nan Xing) and *Pinelliae Rhizoma* (Ban Xia) to resolve phlegm and open orifices; *Gastrodiae Rhizoma* (Tian Ma), *Scorpio* (Quan Xie) and *Bombyx Batryticatus* (Jiang Can) to stop wind and spasm; *Succinum* (Hu Po), *Polygalae Radix* (Yuan Zhi), *Cinnabarite* (Chen Sha) and *Poria cum Ligno Hospite* (Fu Shen) to calm the heart and spirits; *Salviae Miltiorrhizae Radix et Rhizoma Radix* (Dan Shen) to promote blood circulation, and *Ophiopogonis Radix* (Mai Men Dong) to nourish the heart.

方药：定痫丸加减。常用：竹沥、贝母、陈皮、石菖蒲、胆南星、半夏化痰开窍；天麻、全蝎、僵蚕息风止痉；琥珀、远志、辰砂、茯神镇心安神；丹参活血，麦门冬养心。

Modification: For vertigo and strabismus, add *Os Draconis* Crudus (Sheng Long Gu), *Ostreae Concha Crudus* (Sheng Mu Li), *Magnetitum* (Ci Shi) and *Margaritifera Concha* (Zhen Zhu Mu) to suppress and calm the spirits; for sticky phlegm, add *Trichosanthis Fructus* (Gua Lou); for clear away and thin phlegm and drooping, add *Zingiberis Rhizoma* (Gan Jiang) and *Asari Radix et Rhizoma* (Xi Xin).

加减：眩晕、目斜视者，加生龙骨、生牡蛎、磁石、珍珠母重镇安神等；若痰黏，加瓜蒌；若痰涎清稀，加干姜、细辛。

2.2.2 Phlegm-fire Interferes with the Spirits

2.2.2 痰火扰神

Manifestations: Faint, falling to the ground, convulsion, drooping or roar at the attack stage, irritation, restlessness, sleeplessness, difficult expectoration, bitter mouth and dry throat, constipation,

证候：发作时昏仆抽搐，吐涎，或有吼叫，平时急躁易怒，心烦失眠，咳痰不爽，口苦咽干，便秘溲黄，目赤。舌

yellow urine, reddish eyes, red tongue with yellow greasy tongue fur, and taut rolling rapid pulse at ordinary times.

红,苔黄腻,脉弦滑而数。

Treatment: To clear away heat and purge fire, resolve phlegm and open orifices

治法: 清热泻火,化痰开窍。

Formulas and Herbs: *Gentian Liver-Draining Decoction* (Long Dan Xie Gan Tang) and *Phlegm-Cleansing Decoction* (Di Tan Tang), usually comyosed of *Gentianae Radix et Rhizoma* (Long Dan), *Scutellariae Radix* (Huang Qin), *Gardeniae Fructus* (Zhi Zi), *Bupleuri Radix* (Chai Hu) to cleanse the liver and purge fire; *Pinelliae Rhizoma* (Ban Xia), *Arisaematis Rhizoma* (Tian Nan Xing), *Aurantii Fructus Immaturus* (Zhi Shi), *Citri Reticulatae Pericarpium* (Chen Pi) and *Bambusae Caulis in Taenias* (Zhu Ru) to remove phlegm and open orifices.

方药: 龙胆泻肝汤合涤痰汤。常用:龙胆草、黄芩、栀子、柴胡清肝泻火;半夏、天南星、枳实、陈皮、竹茹豁痰开窍。

Modification: For severe convulsion, add *Gastrodiae Rhizoma* (Tian Ma), *Haliotidis Concha* (Shi Jue Ming), *Uncariae Ramulus cum Uncis* (Gou Teng), *Pheretima* (Di Long) and *Scorpio* (Quan Xie) to check the liver and stop wind; for constipation due to phlegm-fire blockage, use *Chlorite- Expelling- Phlegm Pills* (Meng Shi Gun Tan Wan).

加减: 抽搐严重者,加天麻、石决明、钩藤、地龙、全蝎,以平肝息风;痰火壅实而见便秘者,用礞石滚痰丸。

2.2.3 Stasis blocks Collaterals in the Head

2.2.3 瘀阻脑络

Manifestations: Dizziness and headache at ordinary times with fixed pain, usually with one-side body convulsion or facial spasm with bluish lips and complexion; dark red tongue or with stasis spots with thin yellow tongue fur; uneven or taut pulse; usually due to external head injury, partum injury, infection inside the head or congenital atelencephalia.

证候: 平素头晕头痛,痛有定处,常伴单侧肢体抽搐,或一侧面部抽动,颜面口唇青紫。舌质暗红或有瘀斑,舌苔薄白,脉涩或弦。多继发于颅脑外伤、产伤、颅内感染性疾患后,或先天脑发育不全。

Treatment: To promote blood circulation and remove stasis, stop wind and dredge collaterals.

治法: 活血化瘀,息风通络。

Formulas and Herbs: *Orifice-Opening and Blood-Activating Decoction* (Tong Qiao Huo Xue Tang), usually composed of *Persicae Semen* (Tao Ren), *Carthami Flos* (Hong Hua), *Chuanxiong Rhizoma* (Chuan Xiong) and *Paeoniae Radix Rubra* (Chi Shao) to promote blood circulation and remove stasis; *Moschus* (She Xiang) to open orifices and break blockade; *Allium fistulosum* (Da Cong), *Rice Wine* (Huang Jiu) and *Zingiberis Rhizoma Recens* (Sheng Jiang) to accept yang and activate blood.

方药: 通窍活血汤。常用:桃仁、红花、川芎、赤芍药活血化瘀;麝香开窍通闭;大葱、黄酒、生姜通阳活血。

Modification: For severe phlegm and drooping, add *Pinelliae Rhizoma* (Ban Xia), *Arisaematis Rhizoma* (Tian Nan Xing) and *Bambusae Caulis in Taenias* (Zhu Ru); for severe convulsion, *Scolopendra* (Wu Gong) and *Scorpio* (Quan Xie).

加减: 痰涎偏盛者,加半夏、胆南星、竹茹;抽搐严重者,加蜈蚣、全蝎。

2.2.4 Deficiency of the Heart and Spleen

2.2.4 心脾两虚

Manifestations: Frequent attacks with no recovery, lassitude and fatigue, palpitation, short breath, insomnia and dreaminess, pale complexion, emaciation, poor appetite, loose stool; pale tongue with white greasy tongue fur; deep fine weak pulse.

证候: 反复发痫不愈,神疲乏力,心悸气短,失眠多梦,面色苍白,体瘦纳呆,大便溏薄。舌质淡,苔白腻,脉沉细而弱。

Treatment: To supplement and invigorate qi and blood, strengthen the spleen and calm the minds.

治法: 补益气血,健脾宁心。

Formulas and Herbs: *Six Nobles Decoction* (Liu Jun Zi Tang) and *Angelica Splenic Decoction* (Gui Pi Tang), usually composed of *Ginseng Radix et Rhizoma* (Ren Shen), *Scutellariae Radix* (Huang Qin), *Poria* (Fu Ling), *Atractylodis Macrocephalae Rhizoma* (Bai Zhu) and *Glycyrrhizae Radix et Rhizoma Praeparata* (Zhi Gan Cao) to invigorate qi and strengthen the spleen; *Angelicae Sinensis Radix* (Dang Gui), *Salviae Miltiorrhizae Radix et Rhizoma Radix* (Dan Shen), *Rehmanniae Radix Praeparata* (Shu Di Huang) to nourish the heart and nourish

方药: 六君子汤合归脾汤。常用:人参、黄芪、茯苓、白术、炙甘草益气健脾;当归、丹参、熟地黄养心补血;陈皮、半夏理气化湿;酸枣仁、远志、五味子养心安神。

blood; *Citri Reticulatae Pericarpium* (Chen Pi) and *Pinelliae Rhizoma* (Ban Xia) to regulate qi and transform dampness; *Ziziphi Spinosae Semen* (Suan Zao Ren), *Polygalae Radix* (Yuan Zhi) and *Schisandrae Chinensis Fructus* (Wu Wei Zi) to nourish the heart and calm the spirits.

Modification: For serious turbid phlegm, nausea, vomiting phlegm and drooping, add *Arisaema cum Bile* (Dan Nan Xing), *Bambusae Caulis in Taenias* Preparata (Jiang Zhu Ru), *Trichosanthis Fructus* (Gua Lou), *Acori Tatarinowii Rhizoma* (Shi Chang Pu), *Inulae Flos* (Xuan Fu Hua) to resolve phlegm and subtract turbidity; for loose stool, add *Coicis Semen* (Yi Yi Ren) Fried, *Lablab Semen Album* (Bian Dou) Fried, *Zingiberis Rhizoma Recens* (Sheng Jiang) Baked; for sleepwalking, add *Os Draconis* Crudus (Sheng Long Gu), *Ostreae Concha* Crudus (Sheng Mu Li) and *Ferric Oxide* (Sheng Tie Luo) to tranquilize the minds and calm the spirits.

加减：若痰浊盛而恶心呕吐痰涎者，加胆南星、姜竹茹、瓜蒌、石菖蒲、旋覆花化痰降浊；便溏者，加炒薏苡仁、炒扁豆、炮姜等健脾止泻；夜游者，加生龙骨、生牡蛎、生铁落等镇心安神。

2.2.5 Yi-deficiency of the Heart and Kidney

2.2.5 心肾阴虚

Manifestations: Frequent epilepsy attacks, wandering mind, palpitation, forgetfulness, insomnia, dizziness, vertigo, dry eyes, dark complexion, brownish wither helix, soreness in the waist and weakness in the knees, dry stool; pale red tongue; deep fine rapid pulse.

证候：痫病频发，神思恍惚，心悸，健忘失眠，头晕目眩，两目干涩，面色晦暗，耳轮焦枯不泽，腰膝酸软，大便干燥。舌质淡红，脉沉细而数。

Treatment: To supplement and invigorate the heart and kidney, suppress yang and calm the spirits.

治法：补益心肾，潜阳安神。

Formulas and Herbs: *Kidney Pills* (Zuo Gui Wan) to invigorate kidney-yin and stop liver-wind, along with *Celestial Emperor Heart-Supplementing Elixir* (Tian Wang Bu Xin Dan) to calm the spirits and minds.

方药：左归丸合天王补心丹。前方补肾阴，息肝风；后方养心阴，安神志。

Modification: For wandering mind for long, add *Asini Corii Colla* (E Jiao) to supplement heart-blood; for feverish sensation in the heart, add *Gardeniae Fructus* (Zhi Zi) Baked and *Nelumbinis Plumula* (Lian Zi Xin) to cleanse the heart and eliminate irritation; for dry stool, add *Scrophulariae Radix* (Xuan Shen), *Trichosanthis Radix* (Tian Hua Fen), *Angelicae Sinensis Radix* (Dang Gui) and *Cannabis Fructus* (Huo Ma Ren) to nourish yin and moisturize intestines to ease stool.

加减：若神思恍惚，持续时间长者，加阿胶补益心血；心中烦热者，加焦山栀、莲子心清心除烦；大便干燥者，加玄参、天花粉、当归、火麻仁以养阴润肠通便。

Dementia

痴 呆

Dementia is a disease of spiritual and emotional abnormality due to diminishing marrow and withering head, and dysfunction of spirit mechanism, characterized by foolishness and moronism, low IQ and forgetfulness. Indifference, reticence, retardation, forgetfulness are symptoms of light dementia. Silence, or living alone without going out, or murmur but illogical, weird behaviors, laughter or cry, or no desire for food, feeling not hungry even without eating for days, are severe dementia.

痴呆是由髓减脑消，神机失用所导致的一种神志异常的疾病，以呆傻愚笨，智能低下，善忘等为主要临床表现。轻者可见神情淡漠，寡言少语，反应迟钝，善忘；重则表现为终日不语，或闭门独居，或口中喃喃，言辞颠倒，行为失常，忽笑忽哭，或不欲食，数日不知饥饿等。

1 Etiology and Pathogenesis

1 病因病机

The primary cause of dementia is old age and weakness, deterioration due to prolonged illness, internal injury of seven emotions. The pathogenesis is insufficiency of marrow-sea and dysfunction of spirit mechanism.

本病的主要病因是年高体虚、久病耗损、七情内伤。基本病机为髓海不足，神机失用。

1.1 Head and Marrow Lack Nurturing Due to Old Age and Weakness

1.1 年老体虚，脑髓失养

Old age and prolonged illness lead to insufficiency of Essential-Qi in the kidney, deficiency of

年老久病，肾中精气不足，髓海亏虚，神机失用；或

marrow-sea and dysfunction of the mechanism of the spirit. Or the sluggish circulation of qi and blood due to old age brings about the stasis in cerebral collaterals, which also can lead to the dysfunction of spirit mechanism, resulting in dementia.

年高气血运行迟缓,脑络瘀阻,亦可使神机失用,导致本病。

1.2 Injured Emotions and Minds, Phlegm and Stasis Blockade

1.2 情志所伤,痰瘀痹阻

Emotional and spiritual discontent leads to liver-qi depression which in turn, leads to qi-stagnation and blood stasis. Or depressive liver-qi invades the spleen and damages itscontrolance of transportation. Then accumulated dampness turns into phlegm, which along with stasis, obstructs cerebral collaterals, leading to dysfunction of spirit mechanism and then dementia.

情志不畅,肝气郁结,气滞血瘀;或肝郁犯脾,脾失健运,聚湿成痰,痰瘀互结,痹阻脑络,神机失用,发为痴呆。

1.3 Deficiency of Head and Marrow Due to Deterioration by Prolonged Illness

1.3 久病耗损,脑髓空虚

Prolonged diseases like stroke and vertigo damage qi and blood of the liver, kidney, heart and spleen, leading to the lack of nourish of the head and marrow. Or the cerebral collaterals obstruction due to prolonged illness leads to the dysfunction of spirit mechanism and then dementia.

中风、眩晕等病日久,肝、肾、心、脾之气血阴阳损伤,脑髓失养;或久病脑络瘀阻,神机失用,而成痴呆。

In a word, dementia lies in the head but is related to the heart, kidney, liver and spleen. The pathological nature is usually primary deficiency and secondary excess. The former refers to deficiency of yin-essence, qi and blood and the latter refers to obstruction in the head due to qi, fire, phlegm and stasis. It is interchangeable between deficiency and excess, among qi-stagnation, phlegm-turbidity and blood-stasis.

综上所述痴呆的病位在脑,与心、肾、肝、脾均有关系。病理性质多属本虚标实,本虚为阴精、气血亏虚;标实为气、火、痰、瘀内阻于脑。虚实之间及气滞、痰浊、血瘀之间常可相互转化。

2 Syndrome Differentiation and Treatment

2.1 Key Points of Syndrome Differentiation

Doctors should first distinguish congenital dementia from acquired dementia. And then identify deficiency and excess.

Congenital dementia usually starts at tender ages due to congenital defects and can hardly be cured. Acquired dementia is due to old age, weakness and prolonged illness or intoxication and external injuries. It usually starts in adulthood, especiallyin the presenile. Dementia is of primary deficiency and secondary excess and many clinical cases are complication of both deficiency and excess. Dementia of deficiency type has such manifestations as insufficient essential-qi, lusterless complexion, emaciation, slow and powerless speech and behavior. Dementia of excess type has symptoms like intelligence decline, dumb face as well as remarkable changes of emotions, minds and personality to be either overexcited or depressed due to pathogenic excess of turbidity blinding the orifices.

The therapeutic principle should be toresolve depression and expel phlegm, promote blood circulation and open orifices, cleanse the liver and purge fire, supplement deficiency and strengthen healthy qi, supplement marrow and nourish the head. During treatment, in addition to supplementing deficiency and strengthening health qi, supplementing and invigorating kidney-essence, attention should be given to invigorate the spleen and stomach in order to supplement head and marrow which then can be nourished. Meanwhile, doctors should be cautious not to overdo with supplementing deficiency in case

2 辨证论治

2.1 辨治要点

痴呆之证应首先辨先天与后天;再辨虚实。

先天性痴呆多于幼年起病,与禀赋不足有关,治疗大多非常困难。后天性痴呆与年老体虚、久病有关,或与中毒、外伤有关,起病多在成年后,早老期发病尤多。本病乃本虚标实之证,临床上以虚实夹杂者多见。痴呆属虚者,临床主要以神气不足,面色失荣,形体消瘦,言行迟弱为特征;痴呆属实者,除见智能减退、表情反应呆钝外,临床还可见因浊实之邪蒙蔽心窍而引起情志、性格方面或亢奋或抑制的明显改变。

治疗原则以开郁逐痰、活血通窍、平肝泻火治其标,补虚扶正、充髓养脑治其本。治疗时宜在扶正补虚、填补肾精的同时,注意培补后天脾胃,以冀脑髓得充,化源得滋。同时,须注意补虚切忌滋腻太过,以免滋腻损伤脾胃,酿生痰浊。另外,在药物治疗的同时,移情易性,智力和功能训练与锻炼亦不可轻视。

the spleen and stomach are injured by over-nourishing with greasy materials, which can generate phlegm-turbidity. Besides herbstion, emotional diversion and personality change, intelligence and function training and practice should not be overlooked.

2.2 Therapeutic Methods of Different Patterns

2.2.1 Insufficiency of Marrow-sea

Manifestations: Diminishing intelligence, especially remarkable in memory, calculation, direction and judgment, dull expression, inaccuracy, dizziness, tinnitus, laziness and desire for lying down, rotten teeth, withered hair, sore in the waist and knees, difficulty to walk; thin pale tongue with white thin tongue fur; deep fine and weak pulse.

Treatment: To invigorate the kidney and strengthen marrow, supplement essence and nourish spirits.

Formulas and Herbs: *Seven Blessed Decoction* (Qi Fu Yin), usually composed of *Rehmanniae Radix Praeparata* (Shu Di Huang), *Angelicae Sinensis Radix* (Dang Gui) and *Ziziphi Spinosae Semen* (Suan Zao Ren) to nourish yin and nourish blood; *Ginseng Radix et Rhizoma* (Ren Shen), *Atractylodis Macrocephalae Rhizoma* (Bai Zhu) and *Glycyrrhizae Radix et Rhizoma* (Gan Cao) to invigorate qi and strengthen the spleen; *Polygalae Radix* (Yuan Zhi) to resolve phlegm and open orifices.

Modification: For further symptoms of yin-deficiency of the liver and kidney, like soreness in the waist and weakness in the knees, flushed cheeks, night-sweating and tinnitus, add *Achyranthis Bidentatae Radix* (Niu Xi), *Rehmannia Radix* (Sheng Di Huang), *Lycii Fructus* (Gou Qi Zi), *Ligustri*

2.2 分型论治

2.2.1 髓海不足

证候: 智能减退,记忆力、计算力、定向力、判断力明显减退,神情呆钝,语不达意,头晕耳鸣,怠惰思卧,齿枯发焦,腰酸腿软,步履艰难。舌瘦色淡,苔薄白,脉沉细弱。

治法: 补肾益髓,填精养神。

方药: 七福饮。常用:熟地、当归、酸枣仁滋阴养血;人参、白术、甘草益气健脾;远志化痰开窍。

加减: 若兼肝肾阴虚,伴有腰膝酸软,颧红盗汗,耳鸣,加牛膝、生地黄、枸杞子、女贞子、制首乌;若兼肾阳亏虚,见有怯寒肢冷,脚肿气短,加熟附片、巴戟天、益智

Lucidi Fructus (Nü Zhen Zi) and *Polygoni Multiflori Radix Praeparata* (Zhi Shou Wu); for further symptoms of kidney-yang deficiency, like fear of cold, cold limbs, feet edema, short breath, add *Prepared Aconm Lateralis Radix Praeparaia* (Zhi Fu Zi), *Morindae Officinalis Radix* (Ba Ji Tian), *Alpiniae Oxyphyllae Fructus* (Yi Zhi) and *Cistanchis Herba* (Rou Cong Rong); for fatigue and short breath, muscle atrophy, add *Astragali Radix* (Huang Qi), *Codonopsis Radix* (Dang Shen), *Atractylodis Macrocephalae Rhizoma* (Bai Zhu) to invigorate qi and strengthen the spleen.

仁、淫羊藿、肉苁蓉等;若见乏力气短,肌肉萎缩,加黄芪、党参,白术益气健脾。

2.2.2 Deficiency of the Spleen and Kidney

Manifestations: Dumbness, reticence, memory impairment, difficulty of identification and calculation, vague speech, inaccuracy, along with soreness in the waist and weak in the knees, muscle atrophy, little intake, poor appetite, short breath, laziness to talk, drooping or cold limbs, pain in abdomen which is relieved with pressing, diarrhea just before dawn; pale enlarged tongue with white tongue fur or red tongue with little or no tongue fur; deep fine and weak pulse, particularly at two *chi*'s.

Treatment: To invigorate the kidney and strengthen the spleen, supplement qi and generate essence.

Formulas and Herbs: *Rejuvenation Pills* (Huan Shao Dan), usually composed of *Rehmanniae Radix Praeparata* (Shu Di Huang), *Lycii Fructus* (Gou Qi Zi), *Corni Fructus* (Shan Zhu Yu), *Halloysitum Rubrum* (Chu Shi Zi) to supplement and nourish kidney-yin; *Cistanchis Herba* (Rou Cong Rong), *Morindae Officinalis Radix* (Ba Ji Tian), *Foeniculi Fructus* (Xiao Hui Xiang) to warm the kidney and

2.2.2 脾肾两虚

证候: 表情呆滞,沉默寡言,记忆减退,失认失算,口齿含糊,词不达意,伴腰膝酸软,肌肉萎缩,食少纳呆,气短懒言,口涎外溢或四肢不温,腹痛喜按,五更泄泻。舌质淡白,舌体胖大,苔白,或舌红,苔少或无苔,脉沉细弱,双尺尤甚。

治法: 补肾健脾,益气生精。

方药: 还少丹。常用:熟地黄、枸杞子、山茱萸、楮实子滋补肾阴;肉苁蓉、巴戟天、小茴香温肾壮阳;杜仲、怀牛膝补肾壮腰;党参、白术、茯苓、山药、大枣益气健脾;石菖蒲、远志、五味子安神开窍。

strengthen yang; *Eucommiae Cortex* (Du Zhong), *Achyranthis Bidentatae Radix* (Huai Niu Xi) to invigorate the kidney and strengthen the waist; *Codonopsis Radix* (Dang Shen), *Atractylodis Macrocephalae Rhizoma* (Bai Zhu), *Poria* (Fu Ling), *Dioscoreae Rhizoma* (Shan Yao), *Jujubae Fructus* (Da Zao) to invigorate qi and strengthen the spleen; *Acori Tatarinowii Rhizoma* (Shi Chang Pu), *Polygalae Radix* (Yuan Zhi), *Schisandrae Chinensis Fructus* (Wu Wei Zi) to calm the spirits and open orifices.

Modification: For muscle atrophy, add *Placenta Hominis* (Zi He Che), *Asini Corii Colla* (E Jiao), *Dipsaci Radix* (Xu Duan), *Polygoni Multiflori Radix* (Shou Wu) and *Astragali Radix* (Huang Qi); for subtractd intake, abdomen fullness, red tongue with little tongue fur, delete *Cistanchis Herba* (Rou Cong Rong), *Morindae Officinalis Radix* (Ba Ji Tian), *Foeniculi Fructus* (Xiao Hui Xiang), and add *Trichosanthis Radix* (Tian Hua Fen), *Polygonati Odorati Rhizoma* (Yu Zhu), *Ophiopogonis Radix* (Mai Men Dong), *Dendrobii Caulis* (Shi Hu), *Setariae Fructus Germinatus Crudus* (Sheng Gu Ya) and *Hordei Fructus Germinatus Crudus* (Sheng Mai Ya); for further symptoms of yin-deficiency in the liver and kidney, yin-deficiency and fire-excess, like soreness in the waist and weakness in the knees, flushed cheeks, night sweating, tinnitus, change for *Anemarrhena, Phellodendron, and Rehmannia Pills* (Zhi Bai Di Huang Wan) to suppress yang and stop wind.

加减: 若肌肉萎缩,可加紫河车、阿胶、续断、首乌、黄芪;纳减、脘痞,舌红少苔者,可去肉苁蓉、巴戟天、小茴香,加天花粉、玉竹、麦门冬、石斛、生谷芽、生麦芽;伴肝肾阴虚、阴虚火旺,见有腰膝酸软、颧红盗汗、耳鸣,当改用知柏地黄丸,佐以潜阳息风之品。

2.2.3 Phlegm-turbidity Blinds the Orifices

Manifestations: Dull expressions, intelligence decline, capricious cry or laughter, murmur, or si-

2.2.3 痰浊蒙窍

证候: 表情呆钝,智力衰退,或哭笑无常,喃喃自语,

lence all day as dumb as a wooden chicken, no desire for food or drink, distention and pain in abdomen, fullness and discomfort in the stomach, drooping with foam at the mouth, feeling heavy in the head as if being wrapped up; pale tongue with white greasy tongue fur; rolling pulse.

或终日无语，呆若木鸡，伴不思饮食，脘腹胀痛，痞满不适，口多涎沫，头重如裹。舌质淡，苔白腻，脉滑。

Treatment: To resolve phlegm and open orifices; strengthen the spleen and resolve turbidity.

治法：豁痰开窍，健脾化浊。

Formulas and Herbs: *Phlegm-Cleansing Decoction* (Di Tan Tang), usually composed of *Pinelliae Rhizoma* (Ban Xia), *Citri Reticulatae Pericarpium* (Chen Pi), *Poria* (Fu Ling), *Aurantii Fructus Immaturus* (Zhi Shi), *Bambusae Caulis in Taenias* (Zhu Ru), *Arisaematis Rhizoma Preparatum* (Zhi Tian Nan Xing) to resolve phlegm and strengthen the spleen; *Acori Tatarinowii Rhizoma* (Shi Chang Pu), *Polygalae Radix* (Yuan Zhi), *Curcumae Radix* (Yu Jin) to resolve phlegm and open orifices.

方药：涤痰汤。常用：半夏、陈皮、茯苓、枳实、竹茹、制南星化痰健脾；石菖蒲、远志、郁金豁痰开窍。

Modification: For remarkable symptoms of spleen-deficiency, such as fatigue and poor appetite, add *Codonopsis Radix* (Dang Shen), *Atractylodis Macrocephalae Rhizoma* (Bai Zhu), *Hordei Fructus Germinatus* (Mai Ya) and *Amomi Fructus* (Sha Ren); for capricious laughter and cry, murmur, drooping with foam at the mouth, increase the amount of *Citri Reticulatae Pericarpium* (Chen Pi), *Pinelliae Rhizoma* (Ban Xia), *Arisaematis Rhizoma Preparatum* (Zhi Tian Nan Xing) and add *Raphani Semen* (Lai Fu Zi) *Trichosanthis Fructus* (Gua Lou) (whole) and *Fritillariae Thumbergii Bulbus* (Zhe Bei Mu); for live-depression turning into fire that injures the liver-blood and heart-fluid with symptoms like irritation and restlessness, nonsense, endless singing and laughing, use modified

加减：若脾虚明显者，见有乏力纳呆，加党参、白术、麦芽、砂仁等；哭笑无常，喃喃自语，口多涎沫者，重用陈皮、半夏、制南星，并加莱菔子、全瓜蒌、浙贝母；伴有肝郁化火，灼伤肝血心液，症见心烦躁动、言语颠倒、歌笑不休者，宜用转呆汤加味。

Foolishness-Bending Decoction (Zhuan Dai Tang).

2.2.4 Blood-stasis Obstructs Inside

Manifestations: Dull expression, frequent stops in speech, forgetfulness, easiness to be frightened, abnormal thoughts, strange behavior, squamous and dry skin, dry mouth but with no desire for drinking, dark eyes; dark tongue or with stasis spots; fine uneven pulse.

Treatment: To promote blood circulation and eliminate blood stasis; open orifices and waken the mind.

Formulas and Herbs: *Orifice-Dredging and Blood-Activating Decoction* (Tong Qiao Huo Xue Tang), usually composed of *Moschus* (She Xiang) to dredge orifices and waken the spirits; *Persicae Semen* (Tao Ren), *Carthami Flos* (Hong Hua), *Paeoniae Radix Rubra* (Chi ShaoYao), *Chuanxiong Rhizoma* (Chuan Xiong) to eliminate stasis and dredge collaterals; *Bulbus Allii Fistulosi* (Cong Bai), *Zingiberis Rhizoma Recens* (Sheng Jiang) and *Chinese Alcohol* (Bai Jiu) to warm meridians and dredge collaterals.

Modification: For prolonged illness and insufficient qi and blood, with symptoms such as lassitude and fatigue, lusterless face, add *Rehmanniae Radix Praeparata* (Shu Di Huang), *Codonopsis Radix* (Dang Shen), *Astragali Radix* (Huang Qi); for oppression and pain in the chest and hypochondria, obvious squamous and dry skin mainly due to qi-stagnation and blood stasis, use modified *Sanguine Mansion Stasis-Expelling Decoction* (Xue Fu Zhu Yu Tang); for prolonged blood stasis, remarkable deficiency of yin-blood, with symptoms like dizziness and dim eyes, dry throat and mouth, soreness in the

2.2.4 瘀血内阻

证候：表情迟钝，言语不利，善忘，易惊恐，或思维异常，行为古怪，伴肌肤甲错，口干不欲饮，双目晦暗。舌质暗或有瘀点瘀斑，脉细涩。

治法：活血化瘀，开窍醒脑。

方药：通窍活血汤。常用：麝香通窍醒神；桃仁、红花、赤芍药、川芎化瘀通络；葱白、生姜、白酒温经通络。

加减：若久病伴气血不足，症见神疲乏力、面色少华，加熟地黄、党参、黄芪；气滞血瘀为主者，症见胸胁胀痛、肌肤甲错明显，宜用血府逐瘀汤加减；瘀血日久，阴血亏虚明显者，症见头晕眼花、咽干口燥、腰膝酸软，加熟地黄、阿胶、鳖甲、制首乌、女贞子。

waist and weakness in the knees, add *Rehmanniae Radix Praeparata* (Shu Di Huang), *Asini Corii Colla* (E Jiao), *Trionycis Carapax* (Bie Jia), *Polygoni Multiflori Radix* Praeparata (Zhi Shou Wu) and *Ligustri Lucidi Fructus* (Nü Zhen Zi).

Chapter 3 Spleen System Disease

第3章 脾系病证

Stomachache

胃　痛

Stomachache, known as pain in the stomach and abdomen, is a disease of pain located in the area below the heart and above the navel, caused by stomach-qi obstruction and stagnation, characterized by abdomen distension, poor appetite, pantothenic acid, epigastric upset, nausea and vomiting.

胃痛又称胃脘痛，主要因胃气阻滞不通而导致的以心窝部以下、脐以上的胃脘部疼痛为主症，或伴有脘胀、纳呆、泛酸、嘈杂、恶心呕吐等症的一种病证。

1　Etiology and Pathogenesis

1　病因病机

Stomachache is mainly caused by exogenous pathogenic cold, uncontrolled diet, seven-emotion disharmony, weak constitution due to prolonged illness. These factors affect the harmonizing and descending of stomach-qi, leading to unsmooth qi activities. And obstruction results in pain.

胃痛的发生主要是由于外感寒邪、饮食不节、七情失和、久病体虚诸劳等因素，影响了胃气的和降，导致气机不畅，不通则痛。

1.1　Pathogenic Cold Attacks the Stomach and Qi Activity Get Depressed and Stagnated

1.1　寒邪客胃，气机郁滞

Pathogenic cold attacks the stomach and coldness freezes and suppresses yang that leads to unsmooth qi activities. Since cold, which controls gathering and contracting, causes stomach collaterals becoming rigid and qi and blood being unable to flow smoothly. Obstruction leads to pain and stom-

外感寒邪，客于胃腑，寒性凝滞，阳气被遏，气机不畅，寒主收引，胃络拘急，气血不通，不通则痛，故胃痛卒然暴作。

achache, therefore, attacks.

1.2 Uncontrolled Diet Injuring the Stomach

Overeating leads to food retention. Overeating of raw and cold food leads to cold accumulating in the stomach. Overeating of sweat, greasy and spicy food leads to damp-heat obstruction. Or starvation and overeating together hurts the spleen. All the above factors can make damage to the stomach so much as to lead to the disharmony of spleen-qi and stomach-qi, and then stomach-qi stagnation, finally to stomachache.

1.2 饮食不节,脾胃受损

暴饮暴食,宿食停滞;或过食生冷,寒积胃脘;或恣食肥甘辛辣厚味,湿热中阻;或饥饱失常,脾失健运,均可损及脾胃,以致脾胃气机不和,胃气壅滞,遂成胃痛。

1.3 Emotional and Spiritual Dissatisfaction Leads to the Disharmony between the Liver and Stomach

Depression and anger, emotional and spiritual dissatisfaction will result inthe failure of the liver to convey and disperse, which attacks the stomach, bringing about qi stagnation and stomachache.

1.3 情志失畅,肝胃不和

抑郁恼怒,情志不畅,致肝失疏泄,横逆犯胃,气机阻滞,而成胃痛。

1.4 Weak Constitution Due to Prolonged Illness Causes Weak Stomach and Spleen

Congenital defects, or injured stomach and spleen due to prolonged diseases, or overstrain, can lead to weak stomach and spleen. Or cold of deficiency type inzhong jiao causes the stomach's lack in nurturing. Or deficiency of stomach-yin causes the stomach's lack in moisturizing. All these can lead to stomachache.

1.4 体虚久病,脾胃虚弱

禀赋不足,或久病脾胃受损,或劳倦过度,均可导致脾胃虚弱,或为中焦虚寒,胃失温养,或为胃阴不足,胃失濡养,而致胃痛。

Stomachache lies in the stomach, but is closely related to the liver and spleen. Its main pathological feature is that it is obstruction that causes the pain. Any factors such as cold, heat, food retention, qi-stagnation or weakness, that leads to the disharmony of stomach-qi and obstruction, will finally result in stomachache. By pathological nature, it usually

胃痛的病位在胃,与肝脾两脏关系密切。最主要的病机特点是"不通则痛",凡因寒因热因食滞因气滞因虚诸种原因导致胃气失和,阻滞不通,均可产生胃痛。在病理性质上初起多为实证,

begins as excess type, which changes into deficiency type if pain stays. What's more, stomach of deficiency type is likely to be affected by pathogenic factor and therefore becomes a complication of both deficiency type and excess type.

若久痛不愈，或反由实转虚。虚证胃痛又易受邪，而成虚实夹杂之证。

2　Syndrome Differentiation and Treatment

2　辨证论治

2.1　Key Points of Syndrome Differentiation

2.1　辨治要点

Clinically, doctors should distinguish cold from heat, deficiency from excess, qi from blood by identifying the triggering factors, the nature of the pain, aggravating and relieving factors, diet and flavor. Stomachache of excess types should be identified as cold, heat, food retention, qi-stagnation or blood stasis. Stomachache of deficiency type should be identified yin and yang. The treatment should be focused on the principles of regulating qi and relieving pain. Doctors should examine the symptoms carefully and give the right therapeutic methods according to the causes of unsmooth qi activity, such as warming and dispersing, eliminate food retention, dispersing the liver, clear awaying away heat, resolving dampness, promoting blood circulation and warming yang. Doctors should combine supplementing and dredging in a creative way.

临证可从诱发因素、疼痛性质、诱发加重与缓解因素、饮食口味等方面辨别胃痛的寒热虚实、在气在血。实证当分寒、热、食积、气滞和血瘀；虚证应辨阴与阳。治疗上以理气和胃止痛为基本法则，审证求因。根据引起气机不畅的具体病因采用相应的治疗方法，如温散、消食、疏肝、清热、化湿、活血、养阴和温阳等，补通灵活结合。

2.2　Therapeutic Methodsfor Different Patterns

2.2　分型论治

2.2.1　Pathogenic Cold Attacks the Stomach

2.2.1　寒邪客胃

Manifestation: Acute stomachache due to regular intake of raw and cold food or cold attacks, aversion to cold and favor for warmth, pain relieved when it is warm and aggravating when it is cold; pale tongue with thin white tongue fur; taut tight pulse.

证候：常因饮食生冷或受寒而胃痛暴作，恶寒喜暖，得温则减，遇寒则剧。舌淡，苔薄白，脉弦紧。

Treatment: To warm the stomach to dispel cold

治法：温胃散寒，理气止

and regulate qi to stop pain.

痛。

Formulas and Herbs: *Alpiniae Officinarum and Cyperi Pills* (Liang Fu Pills), usually composed of *Alpiniae Officinarum Rhizoma* (Gao Liang Jiang) to warm the stomach and dispel cold; *Cyperi Rhizoma* (Xiang Fu) to regulate qi and stop pain.

方药：良附丸。常用高良姜温胃散寒，香附行气止痛。

Modification: For additional symptoms of physical cold and fever, add *Cyperus Tuber and Perilla Leaf Powder* (Xiang Su San) to dispel wind-cold; for additional symptoms of cold-dampness, like poor appetite and general heaviness, nausea and vomiting and white thin tongue fur, use *Matgnoliae Officinalis Warming Zhong jiao Decoction* (Hou Po Wen Zhong Tang) to dry dampness and warm zhong jiao; for long-depressed pathogenic cold turning into heat and cold complicated with heat with symptoms like bitter dry mouth or burning in the stomach and abdomen with yellow greasy tongue fur, use *Pinellia Purging Stomach-fire Decoction* (Ban Xia Xie Xin Tang) to disperse with acrid herbs and to descend with bitter herbs.

加减：兼见形寒、身热等风寒表证者，可加香苏散以疏散风寒；兼有纳呆、身重、恶心欲吐、苔白腻等寒湿症状，可用厚朴温中汤以温中燥湿；若寒邪郁久化热，寒热错杂，兼见口苦口干，或胃脘有灼热感，苔黄腻等，可用半夏泻心汤辛开苦降、寒热并调。

2.2.2 Uncontrolled Diet Injures the Stomach

2.2.2 饮食伤胃

Manifestations: Distension and pain in the stomach and abdomen after overeating, belching and acid regurgitation, vomiting undigested food, vomiting of food or pain relieved after wind pass, sticky stool; thick greasy tongue fur; rolling pulse.

证候：暴饮暴食后胃脘胀满疼痛，嗳腐吞酸，或呕吐不消化食物，吐食或矢气后痛减，大便不爽。舌苔厚腻，脉滑。

Treatment: To eliminate food retention and stagnation, harmonize the stomach to stop pain.

治法：消食导滞，和胃止痛。

Formulas and Herbs: *Pachyma Compound Digestive Tonic Pills*(Bao He Wan), usually composed of *Crataegi Fructus* (Shan Zha) to promote digestion of greasy food; *Massa Fermentata Medicinalis* (Shen Qu) to promote digestion of alcohol and food,

方药：保和丸。常用：山楂消油腻肉食之积；神曲消酒食之积；莱菔子消谷面之积；半夏、陈皮、茯苓和胃化湿；连翘散结清热。均可加

Raphani Semen (Lai Fu Zi) to promote digestion of grain and flour food; *Pinelliae Rhizoma* (Ban Xia), *Citri Reticulatae Pericarpium* (Chen Pi), *Poria* (Fu Ling) to harmonize the stomach and eliminate dampness; *Forsythiae Fructus* (Lian Qiao) to break and clear away heat. *Setariae Fructus Germinatus* (Gu Ya), *Hordei Fructus Germinatus* (Mai Ya), *Galli Gigerii Endothelium Corneum* (Ji Nei Jin) and others can be added to promote digestion.

入谷芽、麦芽、鸡内金等消食之品。

Modification: For severe distention in abdomen, add *Aurantii Fructus Immaturus* (Zhi Shi), *Amomi Fructus* (Sha Ren) and *Arecae Semen* (Bing Lang) to promote qi flow and eliminate stagnation; for distention in the stomach and abdomen as well as constipation, add *Minor Purgative Decoction* (Xiao Cheng Qi Tang) or change for *Aurantii Immaturus Eliminating Stagnation Pills* (Zhi Shi Dao Zhi Wan) to dredge fu-organs and promote qi flow.

加减: 若脘腹胀甚者,可加枳实、砂仁、槟榔等以行气消滞;若胃脘胀痛而便闭者,可合用小承气汤或改用枳实导滞丸以通腑行气。

2.2.3 Liver-qi Attacks the Stomach

2.2.3 肝气犯胃

Manifestations: Distention and pain in the stomach and abdomen due to emotions and minds, pain stretching to hypochondria, frequent belching, unsmooth stool; thin white tongue fur; taut pulse.

证候: 每因情志因素而胃脘胀闷作痛,脘痛连胁,嗳气频作,大便不畅。苔薄白,脉弦。

Treatment: To disperse the liver and regulate qi, harmonize the stomach and stop pain.

治法: 疏肝理气,和胃止痛。

Formulas and Herbs: *Bupleurum-Dispersing-Liver Powder* (Chai Hu Shu Gan San), usually composed of *Bupleuri Radix* (Chai Hu), *Cyperi Rhizoma* (Xiang Fu) and *Chuanxiong Rhizoma* (Chuan Xiong) to disperse and promote liver-qi to stop pain; aeonia sterniana *Paeoniae Radix Alba* (Bai Shao Yao) to nourish blood and soften the liver to stop pain; *Citri Reticulatae Pericarpium* (Chen Pi) *Aurantii Fructus*(Zhi Qiao), *Glycyrrhizae Radix et*

方药: 柴胡疏肝散。常用:柴胡、香附、川芎疏肝行气止痛;白芍药以养血柔肝止痛;陈皮、枳壳、甘草理气和中。

Rhizoma (Gan Cao) to regulate qi and harmonize zhong jiao.

Modification: For severe pain, add *Toosendan Fructus* (Chuan Lian Zi) and *Corydalis Rhizoma* (Yan Hu Suo) to greatly help to regulate qi and stop pain; for frequent belching, add *Perillae Caulis* (Zi Su Geng), *Inulae Flos* (Xuan Fu Hua), *Kaki Calyx* (Shi Di) to harmonize the stomach and subtract reverse qi-flow; for symptoms of depressed heat in the liver and stomach, such as burning pain in the stomach and abdomen, acid regurgitation and epigastric upset, bitter dry mouth, red tongue with yellow tongue fur, taut or rapid pulse, change for *Liver-Transforming Decoction* (Hua Gan Jian) and *Coptis and evodia Pills* (Zuo Jin Wan) to disperse the liver and purge heat, and regulate qi and harmonize zhong jiao.

加减：若疼痛较甚者，可加川楝子、延胡索以加强理气止痛；若嗳气较频者，可加紫苏梗、旋覆花、柿蒂等以和胃降逆；若见胃脘灼痛，泛酸嘈杂，口干口苦，舌红苔黄，脉弦或数，乃肝胃郁热之证，可改用化肝煎合左金丸，疏肝泄热、理气和胃。

2.2.4 Damp-heat Blocks the Middle

Manifestations: Burning pain in the stomach and abdomen, epigastric upset, poor appetite, nausea and vomiting, bitter dry mouth, thirst but no desire for drink, general heaviness; yellow greasy tongue fur; rapid rolling pulse.

Treatment: To clear away heat and dry dampness, regulate qi and harmonize the stomach.

Formulas and Herbs: *Cleansing the Middle Decoction* (Qing Zhong Tang), usually composed of *Coptidis Rhizoma* (Huang Lian) and *Gardeniae Fructus* (Zhi Zi) to clear away heat and dry dampness; *Pinelliae Rhizoma* (Ban Xia), *Citri Reticulatae Pericarpium* (Chen Pi), *Poria* (Fu Ling), *Glycyrrhizae Radix et Rhizoma Praeparata* (Zhi Gan Cao) and *Amomi Fructus Rotundus* (Dou Kou) to strengthen the spleen, dispel dampness, regulate qi

2.2.4 湿热中阻

证候：胃脘疼痛有灼热感，嘈杂纳呆，恶心欲吐，口干口苦，渴不欲饮，身体困重。舌苔黄腻，脉滑数。

治法：清热化湿，理气和胃。

方药：清中汤。常用：黄连、山栀清热化湿；半夏、陈皮、茯苓、甘草、白豆蔻健脾祛湿，理气和胃。

and harmonized the stomach.

Modification: For severe damp, add *Atractylodis Rhizoma* (Cang Zhu), *Pogostemonis Herba* (Huo Xiang), *Eupatorii Herba* (Pei Lan), *Coicis Semen* (Yi Yi Ren) to regulate qi and eliminate distention; for phlegm-damp obstructing the stomach with symptoms like oppression and distention in the stomach and abdomen, nausea, phlegm vomiting, white greasy or slippery tongue fur, use *Erchen Decoction* (Er Chen Tang) and *Stomach-Calming Powder* (Ping Wei San) to dry dampness, strengthen the spleen, harmonize the stomach and subtract reverse qi flow.

加减: 湿偏重者加苍术、藿香、佩兰、薏苡仁等化湿之品;气滞腹胀者加厚朴、枳壳等以理气消胀;若为痰湿阻胃,症见胃脘胀闷疼痛、恶心、吐痰、苔白腻或滑,可用二陈汤合平胃散,燥湿健脾、和胃降逆。

2.2.5 Blood Stasis Obstructs the Stomach

Manifestations: Sharp pain in the stomach and abdomen in fixed spots, pain felt when pressed, aggravated after food intake and even worse at night; dark purple tongue fur or with stasis spots; uneven pulse.

Treatment: To resolve stasis and dredge collaterals, promote qi flow and stop pain.

Formulas and Herbs: *Great Guffaw Powder* (Shi Xiao San) and *Salviae Miltiorrhizae Drink* (Dan Shen Yin), usually composed of *Typhae Pollen* (Pu Huang), *Faeces Trogopterorum* (Wu Ling Zhi), *Salviae Miltiorrhizae Radix et Rhizoma Radix* (Dan Shen) to promote blood circulation and remove stasis to stop pain; *Santali Albi Lignum* (Tan Xiang), *Amomi Fructus* (Sha Ren) to regulate qi and harmonize the stomach.

Modification: Add *Corydalis Rhizoma* (Yan Hu Suo), *Cyperi Rhizoma* (Xiang Fu), *Curcumae Radix* (Yu Jin), *Aurantii Fructus* (Zhi Qiao) to help to promote blood circulation and qi flow to stop

2.2.5 瘀血阻胃

证候: 病程较长,胃脘疼痛,犹如针刺,痛有定处,按之痛甚,食后加剧,入夜为甚。舌质紫暗或有瘀斑,脉涩。

治法: 化瘀通络,行气止痛。

方药: 失笑散合丹参饮。常用:蒲黄、五灵脂、丹参行血散瘀止痛;檀香、砂仁行气和胃。

加减: 可加延胡索、香附、郁金、枳壳等以加强活血行气止痛之功;如瘀滞较甚,疼痛明显,可加乳香、没药、

pain; for severe stasis and stagnation and considerable pain, add *Olibanum* (Ru Xiang), *Myrrha* (Mo Yao), *Erinaceus* (Ci Wei Pi), *Aspongopus* (Jiu Xiang Chong) to eliminate blood stasis, dredge stagnated qi to stop pain.

刺猬皮、九香虫以祛瘀血、通滞气以止痛。

2.2.6 Deficiency of Stomach-yin

2.2.6 胃阴亏虚

Manifestations: Dull or burning pain in the stomach, dry mouth and throat, emaciation and fatigue, dry stool; red tongue with little fluid; fine rapid pulse.

证候: 胃痛隐隐或灼痛,口干咽燥,消瘦乏力,大便干结。舌红少津,脉细数。

Treatment: *To An Ever Effective Decoction for Nourishing Liver and Kidney* (Yi Guan Jian) and *Paeoniae and Glycyrrhizae Decoction* (Shao Yao Gan Cao Tang), usually composed of *Glehniae Radix* (Bei Sha Shen), *Ophiopogonis Radix* (Mai Men Dong), *Rehmannia Radix* (Sheng Di Huang), *Lycii Fructus* (Gou Qi Zi) to nourish yin and strengthen the stomach; *Angelicae Sinensis Radix* (Dang Gui) along with *Paeoniae Radix Alba* (Bai Shao Yao) to nourish blood and soften the liver; *Paeoniae Radix Alba* (Bai Shao Yao) along with *Glycyrrhizae Radix et Rhizoma* (Gan Cao) to not only relieve acute pain but also nourish yin by acid and sweat herbs combined, *Toosendan Fructus* (Chuan Lian Zi) to regulate qi.

治法: 养阴益胃,和中止痛。

方药: 一贯煎合芍药甘草汤。常用:沙参、麦门冬、生地黄、枸杞子滋阴益胃;当归配白芍药养血柔肝;白芍药配甘草既能缓急止痛,又能酸甘化阴;佐以川楝子行气。

Modification: Add *Citri Fructus* (Xiang Yuan), *Citri Saroodactylis Fructus* (Fo Shou), *Prunus mume var. viridicalyx* (Lü E Mei) to regulate qi without consuming yin; for burning pain in the stomach and abdomen, epigastric upset, acid, add *Coptis and evodia Pills* (Zuo Jin Wan); for yin-deficiency and internal heat, irritation, dry mouth, likeliness to vomit, use *Lophatherum and Gypsum Fibrosum Decoction* (Zhu Ye Shi Gao Tang) to

加减: 可选加香橼、佛手、绿萼梅等药理气而不伤阴;若见胃脘灼痛,嘈杂泛酸者,可配用左金丸;若阴虚兼有内热,烦闷口干,欲呕,可用竹叶石膏汤清胃泄热。

cleanse the stomach and purge heat.

2.2.7 Deficiency Cold of the Spleen and Stomach

Manifestations: Dull pain in the stomach, favor for warmth and pressing, pain aggravated with empty stomach and relieved after intake, fluid regurgitation, tired and fatigue, cold limbs, thin and loose stool; pale tongue or with teeth marks on the edge; white tongue fur; weak pulse.

Treatment: To warm zhong jiao and strengthen the spleen, harmonize the stomach to stop pain.

Formulas and Herbs: *Astragali Strengthening the Middle Decoction* (Huang Qi Jian Zhong Tang), usually composed of *Astragali Radix* (Huang Qi) to invigorate qi and strengthen zhong jiao; *Cinnamomi Ramulus* (Gui Zhi) to promote yang; *Paeoniae Radix Alba* (Bai Shao Yao) and *Glycyrrhizae Radix et Rhizoma* (Gan Cao) to relieve acute pain.

Modification: For frequent fluid regurgitation, add *Zingiberis Rhizoma* (Gan Jiang), *Citri Reticulatae Pericarpium* (Chen Pi), *Pinelliae Rhizoma* (Ban Xia), *Poria* (Fu Ling) to warm the stomach and remove fluid retention; for yang deficiency and excess of cold, cold pain in the stomach and abdomen, vomiting, cold limbs, add *Regulating Zhong jiao Pills* (Li Zhong Wan) to warm zhong jiao and dispel cold; for physical cold along with cold limbs, soreness in the waist and weakness in the knees, use *Aconiti Praeparata-Regulating Zhong jiao Decoction* (Fu Zi Li Zhong Tang) to warm the kidney and spleen, and harmonize the stomach to stop pain; for not enough of cold signs but mainly weak spleen and stomach instead, use *Aucklandia, Amomum and Six Nobles Decoction* (Xiang Sha Liu Jun Zi Tang) to invigorate qi and strengthen the spleen, and to regu-

2.2.7 脾胃虚寒

证候: 胃痛隐隐,喜温喜按,空腹痛甚,得食则减,泛吐清水,体倦乏力,手足不温,大便溏薄。舌淡,或边有齿印,苔白,脉虚弱。

治法: 温中健脾,和胃止痛。

方药: 黄芪建中汤。常用:黄芪益气补中;桂枝通阳;白芍药、甘草缓急止痛。

加减: 泛吐清水较多者,可加干姜、陈皮、半夏、茯苓等以温胃化饮;若阳虚寒甚,胃脘冷痛,呕吐,肢冷,可加理中丸以温中散寒;若兼有形寒肢冷、腰膝酸软,可用附子理中汤温肾暖脾,和胃止痛;若寒象不明显,以脾胃虚弱为主者,可用香砂六君子汤以益气健脾、行气和胃。

late qi and harmonize the stomach.

Vomiting

Vomiting is a disease caused by the stomach's losingcontrolance of harmonizing and descending so that qi flows upward and forces the food to be vomited out of the mouth from the stomach.

1 Etiology and Pathogenesis

The six climatic exogenous pathogenic factors, internal injuries by food, emotional and spiritual disorder and congenital defects can affect the stomach so that the stomach fails to harmonize and descend qi, which flows upwards and leads to vomiting.

1.1 Exogenous Pathogenic Factors Affect the Stomach and Qi Activity Being Depressed and Stagnated

Affected by six pathogenic factors of wind, cold, heat, dampness, dryness, fire or filthy qi, the stomach loses its function of harmonizing and descending. Water, fluid and food move upward with qi and that is vomiting. In different seasons, the pathogenic factors differ. However, cold is more likely to trigger vomiting.

1.2 Uncontrolled Diet Injuring the Spleen and Stomach

Overeating of raw, cold, spicy, sweat, greasy and unclean food, and overdrinking of alcohol will damage the stomach and hinder the spleen, leading to food retention and poor digestion, ascending stomach-qi and in the end, vomiting.

呕 吐

呕吐是指胃失和降，气逆于上，迫使胃中之物从口中吐出的一种病证。

1 病因病机

呕吐的发生主要是由于外感六淫，内伤饮食，情志不调，禀赋不足等因素，影响于胃，使胃失和降，胃气上逆，发生呕吐。

1.1 外邪犯胃，气机郁滞

感受风、寒、暑、湿、燥、火六淫之邪，或秽浊之气，侵犯胃腑，胃失和降之常，水谷随逆气上出，发生呕吐。由于季节的不同，感受的病邪亦会不同，但一般以受寒者居多。

1.2 饮食不节，脾胃受损

饮食过量，暴饮暴食，多食生冷、醇酒辛辣、甘肥及不洁之食物，皆可伤胃滞脾，每易引起食滞不化，胃气不降，上逆而为呕吐。

1.3 Emotional and Spiritual Disorder Leading to Disharmony of the Liver and Stomach

When injured by anger, the liver fails to disperse and affect the stomach nearby, leading to the stomach qi to flow upward. Or the spleen when injured by worry, fails to transport and food is retained which caused the stomach fails to harmonize and descend. Both above situations will lead to vomiting. In addition, when the spleen and stomach is too weak to transfer and transport, fluid and food retained inside which, in case of anger, will throw out along with the reverse flow of qi.

1.3 情志失调，肝胃不和

恼怒伤肝，肝失条达，横逆犯胃，胃气上逆；忧思伤脾，脾失健运，食停难化，胃失和降，均可发生呕吐。亦可因脾胃素虚，运化无力，水谷易于停留，偶因气恼，食随气逆，导致呕吐。

1.4 Weak Spleen and Stomach due to Weak Constitution after Prolonged Illness,

Regular weakness of the spleen and stomach, weaknessof the spleen and stomach after illness, overstrain, or the middle qi consumption and damage, will all be the causes of vomiting. Weakness of the stomach disenables it to contain fluid and food while the weakness of the spleen disenables it to generate essence. Therefore, food retains in the stomach and moves upward, leading to vomiting.

1.4 病后体虚，脾胃虚弱

脾胃素虚，或病后虚弱，劳倦过度，耗伤中气，胃虚不能盛受水谷，脾虚不能化生精微，食滞胃中，上逆成呕。

Vomiting lies in the stomach but is closely related to the liver and spleen. The general pathology is that the stomachfails to harmonize and descend and stomach qi flows upward. The pathological nature is also deficiency and excess. Vomiting of excess type is due to interference by pathogenic factors, stomach-qi obstruction and upward flow of qi. Vomiting of deficiency type is due to deficiency of qi and yin of the spleen and stomach which is too weak to harmonize and descend. Usually at the onset stage, it is of excess type but if vomiting lasts for days, injuring the weak spleen and stomach, excess

呕吐的病位主要在胃，还与肝、脾有密切的关系。其总的发病机制为胃失和降，胃气上逆。病理性质不外虚实两类，实者因邪气所干，胃气痞塞，上逆作呕，虚者由于脾胃气阴亏虚，无力行使和降之职。一般初病多实，若呕吐日久，损伤脾胃，脾胃虚弱，可由实转虚，亦有脾胃素虚，复因饮食所伤，而出现虚实夹杂之证。

will turns into deficiency. Or when weak spleen and stomach are further injured by diet, excess will be complicated by deficiency.

2 Syndrome Differentiation and Treatment

2.1 Key Points of Syndrome Differentiation

Doctors should distinguish deficiency from excess by getting to know about thetriggering factors, duration, pathogenesis, vomitus and manifestations. Generally speaking, vomiting due to cold or eating cold food is exogenous pathogenic factors attacking the stomach. Vomiting due to overeating is food retention in the stomach. Vomiting due to uncontrolled diet and irregular starvation and gluttony is weakness of the spleen and stomach or phlegm and fluid retention. Vomiting triggered by emotions and minds is liver-qi attacking the stomach. Vomiting due to weak constitution after prolonged illness is weakness of the spleen and stomach or complication of both deficiency and excess. Acute attack, short duration, obvious triggering factors, plenty of vomitus, sour and stinking vomitus, sturdy body, replete and energetic pulse characterize excess type. In contrast, slow onset, long duration, intermittence, no obvious triggering factors, little vomitus, no sour or stink, but fatigue and tiredness and weak pulse are features of deficiency type. Sour and stinky vomitus indicates food retained and rotten inside. Vomitus of bitter yellow fluid means gallbladder attacking the stomach. Vomitus of sour green fluid is related to liver-heat attacking the stomach. Vomitus of turbid phlegm, drooping and foam indicates phlegm and fluid retention obstruction. Vomitus of clear away fluid shows the deficiency and cold

2 辨证论治

2.1 辨治要点

呕吐辨证可从起病情况、病程、病因、呕吐物及伴随症状等方面来分别邪正虚实。一般来说：受寒饮冷而吐者，多为外邪犯胃；暴饮暴食而吐者，属食积内停；饮食不节，饥饱无常而致吐者，多为脾胃虚弱，或痰饮内停；由情志诱发者，多属肝气犯胃；久病体虚而吐者，多为脾胃虚弱，或虚实夹杂。起病较急，病程较短，发病因素明显，呕吐量较多，吐出物多酸臭，形体壮实，脉多实而有力者，多为实证；起病较缓，病程较长，或表现为时作时止，发病因素不甚明显，吐出物不多，无酸臭，常伴精神疲乏，倦怠乏力，脉弱无力等症者，多为虚证。呕吐酸腐难闻者，多属食积内腐；呕吐苦水黄水者，多由胆热犯胃；呕吐酸水绿水者，多由肝热犯胃；呕吐浊痰涎沫者，多由痰饮中阻；呕吐清水者，多因脾胃虚寒；泛吐少量黏沫者，多为胃阴不足。治疗上以和胃降逆为总的治则。由外邪、

of the spleen and stomach. Little vomitus of sticky foam means the insufficiency of stomach-yin. The treatment should take as the guiding principle harmonizing the stomach and reducing upward flow. For excess type caused by exogenous pathogenic factors, improper diet, emotional and spiritual disorder, dispelling pathogenic factors is critical. Doctors should focus on dispersing pathogenic qi with purgative herbs, breaking the obstruction and dredging blockade to harmonizing and descending stomach-qi. The actual therapeutic methods should be decided according to the nature of pathogenic factors, including dispersing the exterior, clear awaying away heat, removing dampness, promoting digestion, inducing stagnation, resolve fluid retention and dispersing the liver. The herbs should be of purgative and bitter nature. For vomiting of deficiency type, it is important to strengthen the healthy qi, by invigorating the spleen and stomach, invigorating qi and warming and dredging, nourishing stomach-yin, softening and moisturizing, harmonizing and reducing, respectively. For complication of deficiency and excess, doctors should identify closely the primary symptoms from the secondary symptoms, acuteness from choronicity, the major conflicts from the minor conflicts and then give treatments dialectically.

饮食、情志等引起的实证呕吐,应以祛邪为先,注重辛散邪气,开结宣壅,以达到和降胃气的目的。具体施治时可根据病邪性质的不同而分别采用疏表、清热、利湿、消食、导滞、化饮、疏肝等法,用药应主辛通苦降。虚证呕吐应以扶正为主,分别采用健运脾胃、益气温通和滋养胃阴、柔润和降之法。对于虚实兼夹者,则应细审其标本缓急主次而治之,适当兼顾。

2.2 Therapeutic Methodsfor Different Patterns

2.2 分型论治

2.2.1 Exogenous Pathogenic FactorsInvading the Stomach

2.2.1 外邪犯胃

Manifestations: Sudden vomiting, fullness and oppression in the stomach and abdomen, fever and aversion to cold, headache and pain over body; white greasy tongue fur; slow soft pulse.

证候:突然呕吐,胸脘满闷,发热恶寒,头身疼痛。舌苔白腻,脉濡缓。

Treatment: To disperse the pathogenic factors to relieve the exterior, resolve turbidity and harmonize zhong jiao.

治法: 疏邪解表,化浊和中。

Formulas and Herbs: *Agastachis-Restoring Healthy Energy Syrup* (Huo Xiang Zheng Qi San), usually composed *Perillae Fructus* (Zi Su Zi), *Angelicae Dahuricae Radix*(Bai Zhi) can disperse pathogenic factors and resolve turbidity, and particularly, *Pogostemonis Herba* (Huo Xiang) can remove damp-turbidity in the stomach and intestines as well. Also, *Pinelliae Rhizoma Praeparatum cum Zingibere et Alumine* (Jiang Ban Xia), *Citri Reticulatae Pericarpium* (Chen Pi), *Zingiberis Rhizoma Recens* (Sheng Jiang) can harmonize the stomach and stop vomiting while *Magnoliae Officinalis Cortex* (Hou Pu), *Atractylodis Rhizoma* (Cang Zhu), *Atractylodis Macrocephalae Rhizoma* (Bai Zhu), *Poria* (Fu Ling) can resolve dampness and eliminate fullness to improve the transference and transportation of the stomach and the spleen as well as strengthen *Pogostemonis Herba* (Huo Xiang)'s function of removing dampness with aroma. In addition, *Platycodi Radix* (Jie Geng) can disperse the lung-qi to strengthen *Pogostemonis Herba* (Huo Xiang)'s effects of relieving the exterior.

方药: 藿香正气散。常用:藿香、紫苏、白芷疏邪化浊,藿香又能化胃肠湿浊;姜半夏、陈皮、生姜和胃止呕;厚朴、苍术、白术、茯苓化湿除满,以助脾胃运化功能,加强藿香的芳香化湿作用;桔梗,开宣肺气以加强藿香解表之功。

Modification: For abdomen discomfort and regurgitation of rotten smell, fluid and food retention, delete *Atractylodis Macrocephalae Rhizoma* (Bai Zhu) and add *Galli Gigerii Endothelium Corneum* (Ji Nei Jin) and *Massa Fermentata Medicinalis* (Shen Qu) to promote food digestion; for heavy wind-cold, with symptoms like cold-fever with no sweating, headache and pain over body, add *Schizonepetae Herba* (Jing Jie), *Saposhnikoviae Radix*

加减: 伴见脘痞嗳腐、饮食停滞者,可去白术,加鸡内金、神曲以消食导滞;如风寒偏重,症见寒热无汗、头痛身楚,加荆芥、防风、羌活祛风寒,解表邪;兼气机阻滞,脘闷腹胀者,可酌加木香、枳壳行气消胀;夏令感受暑湿,呕吐而并见心烦口渴者,改用

(Fang Feng) and *Notopterygii Rhizoma et Radix* (Qiang Huo) to dispel wind-cold and relieve the exterior; for qi activity stagnation and oppression in the stomach and distention in the abdomen, add *Aucklandiae Radix* (Mu Xiang) and *Aurantii Fructus*(Zhi Qiao) to promote qi flow and eliminate distention; for summer dampness in summer, vomiting along with irritation and thirst, change for modified *Coptidis and Elsholtziae Decoction* (Huang Lian Xiang Ru Yin).

黄连香薷饮加减。

2. 2. 2 Vomiting Due to Food Retention

Manifestations: Sour and rotten vomitus, distention in the stomach and abdomen which is relieved after vomiting, belching, loss of appetite, loose or dry stool; thick greasy tongue fur; replete rolling pulse.

Treatment: To promote digestion and remove food retention, harmonize the stomach and subtract reverse flow.

Formulas and Herbs: *Pachyma Compound Digestive Tonic Pills* (Bao He Wan), usually composed of *Crataegi Fructus* (Shan Zha), *Massa Fermentata Medicinalis* (Shen Qu) and *Raphani Semen* (Lai Fu Zi) to eliminate food retention and harmonize the stomach; *Citri Reticulatae Pericarpium* (Chen Pi), *Pinelliae Rhizoma* (Ban Xia), *Poria* (Fu Ling) to regulate qi and subtract reverse flow as well as harmonize zhong jiao and stop vomiting; *Forsythiae Fructus* (Lian Qiao) to break obstruction and clear away heat.

Modification: For vomiting due to eating meat, increase the amount of *Crataegi Fructus* (Shan Zha); for vomiting due to eating flour-made food, increase the amount of *Raphani Semen* (Lai Fu Zi);

2. 2. 2 食滞内停

证候：呕吐酸腐，脘腹胀满，吐后得舒，嗳气厌食，大便或溏或结。舌苔厚腻，脉滑实。

治法：消食化滞，和胃降逆。

方药：保和丸。常用：山楂、神曲、莱菔子消食和胃；陈皮、半夏、茯苓理气降逆，和中止呕；连翘散结清热。

加减：若因肉食而吐者，重用山楂；因米食而吐者，加谷芽；因面食而吐者，重用莱菔子，加麦芽；因酒食而吐

for vomiting due to drinking alcohol, add *Amomi Fructus Rotundus* (Bai Dou Kou) and *Flos Puerariae* (Ge Hua) and increase the amount of *Massa Fermentata Medicinalis* (Shen Qu); for vomiting due to eating fish and crab, add *Perillae Folium*(Zi Su Ye) and *Zingiberis Rhizoma Recens* (Sheng Jiang); for vomiting due to eating soybean products, add raw radish juice; for heavy food retention, abdomen fullness and constipation, add *Minor Purgative Decoction* (Xiao Cheng Qi Tang) to induce stagnation and dredge fu-organs.

2.2.3 Obstruction Due to Phlegm and Fluid Retention

Manifestations: Vomitus of clear away fluid, phlegm and drooping, distention in the stomach, loss of appetite, dizziness, palpitation; white greasy tongue fur; rolling pulse.

Treatment: To warm zhong jiao and remove retention, harmonize the stomach and subtract reverse flow.

Formulas and Herbs: *Minor Pinelliae Decoction* (Xiao Ban Xia Tang) and clerotium *Poria, Cinnamomi, Atractylodes and Glycyrrhizae Decoction* (Ling Gui Shu Gan Tang), usually composed of *Pinelliae Rhizoma* (Ban Xia) to resolve retention of phlegm and fluid, harmonize the stomach and stop vomiting; *Zingiberis Rhizoma Recens (Sheng Jiang)* to warm the stomach, dispel cold and stop vomiting; *Poria* (Fu Ling), *Atractylodis Macrocephalae Rhizoma* (Bai Zhu), *Glycyrrhizae Radix et Rhizoma* (Gan Cao) to invigorate the spleen and dry dampness; *Cinnamomi Ramulus* (Gui Zhi) to warmly resolve retention of phlegm and fluid.

Modification: For distention and fullness in the

者,加白蔻仁、葛花,重用神曲;因食鱼、蟹而吐者,加苏叶、生姜;因豆制品而吐者,加生萝卜汁;如积滞较多,腹满便秘,可合用小承气汤以导滞通腑。

2.2.3 痰饮内阻

证候: 呕吐清水痰涎,脘闷不食,头眩心悸。舌苔白腻,脉滑。

治法: 温中化饮,和胃降逆。

方药: 小半夏汤合苓桂术甘汤。常用:半夏化痰饮和胃止呕;生姜温胃散寒而止呕;茯苓、白术、甘草健脾化湿;桂枝温化痰饮。

加减: 脘腹胀满、舌苔厚

stomach and abdomen with thick greasy tongue fur, delete *Atractylodis Macrocephalae Rhizoma* (Bai Zhu) and add *Atractylodis Rhizoma* (Cang Zhu) and *Magnoliae Officinalis Cortex* (Hou Pu) to promote qi flow and remove fullness; for oppression in the stomach and loss of appetite, add *Amomi Fructus Rotundus* (Bai Dou Kou) and *Amomi Fructus* (Sha Ren) to remove turbidity and improve appetite; for irritation and bitter mouth due to phlegm and fluid retention depressed long turning into heat, add *Coptidis Rhizoma* (Huang Lian) and *Scutellariae Radix* (Huang Qin) to clear away heat and remove phlegm or add *Gallbladder-Warming Decoction* (Wen Dan Tang); for dull pain and rumbling stomach, sour rotten vomitus due to obstruction of fu- qi and upward flow of turbid qi, use modified *Stomach-Regulating Purgative Decoction* (Tiao Wei Cheng Qi Tang) to dredge fu-organs and remove turbidity to stop vomiting.

腻者，可去白术，加苍术、厚朴以行气除满；脘闷不食者加白蔻仁、砂仁化浊开胃；若见心烦口苦，为痰饮郁久化热，可加黄连、黄芩等清热化痰，亦可予温胆汤治疗；若腹痛隐隐、肠鸣辘辘、呕吐腐臭，为腑气不通、浊气上逆，可用调胃承气汤加减，通腑泄浊以止呕。

2.2.4 Liver-qi Attacking the Stomach

Manifestations: Vomiting, acid regurgitation, frequent belching, distention and pain in the stomach and abdomen which is worsen with emotional and spiritual stimulation; pale red tongue with thin white tongue fur; taut pulse.

Treatment: To disperse the liver and regulate qi, harmonize the stomach and subtract revere qi flow.

Formulas and Herbs: *Four-Seven Decoction* (Si Qi Tang), usually composed of *Perillae Folium* (Zi Su Ye) and *Magnoliae Officinalis Cortex* (Hou Pu) to regulate qi and release zhong jiao; *Pinelliae Rhizoma* (Ban Xia), *Zingiberis Rhizoma Recens* (Sheng Jiang), *Poria* (Fu Ling), *Jujubae Fructus* (Da

2.2.4 肝气犯胃

证候：呕吐吞酸，嗳气频繁，胸胁胀痛，每遇情志刺激而病情加剧。舌淡红，苔薄白，脉弦。

治法：疏肝理气，和胃降逆。

方药：四七汤。常用：苏叶、厚朴理气宽中；半夏、生姜、茯苓、大枣和胃降逆止呕。

Zao) to harmonize the stomach, subtract reverse flow and stop vomiting.

Modification: For severe distention and pain in the stomach and abdomen, add *Toosendan Fructus* (Chuan Lian Zi), *Curcumae Radix* (Yu Jin), *Cyperi Rhizoma* (Xiang Fu), *Bupleuri Radix* (Chai Hu) to disperse the liver and resolve depression; for vomiting acid fluid, irritation and thirst, add moderately *Coptis and evodia Pills* (Zuo Jin Wan) and *Gardeniae Fructus* (Zhi Zi), *Scutellariae Radix* (Huang Qin) to cleanse the liver and harmonize the stomach with purgative and bitter herbs; for vomiting yellow bitter fluid due to over-spilt bile, add *Paeoniae Radix Alba* (Bai Shao Yao), *Aurantii Fructus*(Zhi Qiao), *Aucklandiae Radix* (Mu Xiang) and *Lysimachiae Herba* (Jin Qian Cao) to disperse the liver and regulate the gallbladder; for vomiting due to liver-yang interfering upward causing disharmony of the stomach and reverse flow, add *Uncariae Ramulus cum Uncis* (Gou Teng), *Haliotidis Concha* Crudes (Sheng Shi Jue Ming) and *Gastrodiae Rhizoma* (Tian Ma) to regulate the liver and suppress yang.

加减：若胸胁胀满疼痛较甚，加川楝子、郁金、香附、柴胡疏肝解郁；如呕吐酸水、心烦口渴，宜清肝和胃、辛开苦降，可酌加左金丸及山栀、黄芩等；若呕吐黄色苦水，则为胆液外溢，可加白芍药、枳壳、木香、金钱草等疏肝利胆；若为肝阳上亢、胃失和降而吐，可加钩藤、生石决明、天麻等平肝潜阳。

2.2.5 Qi-deficiency of the Spleen and Stomach

Manifestations: Poor appetite, poor digestion, nausea, vomiting, discomfort and oppression in the stomach, sticky stool; white and slippery tongue fur; weak taut pulse.

Treatment: To strengthen the spleen and invigorate qi, harmonize the stomach and subtract reverse flow.

Formulas and Herbs: Modified *Aucklandia, Amomum and Six Nobles Decoction* (Xiang Sha Liu Jun Zi Tang), usually composed of *Codonopsis*

2.2.5 脾胃气虚

证候：食欲不振，食入难化，恶心呕吐，脘部痞闷，大便不畅。舌苔白滑，脉象虚弦。

治法：健脾益气，和胃降逆。

方药：香砂六君子汤加减。常用：党参、茯苓、白术、甘草健脾益气；半夏祛痰降

Radix (Dang Shen), *Poria* (Fu Ling), *Atractylodis Macrocephalae Rhizoma* (Bai Zhu), *Glycyrrhizae Radix et Rhizoma* (Gan Cao) to strengthen the spleen and invigorate qi; *Pinelliae Rhizoma* (Ban Xia) to resolve phlegm and subtract reverse flow, harmonize the stomach and stop vomiting; *Citri Reticulatae Pericarpium* (Chen Pi), *Aucklandiae Radix* (Mu Xiang) and *Amomi Fructus* (Sha Ren) to regulate qi and subtract reverse flow.

逆，和胃止呕；陈皮、木香、砂仁理气降逆。

Modification: For frequent vomiting, belching and stomach discomfort, moderately add *Inulae Flos* (Xuan Fu Hua) and *Haematitum* (Zhe Shi) to suppress reverse flow and stop vomiting; for vomiting fair amount of clear away fluid and cold limbs, add *Aconm Lateralis Radix Praeparata* (Fu Zi), *Cinnamomi Cortex* (Rou Gui) and *Euodiae Fructus* (Wu Zhu Yu) to warm the middle, subtract reverse flow and stop vomiting.

加减：若呕吐频作、嗳气脘痞，可酌加旋覆花、代赭石以镇逆止呕；若呕吐清水较多、脘冷肢凉者，可加附子、肉桂、吴茱萸以温中降逆止呕。

2.2.6 Yang-deficiency of Spleen and Stomach

2.2.6 脾胃阳虚

Manifestations: Intermittent vomiting after little extra intake, pale complexion, fatigue and tiredness, favor for warmth and aversion to cold, cold limbs, dry mouth without desire for drink, loose stool; pale tongue; soft weak pulse.

证候：饮食稍多即吐，时作时止，面色㿠白，倦怠乏力，喜暖恶寒，四肢不温，口干而不欲饮，大便溏薄。舌质淡，脉濡弱。

Treatment: To warm zhong jiao and strengthen the spleen, harmonize the stomach and subtract reverse flow.

治法：温中健脾，和胃降逆。

Formulas and Herbs: *Regulating Zhong jiao Decoction* (Li Zhong Tang), usually composed of *Ginseng Radix et Rhizoma* (Ren Shen), *Atractylodis Macrocephalae Rhizoma* (Bai Zhu) to strengthen the spleen and harmonize the stomach, *Zingiberis Rhizoma* (Gan Jiang) and *Glycyrrhizae Radix et Rhizoma* (Gan Cao) to warm gently and harmonize zhong

方药：理中汤。常用：人参、白术健脾和胃；干姜、甘草甘温和中。

jiao.

Modification: For severe vomiting, add *Amomi Fructus* (Sha Ren), *Pinelliae Rhizoma* (Ban Xia) to subtract reverse flow and stop vomiting; for continuous vomiting of clear away fluid, add *Euodiae Fructus* (Wu Zhu Yu) and *Zingiberis Rhizoma Recens* (Sheng Jiang) to warm the middle, subtract reverse flow and stop belching; for continuous vomiting, completely undigested vomitus, sweating, cold limbs, soreness in the waist and weakness in the knees, enlarged pale tongue and deep weak pulse, add *Aconm Lateralis Radix Praeparata processed* (Zhi Fu Zi) and *Cinnamomi Cortex* (Rou Gui) or *Aconiti Praeparata-Regulating Zhong jiao Decoction* (Fu Zi Li Zhong Tang) to warm and supplement yang of the spleen and kidney.

加减：若呕吐甚者，加砂仁、半夏等理气降逆止呕；若呕吐清水不止，可加吴茱萸、生姜以温中降逆止呃；若久呕不止、呕吐之物完谷不化、汗出肢冷、腰膝酸软、舌质淡胖、脉沉细，可加制附子、肉桂或用附子理中汤温补脾肾之阳。

2.2.7 Deficiency of Stomach-yin

2.2.7 胃阴不足

Manifestations: Continuous vomiting or retch at times, feeling hungry but having no desire for food, dry mouth and throat; red tongue with little fluid; fine rapid pulse.

证候：呕吐反复发作，或时作干呕，似饥而不欲食，口燥咽干。舌红少津，脉象细数。

Treatment: To nourish and nourish stomach-yin, subtract reverse flow and stop vomiting.

治法：滋养胃阴，降逆止呕。

Formulas and Herbs: *Ophiopogonis Radix* Decoction (Mai Men Dong Tang), usually composed of *Ginseng Radix et Rhizoma* (Ren Shen), *Ophiopogonis Radix* (Mai Men Dong), *Semen Oryza Sativae* (Jing Mi) and *Glycyrrhizae Radix et Rhizoma* (Gan Cao) to nourish and nourish stomach-yin; *Pinelliae Rhizoma* (Ban Xia) to subtract reverse flow; *Jujubae Fructus* (Da Zao) to invigorate qi and harmonize zhong jiao.

方药：麦门冬汤。常用：人参、麦门冬、粳米、甘草滋养胃阴；半夏降逆止呕；大枣益气和中。

Modification: For severe vomiting, add *Bambusae Caulis in Taenias* (Zhu Ru) and *Eriobotryae*

加减：若呕吐较剧者，可加竹茹、枇杷叶以和降胃气；

Folium (Pi Pa Ye) to harmonize and lower stomach-qi; for dry mouth, red tongue and fever, add *Coptidis Rhizoma* (Huang Lian) to clear away heat and stop vomiting; for dry stool, add *Trichosanthis Semen* (Gua Lou Zi), *Cannabis Fructus* (Huo Ma Ren) and *Mel* (Feng Mi) to moisturize the intestine and ease stool; for fatigue and tiredness, poor appetite and pale tongue, add *Pseudostellariae Radix* (Tai Zi Shen) and *Dioscoreae Rhizoma* (Shan Yao) to invigorate qi and strengthen the spleen.

若口干、舌红、热甚者，加黄连清热止呕；大便干结者，加瓜蒌仁、火麻仁、白蜜以润肠通便；伴倦怠乏力、纳差舌淡，加太子参、山药益气健脾。

Abdominal Pain

腹　痛

Abdominal pain is a disease characterized mainly by pain due to collateral obstruction by qi activities or meridian's lack of nurturing, located in an area below the stomach and above the pubic hair line.

腹痛主要是因气机阻滞脉络或经脉失养而导致的以胃脘以下、耻骨毛际以上部位发生疼痛为主症的病证。

1　Etiology and Pathogenesis

1　病因病机

Abdominal Pain is primarily caused by qi obstruction, collateral blockade or meridian's lack of nurturing due to exogenous pathogenic factors, improper diet, emotional disorder and innate asthenia of yang.

腹痛的发生主要是由于外邪、饮食所伤、情志失调及素体阳虚等因素，导致气机阻滞、脉络痹阻或经脉失养而发生腹痛。

1.1　Seasonal Pathogenic Factors Attacking and Disharmony of the Spleen and Stomach

1.1　外感时邪，脾胃失调

Exogenous pathogenic factors of wind, cold, summer heat, heat, dampness invade into the abdomen, causing dysfunction of the spleen and stomach. The pathogenic factors remain inside, obstructing qi activities and slowing the blood circulation, which leads to pain.

外感风、寒、暑 、热、湿时邪，入侵腹中，脾胃运化功能失调，邪滞于中，气机阻滞，血运不畅，不通则痛。

1.2 Improper Diet Leading to Pathogenic Factors Obstructing zhong jiao

Over-eating and drinking leads to food retention. Or over intake of lard, sweat, greasy or spicy food generates damp-heat. Or uncontrolled intake of raw and cold food results in cold-damp retained inside. All can lead to the pathogenic factors obstructing zhong jiao, causing abdominal pain.

1.2 饮食不节,邪滞中焦

暴饮暴食,饮食停滞;或过食肥甘厚腻或辛辣,酿生湿热;或恣食生冷,寒湿内停,都可使邪滞中焦,引发腹痛。

1.3 Emotional and Spiritual Disorder and the Failure of the Liver to Disperse and Purge

Emotional and spiritual discontent and anger will injure the liver. When the liver fails to disperse and purge, it is depressed and when qi fails to flow freely, it stagnates. Hence, depressed and stagnated liver-qi attacks the stomach nearby and leads to the disharmony between the liver and stomach and unsuccessful flow of qi. And then abdominal pain is resulted in.

1.3 情志失调,肝失疏泄

情志不遂,恼怒伤肝,肝失疏泄,气失条达,肝郁气滞,横逆攻脾,肝脾不和,气机失畅,可引起腹痛。

1.4 Fall and Injury Causing Obstruction of Collateral

Fall and injury, operation in the abdomen will make damage to the meridians and collaterals of zang-fu organs. Blood stasis and qi stagnation then leads to abdominal pain.

1.4 跌仆创伤,络脉痹阻

跌仆创伤,或腹部手术以致脏腑经络受损,气血瘀滞不通而腹痛。

1.5 Roundworm Attacking the Abdomen

The attack of roundworm on the stomach and intestines causes frenetic qi activities and dysfunction of the stomach in harmonizing and descending, resulting in abdominal pain, which comes and goes.

1.5 蛔虫侵袭,脐腹受扰

蛔虫内扰肠胃,以致气机逆乱,胃失和降,故腹痛时作时止。

1.6 Deficiency of Yang and Qi for Long, Zang-fu Organs Lack in Nurturing

Deficiency of yang for long or abdominal pain for long makes damage to the spleen-yang. When the middle-yang weakens, qi and blood go insuffi-

1.6 阳气素虚,脏腑失养

因素体阳虚,或腹痛日久,损及脾阳,中阳衰惫,气血不足,血行迟滞,脏腑经络

cient and when blood circulation slows down, the meridians and collaterals lack in nurturing and abdominal pain comes.

失其温养,腹痛乃作。

Abdominal pain is related to many zang-fu organssuch as the liver, gallbladder, spleen, kidney, intestines, bladder and uterus, and many meridians such as Three Yin Channels of Foot, Foot-Shaoyang, hand-foot-Yangming, Chong, Ren and Dai channels. Its pathology is "pain as the result of obstruction", due to zang-fu qi activities obstruction, unsuccessful circulation of qi and blood, meridian blockade or "pain as the result of weakness" due to zang-fu meridians lacking in nurturing. The pathological factors can be cold accumulation, fire depression, food retention, qi stagnation and blood stasis. The pathological nature is no more than cold, heat, deficiency and excess.

腹痛发病涉及脏腑与经脉较多,包括肝、胆、脾、肾、大小肠、膀胱、胞宫等脏腑,以及足三阴、足少阳、手足阳明、冲、任、带等经脉。基本病机为脏腑气机阻滞,气血运行不畅,经脉痹阻,"不通则痛",或脏腑经脉失养,不荣而痛。病理因素主要有寒凝、火郁、食积、气滞、血瘀。病理性质不外寒、热、虚、实四端。

2 Syndrome Differentiation and Treatment

2 辨证论治

2.1 Key Points of Syndrome Differentiation

2.1 辨治要点

Abdominal pain should be identified to be different nature of cold or heat, deficiency or excess by acuteness or chronicity, nature and location of the pain, relation to diet, stool, triggering, aggravating and relieving factors, syndromes and seasons. Generally speaking, when pain attacks due to cold and is relieved by warming, it is pain of cold type, including deficiency cold and excess cold. In contrast, burning pain is pain of heat. If pain continues and patients favor warmth and pression, it is pain of deficiency while patients refuse to be pressed at the pain spot and pain aggravates after eating, then it is pain of excess. Distentional pain without fixed spots is due to qi stagnation while sharp fixed

腹痛的辨证可从起病的缓急、疼痛的性质和部位、与饮食的关系、大便情况、诱发及加重与缓解因素、伴随症状、发病季节等方面进行虚实寒热的辨别。一般而言:受寒痛作,得温则缓,属寒痛(实寒、虚寒);灼热样痛,属热痛;痛势绵绵,喜温喜按为虚痛;痛处拒按,得食痛增,为实痛;胀痛为主,痛无定处为气滞;腹部刺痛,固定不移为血瘀;吐泻得舒,常为食积。辨别腹痛部位有助了解

pain is due to blood stasis. Pain relief after vomiting is usually due to food retention. Moreover, identification of the location of pain is helpful for grasping the patholgocial changes of zang-fu organs. For example, pain in upper abdomen is usually due to affected spleen, stomach and intestines. Pain in the lower abdomen is due to the liver channel of Jueyin. Pain in the lower abdomen is due to affected kidney and bladder. Pain around navel and clear away vomitus is usually worm affection. "Dredging" is the fundamental treatment principle, based on which, doctors choose appropriate therapeutic methods in line with pattern identification of cold, heat, deficiency and excess to treat both the primary and secondary symptoms. For pain of excess, the focus is on dispelling the pathogenic factors, dispersing and dredging. For pain of deficiency, focus on warming zhong jiao and supplementing deficiency, invigorating qi and nurturing blood. It is important that indiscriminated purging must be avoided. For prolonged pain into collaterals in abdomen, moisturizing with purgative herbs, promoting blood circulation and dredging collaterals can be implemented.

病变脏腑,如痛在大腹,多为脾胃、大小肠受病;痛在少腹,多为厥阴肝经之病;痛在小腹,多为肾与膀胱受病;痛在脐腹,喜吐清水,多为虫扰。治疗上多以“通”字立法,应根据辨证的虚实寒热,在气在血,确立相应治法,在通法的基础上,结合审证求因,标本兼治。属实证者,重在祛邪疏导;对虚痛,应温中补虚,益气养血,不可滥施攻下,对于久痛入络,绵绵不愈之腹痛,可采取辛润活血通络之法。

2.2 Therapeutic Methods of Different Types of Abdominal Pain

2.2 分型论治

2.2.1 Cold Pathogenic Factor Obstructs Inside

2.2.1 寒邪内阻

Manifestations: Acute abdominal pain, aggravated by cold and relieved by warming, tastelessness, no thirst, physical cold and cold limbs, long and clear away urine, loose stool or constipation; pale tongue with white greasy tongue fur; deep tight pulse.

证候: 腹痛拘急,遇寒痛甚,得温痛减,口淡不渴,形寒肢冷,小便清长,便清稀或秘结。舌质淡,苔白腻,脉沉紧。

Treatment: To disperse cold and warm the interior, regulate qi and stop pain.

治法: 散寒温里,理气止痛。

Formulas and Herbs: Alpiniae Officinarum and Cyperi Pills (Liang Fu Pills) and Aromatic Restoring Healthy Qi Powder (Zheng Qi Tian Xiang San), usually composed of *Alpiniae Officinarum Rhizoma* (Gao Liang Jiang), *Zingiberis Rhizoma* (Gan Jiang) and *Perillae Fructus* (Zi Su Zi) to warm zhong jiao and disperse cold; *Linderae Radix* (Wu Yao), *Cyperi Rhizoma* (Xiang Fu) and *Citri Reticulatae Pericarpium* (Chen Pi) to regulate qi and stop pain.

方药：良附丸合正气天香散。常用：高良姜、干姜、紫苏温中散寒；乌药、香附、陈皮理气止痛。

Modification: For sharp and groaning pain in the abdomen due to upward flowing of cold qi with vomiting due to fullness in the chest and hypochondria, use Aconiti and Oryza Sativae Decoction (Fu Zi Jing Mi Tang) to warm zhong jiao and subtract reverse flow of qi; for cold pain in the abdomen and sore over body, feeling cold outside and inside, use Aconite Main Tuber and Cinnamomi Decoction (Wu Tou Gui Zhi Tang) to warm the interior and disperse cold; for acute and cold pain in the lower abdomen due to cold stagnation, use Liver-Warming Decoction (Nuan Gan Jian) and Meridian-Warming Powder (Wen Jing San) to disperse cold; for accumulation of excess cold, acute adominal pain and constipation, use *Rhei and Aconiti Praeparata Decoction* (Da Huang Fu Zi Tang) to warm and purge accumulated cold; for affection by cold-damp in summer with symptoms like nausea, vomiting, distention in the chest, poor appetite, general heaviness, fatigue and white greasy tongue fur, add moderately *Pogostemonis Herba* (Huo Xiang), *Atractylodis Rhizoma* (Cang Zhu), *Magnoliae Officinalis Cortex* (Hou Po), *Amomi Fructus Rotundus* (Bai Dou Kou) and *Pinelliae Rhizoma* (Ban Xia) to

加减：如寒气上逆致腹中切痛雷鸣、胸胁逆满呕吐，用附子粳米汤温中降逆；腹中冷痛、身体疼痛、内外皆寒者，用乌头桂枝汤温里散寒；若少腹拘急冷痛，属肝脉寒滞，用暖肝煎温经散寒；若寒实积聚，腹痛拘急、大便不通，用大黄附子汤温泻寒积；夏日感受寒湿，伴见恶心呕吐、胸闷、纳呆、身重、倦怠、舌苔白腻者，可酌加藿香、苍术、厚朴、白蔻仁、半夏，以温中散寒，化湿运脾。

warm the middle to disperse cold and dry dampness to invigorate spleen.

2.2.2 Damp-heat Blocks and Stagnates

Manifestations: Abdominal pain that denies pressing, irritation, thirst for drinking, dry stool or loose sticky stool, yellow short urine; red tongue with yellow dry tongue fur or yellow greasy tongue fur; rapid rolling pulse.

Treatment: To purge heat and dredge fu-organs, promote qi and resolve stagnation.

Formulas and Herbs: *Major Purgative Decoction* (Da Cheng Qi Tang), usually composed of *Rhei Radix et Rhizoma* (Da Huang) to discharge dry stool; *Natrii Sulfas* (Mang Xiao) to purge heat with salty cold herbs as well as softening solidity and resolving clots; *Magnoliae Officinalis Cortex* (Hou Po) and *Aurantii Fructus* (Zhi Qiao) to remove stagnation and eliminate discomfort.

Modification: For not serious feverish sensentaion with heavy damp-heat and sticky stool, subtract *Natrii Sulfas* (Mang Xiao) and add *Gardeniae Fructus* (Zhi Zi) and *Scutellariae Radix* (Huang Qin); for pain stretching to the hypochondria, add *Curcumae Radix* (Yu Jin) and *Bupleuri Radix* (Chai Hu); for sharp abdominal pain, interchanging cold and heat, nausea and vomiting, constipation, use *Major Bupleurum Decoction* (Da Chai Hu Tang) to relieve both the exterior and interior.

2.2.2 湿热壅滞

证候：腹痛拒按，烦渴引饮，大便秘结，或溏滞不爽，潮热汗出，小便短黄。舌质红，苔黄燥或黄腻，脉滑数。

治法：泄热通腑，行气导滞。

方药：大承气汤。常用：大黄攻下燥屎；芒硝咸寒泄热，软坚散结；厚朴、枳实导滞消痞。

加减：若燥热不甚，湿热偏重，大便不爽者，可去芒硝，加栀子、黄芩等；若痛引两胁，可加郁金、柴胡；如腹痛剧烈、寒热往来、恶心呕吐、大便秘结者，改用大柴胡汤表里双解。

2.2.3 Food Retention Stagnates

Manifestations: Distention and fullness in the stomach and abdomen, pain resisting pressing, belching and acid regurgitation, loss of appetitie, vomiting and nausea, pain for diarrhea and relief after diarrhea, or constipation; thick greasy tongue fur;

2.2.3 饮食积滞

证候：脘腹胀满，疼痛拒按，嗳腐吞酸，厌食呕恶，痛而欲泻，泻后痛减，或大便秘结。舌苔厚腻，脉滑。

rolling pulse.

Treatment: To remove food retention and resolve stagnation; regulate qi and stop pain.

Formulas and Herbs: *Aurantii Immaturus Eliminating Stagnation Pills* (Zhi Shi Dao Zhi Wan), usually composed of *Rhei Radix et Rhizoma* (Da Huang), *Aurantii Fructus Immaturus* (Zhi Shi), *Massa Fermentata Medicinalis* (Shen Qu) to remove food retention and eliminate stagnation, *Scutellariae Radix* (Huang Qin), *Coptidis Rhizoma* (Huang Lian) and *Alismatis Rhizoma* (Ze Xie) to clear away heat and dry dampness; *Atractylodis Macrocephalae Rhizoma* (Bai Zhu) and *Poria* (Fu Ling) to invigorate the spleen to promote transportation.

Modification: For abdominal pain and distentions and fullness, add *Magnoliae Officinalis Cortex* (Hou Pu) and *Aucklandiae Radix* (Mu Xiang) to promote qi flow to stop pain; for severe diarrhea, use *Aucklandiae and Arecae Pills* (Mu Xiang Bing Lang Wan) to remove food retention, eliminate stagnation, clear away heat and dry dampness; for light food retention and abdominal pain, use *Pachyma Compound Digestive Tonic Pills* (Bao He Wan).

2. 2. 4　Depressed Liver-qi Stagnates

Manifestations: Distention and oppression in the abdomen with no fixed spots, intermittent pain stretching to the lower abdomen or to the hypochondria, pain relieved after belching or passing gas, pain aggravated with worry and anger; red tongue with white thin tongue fur; taut pulse.

Treatment: To disperse the liver to resolve depression; regulate qi and stop pain.

Formulas and Herbs: *Bupleurum-Dispersing-Liver Powder* (Chai Hu Shu Gan San), usually com-

治法：消食导滞，理气止痛。

方药：枳实导滞丸。常用：大黄、枳实、神曲消食导滞；黄芩、黄连、泽泻清热化湿；白术、茯苓健脾助运。

加减：若腹痛胀满者，加厚朴、木香行气止痛；若兼下痢后重者，可用木香槟榔丸消食导滞、清热利湿；如食滞不重、腹痛较轻者，用保和丸。

2. 2. 4　肝郁气滞

证候：腹痛胀闷，痛无定处，痛引少腹，或兼痛窜两胁，时作时止，得嗳气或矢气则舒，遇忧思恼怒则剧。舌质红，苔薄白，脉弦。

治法：疏肝解郁，理气止痛。

方药：柴胡疏肝散。常用：柴胡、枳壳、香附、陈皮疏

posed of *Bupleuri Radix* (Chai Hu), *Aurantii Fructus*(Zhi Qiao), *Cyperi Rhizoma* (Xiang Fu) and *Citri Reticulatae Pericarpium* (Chen Pi) to disperse the liver and regulate qi; *Paeoniae Radix Alba* (Bai Shao Yao) and *Glycyrrhizae Radix et Rhizoma* (Gan Cao) to relieve acute pain; *Chuanxiong Rhizoma* (Chuan Xiong) to promote qi flow and blood circulation.

肝理气;白芍药、甘草缓急止痛,川芎行气活血。

Modification: For severe qi stagnation and distention and pain in chest and hypochondria, add *Toosendan Fructus* (Chuan Lian Zi) and *Curcumae Radix* (Yu Jin); for pain stretching to the lower abdomen and testicle, and hernia of intestines, add *Citri Reticulatae Semen* (Ju He) and *Litchi Semen* (Li Zhi He) or use *Tiantai Lindera Powder* (Tian Tai Wu Yao San); for abdominal pain and bowel sounds, qi stagnation and diarrhea, use *Important Formula for Pain and Diarrhea* (Tong Xie Yao Fang); for prolonged liver depression turning into heat, add *Moutan Cortex* (Mu Dan Pi) and *Gardeniae Fructus* (Zhi Zi) to clear away heat and purge the liver.

加减: 若气滞较重,胸肋胀痛者,加川楝子、郁金;若痛引少腹、睾丸,小肠疝气者,加橘核、荔枝核,或予天台乌药散;若腹痛肠鸣、气滞腹泻者,可用痛泻要方;肝郁日久化热者,加牡丹皮、山栀子清肝泄热。

2.2.5 Blood Stasis Retains Inside

2.2.5 瘀血内停

Manifestations: Sharp needling-like abodominal pain on fixed spots with no way to be relieved or cured; purple dark tongue; fine uneven pulse.

证候: 腹痛较剧,痛如针刺,痛处固定,经久不愈。舌质紫黯,脉细涩。

Treatment: To promote blood circulation and remove blood stasis; harmonize the collaterals and stop pain.

治法: 活血化瘀,和络止痛。

Formulas and Herbs: *Lower abdomen Stasis-Expelling Decoction* (Shao Fu Zhu Yu Tang), usually composed of *Angelicae Sinensis Radix* (Dang Gui), *Imperatae Rhizoma* (Chuan Xiong), *Paeoniae Radix Rubra* (Chi Shao) and *Glycyrrhizae Radix et*

方药: 少腹逐瘀汤。常用:当归、川芎、赤芍药、甘草养血和营;延胡索、蒲黄、五灵脂化瘀止痛;肉桂、干姜、小茴香温经止痛。

Rhizoma (Gan Cao) to nourish blood and harmonize ying-qi; *Corydalis Rhizoma* (Yan Hu Suo, Yuan Hu), *Typhae Pollen* (Pu Huang), *Faeces Trogopterorum* (Wu Ling Zhi) to remove stasis and stop pain; *Cinnamomi Cortex* (Rou Gui), *Zingiberis Rhizoma* (Gan Jiang) and *Foeniculi Fructus* (Xiao Hui Xiang) to warm meridians and stop pain.

Modification: For abdominal pain after operation or falling, add *Lycopi Herba* (Ze Lan), *Myrrha* (Mo Yao), *Notoginseng Radix et Rhizoma* (San Qi); for abdominal pain with qi stagnation, add *Cyperi Rhizoma* (Xiang Fu) and *Bupleuri Radix* (Chai Hu); for blood accumulated in xia jiao and black stool, use *Peach-pit Purgative Decoction* (Tao He Cheng Qi Tang).

加减: 若腹部术后作痛,或跌仆损伤作痛,可加泽兰、没药、三七;若腹痛兼气滞者,加香附、柴胡;若下焦蓄血,大便色黑,可用桃核承气汤。

2.2.6 Roundworm Interferes Inside

2.2.6 蛔虫内扰

Manifestations: Intemitent abdominal pain around navel, favor warmth and pressing, epigastric upset, irritation and vomiting, even worms in vomitus and stool, abdominal enterozoic mass.

证候: 脐周腹痛,时作时止,喜温喜按,胃脘嘈杂,心烦喜呕,甚或吐虫、便虫、腹中虫瘕。

Treatment: To dispel roundworms; regulate the spleen and stomach.

治法: 驱除蛔虫,调理脾胃。

Formulas and Herbs: First use *Black Plum Pills* (Wu Mei Wan) to calm down roundworms to stop pain, when pain is relieved, use *Worm-Dispelling Pills* (Hua Chong Wan). *Mume Fructus* (Wu Mei), *Sichuan Pepper* (Chuan Jiao) and *Asari Radix et Rhizoma* (Xi Xin) can calm down the roundworm with sour and purgative herbs while *Coptidis Rhizoma* (Huang Lian) and *Phellodendri Chinensis Cortex* (Huang Bo) can dispel roundworm with bitterness as well as clear away heat. *Zingiberis Rhizoma* (Gan Jiang), *Aconm Lateralis Radix Praeparata* (Fu Zi), *Cinnamomi Ramulus* (Gui Zhi) can warm

方药: 先用乌梅丸安蛔定痛,待腹痛缓解予化虫丸驱除蛔虫。常用:乌梅、川椒、细辛酸辛安蛔;黄连、黄柏苦可下蛔,寒可清热;干姜、附子、桂枝温脏祛寒;人参、当归补气养血;鹤虱、苦楝根皮、槟榔、芜荑、使君子等驱除蛔虫。

the organs and dispel cold while *Ginseng Radix et Rhizoma* (Ren Shen) and *Angelicae Sinensis Radix* (Dang Gui) to supplement qi and nourish blood. *Fructus Carpesii* (He Shi), *Radix Melia Azedarach* (Ku Lian Gen) and *Meliae Cortex* (Ku Lian Pi), *Arecae Semen* (Bing Lang), *Fructus Ulmi Macrocarpae* (Wu Yi) and *Quisqualis Fructus* (Shi Jun Zi) can dispel roundworms.

Modification: For abdominal bulging pain, vomiting, constipation, passing gas and abdominal enterozoic mass with thin greasy or yellow greasy tongue fur and taut pulse due to intangled roundworms blocking fu-qi, use modified *Major Purgative Decoction* (Da Cheng Qi Tang) to dredge and purge.

加减：若虫结成团，腑气闭结，症见腹部攻撑作痛、呕吐、便秘、矢气，并有虫瘕，苔薄腻或黄腻，脉弦，宜通里攻下，用大承气汤加减。

2.2.7 Deficiency inzhong jiao and Visceral Cold

2.2.7 中虚脏寒

Manifestations: Intermittent dull abdominal pain, favor warmth and pressing, physical cold and cold limbs, fatigue and tiredness, short breath and laziness to talk, poor appetite, lusterless face and loose stool; pale tongue with thin white tongue fur; deep fine pulse.

证候：腹痛绵绵，时作时止，喜温喜按，形寒肢冷，神疲乏力，气短懒言，胃纳不佳，面色无华，大便溏薄。舌质淡，苔薄白，脉沉细。

Treatment: To warm zhong jiao and supplement deficiency; relieve spasm and stop pain.

治法：温中补虚，缓急止痛。

Formulas and Herbs: *Minor Center-Fortifying Decoction* (Xiao Jian Zhong Tang), usually composed of *Cinnamomi Ramulus* (Gui Zhi) and *Zingiberis Rhizoma Recens* (Sheng Jiang) to warm yang and dispel cold; *Paeoniae Radix Alba* (Bai Shao Yao) and *Glycyrrhizae Radix et Rhizoma Praeparata* (Zhi Gan Cao) to relieve spasm and stop abdominal pain; *Caramels* (Yi Tang) and *Jujubae Fructus* (Da Zao) to warm and invigorate zhong jiao.

方药：小建中汤。常用：桂枝、生姜温阳散寒；白芍药、炙甘草缓急止痛；饴糖、大枣甘温补中。

Modification: For heavy cold in the abdomen,

加减：腹中大寒，呕吐肢

vomiting and cold limbs, use *Major Center-Fortifying Decoction* (Da Jian Zhong Tang) to warm the middle and dispel cold; for abdominal pain and diarrhea, weak pulse, cold limbs and yang-deficiency in the spleen and stomach, use *Aconiti Praeparata-Regulating Zhong jiao Decoction* (Fu Zi Li Zhong Tang); for deficiency-cold in the large intestines, accumulated cold and constipation, use *Spleen-Warming Decoction* (Wen Pi Tang); for extreme deficiency of the middle qi, short breath and laziness to talk, use *Center-Supplementing qi-Boosting Decoction* (Bu Zhong Yi Qi Tang) or *Angelicae Sinensis-Four Disorder Decoction* (Dang Gui Si Ni Tang) or *Astragali Strengthening the Middle Decoction* (Huang Qi Jian Zhong Tang).

冷,可用大建中汤温中散寒;若腹痛下利、脉微肢冷,脾肾阳虚者,可用附子理中汤;若大肠虚寒,积冷便秘者,可用温脾汤;若中气大虚,少气懒言,可用补中益气汤,还可选用当归四逆汤、黄芪建中汤等。

Diarrhea

泄　泻

Diarrhea is a kind of diseases characterized by loose stool with undigested grains or water-like stool and increasing times of stool, mainly due to dysfunction of thespleen and stomach and fluid-dampness penetrating downward.

泄泻主要是因脾胃运化失常,水湿下渗,而出现以粪便稀薄,或完谷不化,甚至泻出如水样,并多伴有排便次数增多为特征的一类病证。

1　Etiology and Pathogenesis

1　病因病机

Diarrhea is primarily due to dysfuntion of the spleen and stomach and fluid-dampness penetrating downward, which can be caused by exogenous pathogenic factors, improper diet, disharmony of the seven emotions and weak zang-fu organs.

泄泻的发生主要是由于感受外邪、饮食所伤、七情不和及脏腑虚弱等因素,导致脾胃功能失常,水湿下渗而产生本病。

1.1　Exogenous Pathogenic Factors with Dampness Invade inside and Encumber the Spleen

1.1　外邪夹湿,内侵困脾

Any of the six pathogenic factors can cause di-

六淫之邪,均能使人发

arrhea. Among them, summer heat, dampness and (wind-) cold are the most common causes, and dampness in particular. The spleen favors dryness and averts dampness. Exogenous pathogenic dampness is most likely to affect the spleen which fails to transport and distinguish turbidity from clarity so that fluid and grain move downward indiscriminatedly, leading to diarrhea. Clinical manifestations are usually complications of pathogenic dampness with other pathogenic factors, namely, summer-heat dampness, cold-dampness, wind-cold dampness and damp-heat. The pathological keypoint is pathogenic dampness predominance.

生泄泻,其中以暑、湿、(风)寒、热较为常见,尤以感受湿邪致泻者为最多。脾喜燥而恶湿,外来湿邪最易困阻脾土,以致脾运失司,清浊不分,水谷混杂而下,发生泄泻。临证往往为诸邪与湿邪夹杂,合为暑湿、寒湿、风寒湿、湿热等内侵于人。病机的关键在于湿邪偏胜。

1.2 Emotional and Spiritual Injuries Causes the Disharmony between the Liver and Spleen

Worry and anger, emotional and spiritual injuries will depress liver-qi which fails to flow smoothly, affecting the nearby stomach. Over worry indirectly affects spleen-qi, causing the spleen fails to transport and fluid and grain are excreted indiscriminately, leading to diarrhea. Clinincally, innate weakness and deficiency of spleen-qi can easily result in exuberance of liver-wood. The conditioned, once disturbed, will lead to the trap of earth-qi and affection of both the liver and spleen, causing diarrhea.

1.2 情志所伤,肝脾不和

忧郁恼怒,情志所伤,肝气郁结,失于条达,横逆乘脾;或思虑太过,暗耗脾气,脾运失职,水谷不分,混杂而下,变为泄泻。临证亦有素体脾气虚弱,土虚而肝木易于相对偏旺,一有变动,便可招致土气受困,肝脾两病而发为泄泻。

1.3 Food Retention Damaging the Spleen and Stomach

Over-eating causes food retention while over intake of greasy and sweat food will produce damp-heat. Cold-dampness will attackzhong jiao due to over intake of raw and cold food. Or intake of unclean food by mistake will generate pathogenic turbidity. The key pathology is improper diet dama-

1.3 饮食积滞,脾胃受伤

饮食过量,化为积滞;或恣食肥甘,滋生湿热;或过食生冷,寒湿伤中;或误食不洁,化生浊邪等,病机之关键是饮食伤脾。

ging the spleen.

1.4 Over-strain Hurting the Spleen and Spleen-qi and Lucid Yang Failing to Rise

Irregular diet for long, overstrain and internal injuries, excess of worry, prolonged illness, weak constitution, or wrong use of laxative can all lead to weak spleen and stomach and lucid yang's failure to rise. The spleen and stomach can no longer receive, gather, transport or transfer fluid and grain so that dampness retains inside and clarity mixes with turbidty, leading to diarrhea.

1.5 Deficiency and Exhaustion due to Old Age Leading to Weak Fire of the Vital Gate

Weakness due to old age, deficiency of yang and qi, prolonged illness or imtemperance in sexual life will injury kidney-yang and fire of the vital gate, causing the spleen to fail to warm, transport and transfer. Then, occurs diarrhea.

The pathological location is the spleen and stomach, small and large intestines, but also have relation to the liver and kidney. The main pathological feature is weak spleen and dampness predominance. Respectively, for diarrhea due to exogenous pathogenic factors, dampness is critical and other pathogenic factors, only complicated with dampness, will cause diarrhea. For diarrhea due to endogenous factors, weak spleen is critical. The pathological nature of diarrhea comes into two types: deficiency and excess. Generally, acute severe diarrhea is of excess type, due to predominance of dampness damaging the spleen or dampness due to food stagnation blocking zhong jiao and affecting the spleen. Meanwhile, prolonged diarrhea is of deficiency type due to that the spleen is too weak to

1.4 劳倦伤脾，脾气清阳不升

若长期饮食失调，或劳倦内伤，或思虑过度，或久病缠绵，或素体不足，或误用泻下之剂，均可导致脾胃虚弱，清阳不升，不能受纳水谷和运化精微，湿滞内生，清浊不分，遂成泄泻。

1.5 年老虚损，命门火衰

年老体衰、阳气不足，或久病之后，或房室无度，多可肾阳受损、命门火衰，而致脾失温煦、运化失权而成泄泻。

泄泻的病位在脾胃、大肠、小肠，同时与肝肾有关。泄泻最主要的病机特点是脾虚湿胜。分而言之，外邪致泻以湿邪最为重要，其他诸多邪气需与湿邪兼夹，方易成泻；内因则以脾虚最为关键。病理性质有虚实之分。一般来说：暴泻以湿盛为主，多因湿盛伤脾，或食滞生湿，壅滞中焦，脾为湿困所致，病属实证；久泻多偏于虚证，由脾虚不运而生湿，或他脏及脾，如肝木克脾，或肾虚火不暖脾，水谷不化所致。而湿邪与脾病，往往相互影响，互

transport so that dampness is generated, or due to that the spleen is affected by other zang-organs such as liver-wood suppressing the spleen or weak kidney-fire's inability to warm the spleen that fails to transfer fluid and grains. Pathogenic dampness and spleen diseases affect each other or are interdetermined. Excess of dampness can suppress the spleen's controlance of transportation while spleen weakness, in turn, will generate dampness. Moreover, deficiency and excess are interchangeable and complicated.

为因果,湿盛可困遏脾运,脾虚又可生湿。虚实之间又可相互转化夹杂。

2 Syndrome Differentiation and Treatment

2.1 Key Points of Syndrome Differentiation

Diarrhea should be identified according to the pathogenesis, duration, quality of stool and abodominal pain along with other accompanying syndromes and seasonal factors. Acute diarrhea attacks suddenly but lastsfor short time or sometimes with secondary symptoms, primarily due to predominance of excessive dampness and excess of pathogenic factors. While prolonged diarrhea takes on gradually and lasts long, primarily due to spleen deficiency, liver and spleen being affected, or spleen and kidney being affected at the same time, caused frequently by improper diet, overstrain and fatigue, emotional and spiritual disorders. Clinically, prolonged diarrhea can be manifested by the symptoms of both deficiency and excess, but spleen deficiency is primary. Thin, clear away and water-like stool with a little smell is mostly due to cold-dampness. Loose yellowish brown smelly stool with acute excretion and buring annus is due to damp-heat. Smelly stool like stinky eggs is due to food stagna-

2 辨证论治

2.1 辨治要点

泄泻的辨证应着重围绕其发病、病程、粪质、腹痛等情况,结合其他伴随症状和季节因素来进行。暴泻多发病急、病程短,或兼见表证,多以湿盛邪实为主。久泻多发病缓慢,病程较长,易因饮食、劳倦、情志而复发,常以脾虚为主,或肝脾两病,或脾肾同病等,临床上亦可表现为虚实夹杂之证,但总以脾虚为要。大便清稀,或如水样,气味略腥者,多是寒湿为患;大便或稀或溏,其色黄褐,气味臭秽,泻下急迫,肛门灼热者,多是湿热为患;大便臭如败卵者,多为伤食积滞;大便稀溏,甚则完谷不化,无腥臭,多为虚寒之证。治疗上以运脾化湿为原则:

tion while loose stool with undigested whole grains without smell is mostly due to deficiency-cold. The treatment guideline is to resolve the dampness and invigorate the spleen. For acute diarrhea due to predominace of damp-heat, focus on resolving dampness along with removing dampness with diuresis, and use warming to resolve cold-dampness and cleansing to remove damp-heat respectively in line with cold-dampness or damp-heat. For complication with exterior pathogenic factors, resolve dampness along with dispersing. For complication with summer-heat, resolve dampness as well as clear away summer heat. For improper diet, resolve dampness with eliminating food retention. For prolonged diarrhea due to spleen deficiency, focus on invigorating the spleen. For liver-qi subjugating the spleen, it is better to suppress the liver and strengthen the spleen. For kidney-yang deficiency and weakness, it is better to warm the kidney and invigorate the spleen. For descending middle-qi, it is better to boost it. For prolonged diarrhea that cannot be relieved, it is better to strenghthen astringency. However, strenghtening astringency cannot be applied to acute diarrhea in order to avoid blocking the gate and retaing the pathogenic factors. At the same time, promoting diuresis cannot be applied to prolonged diarrhea in case of yin and fluid leakage.

急性泄泻多以湿盛为主，重在化湿，佐以分利，再根据寒湿和湿热的不同，分别采用温化寒湿与清化湿热之法，夹有表邪者，佐以疏解；夹有暑邪者，佐以清暑；兼有伤食者，佐以消导。久泻以脾虚为主，当以健脾。因肝气乘脾者，宜抑肝扶脾。因肾阳虚衰者，宜温肾健脾。中气下陷者，宜升提。久泄不止者，宜固涩。暴泻不可骤用补涩，以免闭门留寇；久泻不可分利太过，以防劫其阴液。

2.2 Therapeutic Methodsfor Different Patterns

2.2.1 Cold-dampness Seizes the Spleen

Manifestations: Diarrhea with clear away, thin, or even water-like stool with abdominal pain and rumbling sound in the intestines, oppression in the stomach, little intake; white greasy tongue fur; soft slow pulse. When complicated with cold, diarrhea

2.2 分型论治

2.2.1 寒湿困脾

证候：泄泻清稀，甚如水样，腹痛肠鸣，脘闷食少。苔白腻，脉濡缓。若兼外感风寒，则泄泻暴起，恶寒发热，头痛，肢体酸痛。苔薄白，脉

attacks suddenly with aversion to cold, fever, sore over body, thin white tongue fur and floating pulse.

浮。

Treatment: To dry dampness with fragant and aromatic herbs; relieve the exterior and disperse cold.

治法: 芳香化湿,解表散寒。

Formulas and Herbs: *Agastachis-Restoring Healthy Energy Powder* (Huo Xiang Zheng Qi San), usually composed of *Pogostemonis Herba* (Huo Xiang) to dispel cold with its acrid-warm nature as well as resolve turbidity with its fragrant and aromatic nature; *Atractylodis Rhizoma* (Cang Zhu), *Poria* (Fu Ling), *Pinelliae Rhizoma* (Ban Xia), *Citri Reticulatae Pericarpium* (Chen Pi) to invigorate the spleen and dispel dampness as well as harmonize zhong jiao and stop vomiting; *Magnoliae Officinalis Cortex* (Hou Pu) and *Arecae Pericarpium* (Da Fu Pi) to regulate qi and eliminate fullness; *Perillae Fructus* (Zi Su Zi), *Angelicae Dahuricae Radix*(Bai Zhi), *Platycodi Radix*(Jie Geng) to relieve the exterior and dispel cold as well as disperse and induce qi activity, *Aucklandiae Radix* (Mu Xiang) to regulate qi and stop pain.

方药: 藿香正气散。常用:藿香辛温散寒,芳香化浊;苍术、茯苓、半夏、陈皮健脾祛湿,和中止呕;厚朴、大腹皮理气除满;紫苏、白芷、桔梗解表散寒、疏利气机,加木香理气止痛。

Modification: For severe exterior pathogenic factors and remarkable cold and fever with sore body, add *Schizonepetae Herba* (Jing Jie) and *Saposhnikoviae Radix*(Fang Feng) or *Schizonepeta and Ledebouriella Detoxifying Powder* (Jing Fang Bai Du San); for heavy pathogenic cold, add *Pure-Yang Correcting Qi Pills* (Chun Yang Zheng Qi Wan); for heavy pathogenic dampness, abdominal fullness and rumbling sounds in the intestines, difficult urination, use *Poria Stomach Decoction* (Wei Ling Tang) to invigorate the spleen, promote qi flow and dispel dampness.

加减: 若表邪偏重、寒热身痛显著者,可加荆芥、防风,或与荆防败毒散合用;寒邪重者,可合用纯阳正气丸;若湿邪偏重,腹满肠鸣、小便不利,可改用胃苓汤健脾行气祛湿。

2.2.2 Damp-heat Blocks Inside

Manifestations: Abdominal pain and diarrhea attack in turn, urgent diarrhea or sticky diarrhea, thin or loose stool, yellowish brown and stinky stool, buring annus, irrtition, feverish sensation, short and dark urine; yellow greasy tongue fur; soft rapid pulse or slippery rolling pulse.

Treatment: To clear away heat and eliminate dampness; promote clarity and subtract turbidity.

Formulas and Herbs: *Peucedani, Scutellariae and Coptidis Decoction* (Ge Gen Qin Lian Tang), usually composed of *Scutellariae Radix* (Huang Qin), *Coptidis Rhizoma* (Huang Lian) to clear away heat and dry dampness with bitter and cool herbs; *Puerariae Lobatae Radix* (Ge Gen) to clear away heat and enable the spleen to promote clarity; *Glycyrrhizae Radix et Rhizoma* (Gan Cao) to harmonize zhong jiao gently.

Modification: For heavy pathogenic heat, abdominal pain and diarrhea in turns, bitter and dry mouth, moderately add *Taraxaci Herba* (Pu Gong Ying), *Forsythiae Fructus* (Lian Qiao), *Lonicerae Japonicae Flos* (Jin Yin Hua) and *Sophorae Flavescentis Radix* (Ku Shen) to clear away heat and detoxify or change for Pulsatillae Decoction (Bai Tou Weng Tang); for heavy pathogenic dampness, fullness and oppression in the chest and abdomen, no thirst or thirst but with no desire for drink, yellowish thick greasy tongue fur, add *Stomach-Calming Powder* (Ping Wei San) to dry dampness and relieve zhong jiao; for diarrhea of complicated cold and heat due to damp-heat, without cure, bitter mouth and hiccup, cold pain in the abdomen which gets worse when eating cold food and diarrhea gets

2.2.2 湿热内蕴

证候:腹痛泄泻交作,泻下急迫,或泻而不爽,大便质或稀或溏,大便色黄褐而臭,肛门灼热,烦热口渴,小便短赤。舌苔黄腻,脉濡数或滑数。

治法:清热利湿,升清降浊。

方药:葛根芩连汤。常用:黄芩、黄连苦寒清热燥湿,配以葛根既有清热之功,又可助脾升清;甘草甘缓和中。

加减:若热邪偏甚、痛泻交作,口苦口干重者,可酌加蒲公英、连翘、金银花、苦参等以清热解毒,或改用白头翁汤;若湿邪偏重、胸腹满闷、口不渴或渴不欲饮、舌苔微黄厚腻者,宜合平胃散,以燥湿宽中;如湿热泄泻,日久不愈,症见口苦干呕、腹部冷痛、饮冷则泄泻更甚、苔薄黄腻等寒热错杂之证,可予乌梅丸,辛开苦降、寒热并调;若外有风寒表邪,内有湿热入侵,见发热恶寒、头痛身重、烦渴自汗、面垢、小便短赤者,可选用新加香薷饮合

worse as well, thin yellow greasy tongue fur, apply *Black Plum Pills* (Wu Mei Wan) to open with acridity and downbear with bitterness and regulate cold and heat at the same time; for exterior pathogenic factors like wind-cold and damp-heat inside with symptoms like fever, aversion to cold, general heaviness, headache, irritation, thirst, spontaneous sweating, dirty complexion and short dark urine, use *Newly Added Elsholtziae Decoction* (Xin Jia Xiang Ru Yin) and *Six-To-One power* (Liu Yi San) to relieve both the exterior and interior, clear away summer heat and resolve dampness; for diarrhea due to cold-dampness caused by overeating cool, raw and cold food in summer, use *Agastachis-Restoring Healthy Energy Powder* (Huo Xiang Zheng Qi San) or *Pure-Yang Correcting Qi Pills* (Chun Yang Zheng Qi Wan).

六一散以表里双解、清暑化湿;暑令亦可因贪凉、过食生冷等引起寒湿泄泻,可予藿香正气散或纯阳正气丸。

2.2.3 Food Stagnates in the Intestines and Stomach

Manifestations: Abdominal pain, rumbling sounds in the intestines, stool smelling like stinky eggs with whole undigested grains, pain relieved after diarrhea, distention and fullness in the stomach and abdomen, sour stinky belching, loss of appetite; dirty yellow or thin greasy tongue fur; rolling pulse.

Treatment: To eliminate food retention and induce stagnation; treating diarrhea with purgative

Formulas and Herbs: *Aurantii Immaturus Eliminating Stagnation Pills* (Zhi Shi Dao Zhi Wan), usually composed of *Rhei Radix et Rhizoma* (Da Huang) and *Aurantii Fructus Immaturus* (Zhi Shi) to push out food retention; *Scutellariae Radix* (Huang Qin) and *Forsythiae Fructus* (Lian Qiao) to clear away heat and dry dampness, as well as solidi-

2.2.3 食滞肠胃

证候: 腹痛肠鸣,泻下粪便臭如败卵,并夹有完谷,泻后痛减,伴有脘腹胀满,嗳腐酸臭,不思饮食。苔垢黄或厚腻,脉滑。

治法: 消食导滞,通因通用。

方药: 枳实导滞丸合保和丸。常用:大黄、枳实等推荡积滞,佐以黄芩、黄连清热燥湿、厚肠止泻,茯苓、泽泻利水渗湿,白术健脾;再以保和丸助其运化、消其积滞。

fy the intestines to stop diarrhea; *Poria* (Fu Ling), *Alismatis Rhizoma* (Ze Xie) to induce fluid and dampness; *Atractylodis Macrocephalae Rhizoma* (Bai Zhu) to invigorate the spleen, and then use *Pachyma Compound Digestive Tonic Pills* (Bao He Wan) to promote transportation and transference to eliminate retention and stagnation.

Modification: For food retention turing into heat, add *Coptidis Rhizoma* (Huang Lian) to clear away heat, dry dampness and stop diarrhea; for spleen-deficiency, add *Atractylodis Macrocephalae Rhizoma* (Bai Zhu) and *Lablab Semen Album* (Bian Dou) to strengthen the spleen and dispel dampness.

加减: 食积化热可加黄连清热燥湿止泻;兼脾虚可加白术、扁豆健脾祛湿。

2.2.4 Liver-qi Restricts the Spleen

2.2.4 肝气乘脾

Manifestations: Abdominal pain and diarrhea with thundering sounds in the abdomen, dashing pain, frequent passing gas, likeliness to be triggered by depressive, angry emotions and tense, distention and oppression in the chest and hypochondria at ordinary times, belching and little intake; pale red tongue with thin tongue fur; taut pulse.

证候: 腹痛而泻,伴有腹中雷鸣、攻窜作痛、矢气频作,每于抑郁恼怒或情志紧张之时诱发,平素亦多胸胁胀闷、嗳气食少。舌淡红,苔薄,脉弦。

Treatment: To depress the liver and calm the spirits; strengthen the spleen and boost earth.

治法: 抑肝宁神,健脾扶土。

Formulas and Herbs: *Pain and Diarrhea Formula* (Tong Xie Yao Fang) and *Counterflow Cold Powder* (Si Ni San), usually composed of *Atractylodis Macrocephalae Rhizoma* (Bai Zhu) to invogirate the spleen and supplement deficiency; *Paeoniae Radix Alba* (Bai Shao Yao) to nourish blood and soften the liver; *Citri Reticulatae Pericarpium* (Chen Pi) to regulate qi and enliven the spleen, *Saposhnikoviae Radix*(Fang Feng) to raise the clear away and stop diarrhea; *Bupleuri Radix*, (Chai Hu) *Aurantii Fructus* (Zhi Qiao) and *Glycyrrhizae Radix et*

方药: 痛泻要方合四逆散。常用白术健脾补虚,白芍药养血柔肝,陈皮理气醒脾,防风升清止泻,柴胡、枳壳、甘草疏肝理气和中。

Rhizoma (Gan Cao) to disperse the liver, regulate qi and harmonize zhong jiao.

Modification: For constitutional spleen and stomach deficiency so that liver-wood restriction and counter-restriction, add *Codonopsis Radix* (Dang Shen), *Dioscoreae Rhizoma* (Shan Yao), *Lablab Semen Album* (Bian Dou) and *Poria* (Fu Ling) to strengthen the spleen and boost earth; for severe abdominal twisting pain, add *Corydalis Rhizoma* (Yan Hu Suo) and *Liquidambaris Fructus* (Lu Lu Tong) to help to relieve pain; for severe diarrhea, add *Puerariae Lobatae Radix* (Ge Gen) and Cortex Pericarpium Granati (Shi Liu Pi) to raise the clear away, astrict and stop diarrhea.

加减：若为脾胃素虚、肝木乘侮者，常需合用党参、山药、扁豆、茯苓等健脾扶土之品；若见腹痛明显、阵阵绞痛者，可加延胡索、路路通等加强止痛之功；泻甚者，可再入葛根、石榴皮等升清、收涩止泻之品。

2.2.5 Weakness and Deficiency of the Spleen and Stomach

2.2.5 脾胃虚弱

Manifestations: Recurrent loose stool or diarrhea with undigested whole grains in the excretion, decreasing food intake, discomfort and oppression in the stomach after eating, remarkable increasing times of stool with a little greasy food, withering yellow complextion, fatigue and tiredness; pale tongue with white tongue fur; fine weak pulse.

证候：大便时溏时泻，迁延反复，完谷不化，饮食减少，食后脘闷不舒，稍进油腻食物则大便次数明显增加，面色萎黄，神疲倦怠。舌淡苔白，脉细弱。

Treatment: To strengthen the spleen and percolate dampness; boost qi and stop diarrhea.

治法：健脾渗湿，益气止泻。

Formulas and Herbs: *Ginseng, Poria and Atractylodes Powder* (Shen Ling Bai Zhu San), usually composed of *Ginseng Radix et Rhizoma* (Ren Shen), *Atractylodis Macrocephalae Rhizoma* (Bai Zhu), *Poria* (Fu Ling) and *Glycyrrhizae Radix et Rhizoma* (Gan Cao) to strengthen the spleen and boost qi; *Amomi Fructus* (Sha Ren), *Citri Reticulatae Pericarpium* (Chen Pi) *Platycodi Radix* (Jie Geng), *Lablab Semen Album* (Bian Dou) *Dioscoreae Rhizoma*

方药：参苓白术散。常用：人参、白术、茯苓、甘草健脾益气；砂仁、陈皮、桔梗、扁豆、山药、莲子肉、薏苡仁理气健脾化湿。

(Shan Yao), *Nelumbinis Semen* (Lian Zi) and *Coicis Semen* (Yi Yi Ren) to regulate qi, strengthen the spleen and dry dampness.

Modification: For abdominal cold and pain due to spleen-yang deficiency and exhaustion and yin-cold excess, add *Aconiti Praeparata-Regulating Zhong jiao Decoction* (Fu Zi Li Zhong Tang); for complicated dampness excess, use modified *Yang-Raising and Dampness-Dispersing Decoction* (Sheng Yang Chu Shi Tang); for prolonged diarrhea, middle-qi descending and prolapse of the anus, use *Center-Supplementing qi-Boosting Decoction* (Bu Zhong Yi Qi Tang) to boost qi, raise yang and lift the prolapse; for continuous excessive diarrhea that cannot stop, add *Chebulae Fructus Simmered* (Wei He Zi), *Nutmeg Simmered* (Wei Rou Guo) and *Corni Fructus* (Shan Zhu Yu) to warm and astrict to stop diarrhea.

加减: 若脾阳虚衰、阴寒内盛腹中冷痛者,可合用附子理中丸;夹有湿盛者,可用升阳除湿汤加减;若久泻、中气下陷脱肛者,可用补中益气汤益气升阳举陷;若久泻不止、泄泻无度、次数频繁者,可入煨诃子、煨肉果、山茱萸等温涩止泻之品。

2.2.6 Kidney Fails to Astrict Due to Deficiency

2.2.6 肾虚不涩

Manifestations: Abdominal pain, rumbling sounds in the intestines and diarrhea with undigested whole grains before dawn, relief after diarrhea, cold body and limbs, soreness in the waist and weakness in the knees; pale tongue with white tongue fur; deep fine pulse.

证候: 黎明五更之前腹痛肠鸣即泻,泻下完谷,泻后则安,形寒肢冷,腰膝酸软。舌淡苔白,脉沉细。

Treatment: To warm and supplement the spleen and kidney; strengthen astringency to stop diarrhea.

治法: 温补脾肾,固涩止泻。

Formulas and Herbs: *Four Divinities Pills* (Si Shen Wan), usually composed of *Psoraleae Fructus* (Bu Gu Zhi) to warm and supplement kidney-yang; *Myristicae Semen* (Rou Dou Kou) and *Euodiae Fructus* (Wu Zhu Yu) to warm zhong jiao and disperse cold; *Schisandrae Chinensis Fructus* (Wu Wei

方药: 四神丸。常用:补骨脂温补肾阳;肉豆蔻、吴茱萸温中散寒;五味子收敛止泻。

Zi) to astrict and stop diarrhea.

Modification: For remarkable spleen deficiency, add *Codonopsis Radix* (Dang Shen) and *Atractylodis Macrocephalae Rhizoma* (Bai Zhu) to boost qi and strengthen the spleen; for fire weakness of the vital gate and yin-cold excess accumulated, add *Aconiti Praeparata-Regulating Zhong jiao Decoction* (Fu Zi Li Zhong Tang); for diarrhea that cannot help, or hard trying to excrete stool in vain, change for *True Man Viscus-Nourishing Decoction* (Zhen Ren Yang Zang Tang) to astrict the intestines and stop diarrhea; for complications of both deficiency and excess with unremarkable spleen deficiency and kidney-cold such as irritation or epigastric upset, sticky frozen stool, change for *Black Plum Pills* (Wu Mei Wan).

加减：脾虚甚者，可加党参、白术等益气健脾；命门火衰、阴寒内盛者，可合用附子理中丸；若泻下滑脱不禁，或需坐努责者，可改用真人养脏汤涩肠止泻；若脾虚肾寒不著，反见心烦嘈杂、大便夹有黏冻等寒热错杂证候，可改服乌梅丸。

Dysentery

痢　疾

Dysentery is a kind of disease characterized by abdominal pain, tenesmus, and red and white pus and blood due to the intestine's failure of controlance as transportation, damage of the intestinal membrane, rotten flesh and decayed blood caused by pathogenic factors stagnated in the intestines, qi and blood obstruction.

痢疾主要是因邪滞于肠，气血壅滞，肠道传导失司，脂络受损，肉败血腐而出现以腹痛、里急后重、下痢赤白脓血为主要临床表现的一类病证。

1 Etiology and Pathogenesis

1 病因病机

Dysentery is mainly casued by exogenous pathogenic factors or improper diet, which leads to pathogenic factors hidden in the intestines, qi ang blood obstruction, the intestines failure to transport and damage of the intestinal membrane. For patients of constitutional weakness who are likely to be affected by

痢疾的发生主要是由于感受外邪或饮食所伤等因素，以致邪蕴肠腑，气血壅滞，传导失司，脂络受伤而成痢。而素体脾胃虚弱多易感邪致病，或导致邪恋而下利

pathogenic factors, pathogenic factors tend to linger and move downward which make it hard to be cured.

迁延难愈。

1.1 Noxious Dampness Affects and Rivals against Qi and Blood

1.1 感受湿毒，搏结气血

Pathogenic damp-heat, sometimes along with food retention, accumulates in the intestines and rivals against qi and blood, cauing obstruction in the intestines which failsto transport, leading to damage of the intestinal membrane, qi-blood stagnation and rotten flesh turning into pus and blood, and finally dysentery with red and white excretion. However, if the dysentery is caused by epidemic pathogenic factors, itwill develop quickly, suddenly and seriouly.

湿热之邪，或与食积相合，积于肠腑，与气血搏结，壅塞肠道，使其传导失常，导致脂络受伤，气血凝滞，腐败化为脓血而痢下赤白。若感受疫毒之邪，则伤人最速，发病骤急，其势深重。

1.2 Frequent Dysentery Due to Weak Constitution; Healthy Qi Defeciency and Pathogenic Factors Linger

1.2 体虚久利，正亏邪恋

Too early astringency results in the lingering of pathogenic factors which, if for long, will damage the spleen-qi and stomach-qi. Or sometimes pathogenic factors attack due to weak constitution. In spite of several "fights", parts of the pathogenic factors still remain. Both the above two circumstances can lead to manifestation of healthy qi deficiency, lingering pathogenic factors and complication of heat and cold. And dysentery goes and comes and takes for long. Lingering pathogenic factors due to damp-heat, if not radically eliminated, will cause dysentery relapse at times of over-strain or improper diet or new pathogenic factor attacks. Meanwhile, spleen and stomach damage will allow pathogenic epidemic factors to invade inside the body which results in retention and stagnation, which turns into damp-heat and causes dysentery.

下痢收涩过早，邪留日久而伤脾胃之气；或体虚感邪，虽经攻伐，仍余邪不尽，均可导致正虚邪恋、寒热夹杂之证，则有下痢时发时止，日久缠绵难愈。因湿热余邪留恋不去，病根未除，故一遇劳作，或饮食稍有不慎，或新感外邪，均可死灰复燃，再次发生腹痛里急后重，痢下赤白等症。同时，脾胃损伤也可进而导致时邪疫毒乘虚入侵或积滞内生，蕴为湿热而变生久痢。

Dysentery, pathogocially, lies in the intestines,

痢疾的病位在肠，与脾

but is closely related to the spleen, stomach and kidney. The pathological mechanism is that pathogenic factors remaining in the intestines, and qi and blood blockade make the intestine incapable of transportation and transference. Then the intestinal membrane is injured and get rotten into pus and blood and that comes dysentery. Among all, dampness stagnation with pathogenic epidemic factors is the main pathological factor in all stages of the disease. Meanwhile, the excess and weakenss of yin and yang, qi, and blood, specifically in an individual is usuall the key to pathological changes. Of all the epidemic pathogenic factors, damp-heat is the most common and is most likely to lead to a lingering and tangled state. In addition, as dysentery is caused by stagnation of pathogenic factors rivaling against qi and blood, thence, qi-stagnation and blood stasis should be given due attention to in treatment. Especially for patients with dysentery for long, stasis prodominates, which when tangled with dampness stagntion, makes it even more difficult and complicated.

胃肾的关系密切,病机主要是邪滞于肠,气血壅滞,肠道传化失司,脂络受伤,腐败化为脓血而为痢。其中湿滞疫毒是主要的病理因素,并贯穿发病始终,而人体体质阴阳气血的盛衰又是病机转化的关键。在湿滞疫毒诸邪中尤以湿热为最多,也最容易造成留恋胶结之势。此外,痢疾是由邪滞与气血相搏而发病,故应注意气滞血瘀这一病理因素,尤其是久痢之人其瘀更甚,常与湿滞胶结,病势更趋缠绵难愈,这也是造成病情复杂的重要原因。

2 Syndrome Differentiation and Treatment

2 辨证论治

2.1 Key Points of Syndrome Differentiation

2.1 辨治要点

Doctors should first distinguish new diseases from old diseases, deficiency from excess. Acute dysentery sets on suddenly but lasts for a short time, with abdominal pain and fullness. Patients refuse to be pressed on the abdomen and can hardly hold stool when pain comes. After the stool, patients have tenesmus and temporary relief. That is malaris of excess type. In contrast, chronic dysentery sets on gradually, worse or less, and lasts long with continuous pain which is relieved when pressed on. Pa-

首先当分新久虚实:暴痢发病急,病程短,腹痛胀满,痛而拒按,痛时窘迫欲便,便后里急后重暂时减轻者为实;久痢发病慢,时轻时重,病程长,腹痛绵绵,痛而喜按,便后里急后重不减,坠胀甚者,常为虚中夹实。其次辨别寒热:大便脓血,赤多白少,或纯出脓血色鲜红,甚

tients will not have tenesumus after stool. That is dysentery of deficiency type. Secondly, doctors should tell cold from heat. Dysentery of heat type has the manifestations such as stool with pus and blood, with more darkness than whiteness in it, or pus and blood only with scarlet or purple color, abodominal pain, apparent tenusmus, burning anus, thirst and favor for cool drinks, bad mouth smell, dark and short urine, red tongue with yellow greasy tongue fur, and rapid rolling pulse. Dysentery of cold type features more whiteness than darkness in stool or white glue-like stool, abdominal pain that desires for pressing, no apparent tenesmus, pale complexion, cold limbs and physical coldness, deep fine pulse. The treatment principles should be in accordance with pattern identification of cold or heat, deficinecy or excess. Use cleansing methods for heat type and warming methods for cold type. Use dredging for excess type and supplementing methods for defeciency type. Use cleansing and warming methods together for compliaction of cold and heat. Use suppressing and supplementing for complication of deficiency and excess. In the onset stage, it is more likely to belong to excess and heat type, which can be treated by clear awaying away heat and drying dampness to detoxify while for chronic dysentery of deficiency and cold type, it is better to supplement deficiency and and warm zhong jiao, regulate the spleen and stomach as well as cleanse the intestines to astringe and arrest prolapsus. Regulating qi and harmonizing blood should be go through the whole treatment process.

或鲜紫，腹痛，里急后重感明显，肛门灼痛，兼渴喜冷饮，口臭，小便短赤，舌质红，苔黄腻，脉滑数者为热；大便白多赤少，或全为白冻黏液，腹痛喜温喜按，里急后重不明显，兼有面色皖白肢冷形寒，舌淡苔白，脉沉细者为寒。治疗上应根据其病证的寒热虚实，而确定治疗原则。热痢清之，寒痢温之，初痢实则通之，久痢虚则补之，寒热交错者清温并用，虚实夹杂者攻补兼施。痢疾初起之时，以实证、热证多见，宜清热化湿解毒，久痢虚证、寒证，应以补虚温中，调理脾胃，兼以清肠，收涩固脱。而调气和血的治则贯穿始终。

2.2 Therapeutic Methods for Different Patterns

2.2.1 Dysentery of Damp-Heat

Manifestations: Fever, abdominal pain that resists pressing, dysentery with dark and white pus and blood, as sticky as glue, stingy, burning pain in the anus, tenesmus, dark and short urine; yellow greasy tongue fur; rapid rolling pule.

Treatment: To clear away heat and dry dampness; detoxify, regulate qi and promote blood circulation.

Formulas and Herbs: *Peony Root Decoction* (Shao Yao Tang), usually composed of *Paeoniae Radix Alba* (Bai Shao), *Glycyrrhizae Radix et Rhizoma* (Gan Cao) and *Angelicae Sinensis Radix* (Dang Gui) to treat pus and blood by harmonizing and defending; *Aucklandiae Radix* (Mu Xiang), *Arecae Semen* (Bing Lang) to regulate qi and eliminate anal bulging; *Coptidis Rhizoma* (Huang Lian) and *Rhei Radix et Rhizoma* (Da Huang) to clear away heat and detoxify; *Cinnamomi Cortex* (Rou Gui) to purge and resolve clots as well as contradict the bitterness and cold of other herbs.

Modification: For heat rivaling over dampness with more darkness than whiteness, add moderately *Pulsatillae Radix* (Bai Tou Weng), *Fraxini Cortex* (Qin Pi) and *Phellodendri Chinensis Cortex* (Huang Bo); for fresh blood only, add *Sanguisorbiae Radix Preparata* (Di Yu Tan), *Platycladi Cacumen Preparata* (Ce Bai Ye), *Lonicerae Japonicae Flos Preparata* (Yin Hua Tan), *Moutan Cortex* (Mu Dan Pi) and *Sophorae Flos Immaturus* (Huai Mi) to help cleanse the intestines and cool blood; for dampness rivaling over heat, more whiteness than darkness, subtract herbs of bitter and cool nature, such as

2.2 分型论治

2.2.1 湿热痢

证候：身热腹痛，痛而拒按，痢下赤白脓血相杂，黏稠如胶冻，腥臭；肛门灼热，里急后重，小便短赤。舌苔黄腻，脉滑数。

治法：清热化湿、解毒，调气行血。

方药：芍药汤。常用：白芍药、甘草、当归和营以治脓血；木香、槟榔行气以除后重；黄芩、黄连、大黄清热解毒；肉桂既取辛能散结，又制诸药苦寒太过。

加减：若热重于湿，痢下赤多白少者可酌加白头翁、秦皮、黄柏；若痢下纯血鲜红者，可加用地榆炭、侧柏叶、银花炭、牡丹皮、槐米等以增强清肠凉血之功；若湿重于热，痢下白多赤少者，可去黄芩、大黄等苦寒之品，加入茯苓、苍术、厚朴等健脾燥湿之属；若痢疾初起，兼见表证，恶寒发热、头痛身重者，可选用《活人》败毒散；若身热汗

Scutellariae Radix (Huang Qin), *Rhei Radix et Rhizoma* (Da Huang), and add *Poria* (Fu Ling), *Atractylodis Rhizoma* (Cang Zhu) and *Magnoliae Officinalis Cortex* (Hou Po) to strengthen the spleen and dry dampness; for dysentery in the onset stage, with symptoms like aversion to cold and fever, headache and general heaviness, use *Detoxifying Powder* (Bai Du San); for fever and sweating, rapid pulse, exterior that has not be totally relieved, excess heat inside, use *Puerariae, Scutellariae and Coptidis Decoction* (Ge Gen Qin Lian Tang) to reliever the exterior and cleanse the interior; for relieved exterior and unrelieved dysentery, use *Aucklandia and Coptis Pill* (Xiang Lian Wan) to regulate qi, clear away heat and clean up.

出、脉数,表未尽解而里热已盛者,宜用葛根芩连汤解表清里;若表证已减而痢犹未止者,则可以香连丸调气清热善后。

2.2.2 Dysentery of Epidemic Pathogenic Factors

Manifestations: Sudden attacks, purple pus and blood in the dysentery, severe abodominal pain, apparent tenesmus, strong heat and thirst, headache and irritation, nausea and vomitting even losing consciousness and convulsion; red tongue with yellow dry tongue fur; rapid rolling pulse or weak or even disappearing pulse.

Treatment: To clear away heat, detoxify and cool blood.

Formulas and Herbs: *Pulsatillae Decoction* (Bai Tou Weng Tang), usually composed of *Pulsatillae Radix* (Bai Tou Weng) to cool blood and detoxify; *Coptidis Rhizoma* (Huang Lian), *Phellodendri Chinensis Cortex* (Huang Bo), *Fraxini Cortex* (Qin Pi) to clear away heat and dry dampness.

Modification: For heat-toxin into the defensive blood and high fever, with manfestations like unconsciousness and gibberish, or even convulsion,

2.2.2 疫毒痢

证候: 起病急骤,痢下鲜紫脓血,腹痛剧烈,后重感特著,壮热口渴,头痛烦躁,恶心呕吐,甚者神昏惊厥。舌质红绛,舌苔黄燥,脉滑数或微欲绝。

治法: 清热解毒凉血。

方药: 白头翁汤。常用:白头翁凉血解毒为主;黄连、黄柏、秦皮清热化湿。

加减: 神昏谵语甚则惊厥、舌质红、苔黄糙、脉细数,属热毒深入营血,用犀角地

red tongue with yellow coarse tongue fur, rapid fine pulse, use *Rhinocetos Horn and Rehmannia Decoction* (Xi Jiao Di Huang Tang) and *Purple Snow Elixir* (Zi Xue Dan) to clear away ying heat and cool blood and open orifices; for collapse due to acute dysentery with manifestations like pale complexion, sweating, cold limbs, purple dark tongue and lips, little urine, weak disappearing pulse, use *immediately Ginseng Decoction* (Du Shen Tang) or *Ginseng and Aconite Decoction* (Shen Fu Tang).

黄汤、紫雪丹以清营凉血开窍;若暴痢致脱,症见面色苍白、汗出肢冷、唇舌紫黯、尿少、脉微欲绝者,应急服独参汤或参附汤。

2.2.3 Dysentery of Cold-Dampness

Manifestations: Abdominal pain, difficult to hold stool, red and white materials or more whiteness than darkness or white gluelike only, tenesmus, distention in the stomach and fullness in the abdomen, general fatigue and heaviness over the head and torso, poor appetite; white greasy tongue fur; soft slow pulse.

Treatment: To warm zhong jiao and dry dampness; regulate qi and harmonize blood.

Formulas and Herbs: *Priceless Health Restoring Powder* (Bu Huan Jin Zheng Qi San), usually composed of *Pogostemonis Herba* (Huo Xiang) to resolve dampness with its frangrant nature; *Atractylodis Rhizoma* (Cang Zhu), *Pinelliae Rhizoma* (Ban Xia), *Magnoliae Officinalis Cortex* (Hou Po) to invigorate the spleen and dry dampness; *Zingiberis Rhizoma Recens* (Sheng Jiang) to warm the middle and disperse cold; *Citri Reticulatae Pericarpium* (Chen Pi), *Jujubae Fructus* (Da Zao) and *Glycyrrhizae Radix et Rhizoma* (Gan Cao) to regulate qi and resolve fulness as well as strengthen the spleen and harmonize zhong jiao.

Modification: For predominance of pathogenic

2.2.3 寒湿痢

证候: 腹痛拘急,痢下赤白,白多赤少或纯为白冻,里急后重,脘胀腹满,头身困重,饮食乏味。舌苔白腻,脉濡缓。

治法: 温中燥湿,调气和血。

方药: 不换金正气散。常用:藿香芳香化湿;苍术、半夏、厚朴运脾燥湿;生姜温中散寒;陈皮、大枣、甘草行气散满,健脾和中。

加减: 若湿邪偏重,白痢

dampnessd with symptoms as white glue-like stool and severe tenusmus, change for *Poria Stomach Decoction* (Wei Ling Tang) and *Paeoniae Radix Alba* (Bai Shao), *Angelicae Sinensis Radix* (Dang Gui), *Arecae Semen* (Bing Lang) and *Aucklandiae Radix* (Mu Xiang); for spleen deficiency and poor appetite, add *Atractylodis Macrocephalae Rhizoma* (Bai Zhu) and *Massa Fermentata Medicinalis* (Shen Qu) to strenghthen the spleen and promote appetite; for cold accumulation and retention inside with symptoms as abdominal pain, sluggish diarrhea with uncomfortable sensation, add *Arecae Semen* (Binglang), *Rhei Radix et Rhizoma* (Da Huang), *Zingiberis Rhizoma* Preparata (Pao Jiang), *Cinnamomi Cortex* (Rou Gui) to warm and dredge; for dysentery of cold-dampness in summer, use modified *Agastachis-Restoring Healthy Energy Powder* (Huo Xiang Zheng Qi San) to dispel summer heat and cold, dry dampness and stop dysentery.

如胶冻、鼻涕之状，里急后重甚者，可改用胃苓汤合白芍药、当归、槟榔、木香等为治；脾虚纳呆者加白术、神曲健脾开胃；寒积内停，腹痛、痢下滞而不爽，加大黄、槟榔，配炮姜、肉桂，温通导滞；暑天感寒湿而痢者，可用藿香正气散加减，以祛暑散寒、化湿止痢。

2.2.4　Dysentery of Deficiency and Cold

Manifestations: Prolonged dull pain in the abdomen which desires for warmth and pressing, dark and white clear away materials with no smell, or white glue-like materials even fecal incontinence, anal bulging which worsens after stool, physical cold and aversion to cold, cold limbs, little intake and lassitude, soreness and weakness in the waist and knees; pale tongue with white thin tongue fur; deep fine weak pulse.

Treatment: To warm and invigorate spleen and kidney; astringe and arrest proptosis.

Formulas and Herbs: *Peach Blossom Decoction* (Tao Hua Tang) and *True Man Viscus-Nourishing Decoction* (Zhen Ren Yang Zang Tang), usually

2.2.4　虚寒痢

证候：腹部隐痛，缠绵不已，喜温喜按，痢下赤白清稀，无腥臭，或为白冻，甚则滑脱不禁，肛门坠胀，便后更甚，形寒畏冷，四肢不温，食少神疲，腰膝酸软。舌淡苔薄白，脉沉细而弱。

治法：温补脾肾，收涩固脱。

方药：桃花汤合真人养脏汤。常用：人参、白术、干姜、肉桂温肾暖脾；粳米、炙

composed of *Ginseng Radix et Rhizoma* (Ren Shen), *Atractylodis Macrocephalae Rhizoma* (Bai Zhu), *Zingiberis Rhizoma* (Gan Jiang), *Cinnamomi Cortex* (Rou Gui) to warm the kidney and spleen; *Semen Oryza Sativae* (Jing Mi), *Glycyrrhizae Radix et Rhizoma Praeparata* (Zhi Gan Cao) to warm the middle and supplement the spleen; *Chebulae Fructus* (He Zi), Pericarpium papaveris (Ying Su Ke), *Myristicae Semen* (Rou Dou Kou), *Halloysitum Rubrum* (Chi Shi Zhi) to astringe the intestines and arrest proptosis; *Angelicae Sinensis Radix* (Dang Gui), *Paeoniae Radix Alba* (Bai Shao) to nourish blood and promote blood circulation; *Aucklandiae Radix* (Mu Xiang) to promote qi flow and stop pain.

甘草温中补脾;诃子、罂粟壳、肉豆蔻、赤石脂收涩固脱;当归、白芍药养血行血;木香行气止痛。

Modification: For unresolved retention and stagnation, apply a small amount of retention-resolving herbs, such as *Aurantii Fructus* (Zhi Qiao), *Crataegi Fructus* (Shan Zha) and *Massa Fermentata Medicinalis* (Shen Qu); for spleen deficiency and descending qi due to prolonged dysentery, which causes qi shortage and rectocele, add *Astragali Radix* (Huang Qi), *Bupleuri Radix* (Chai Hu), *Cimicifugae Rhizoma* (Sheng Ma), *Codonopsis Radix* (Dang Shen) to supplement the middle and boost qi, raise clarity and uphold the descending.

加减: 若积滞未尽,应少佐消导积滞之品,如枳壳、山楂、神曲等;若痢久脾虚气陷,导致少气脱肛,可加黄芪、柴胡、升麻、党参以补中益气、升清举陷。

2.2.5 Dysentery of Yin Deficiency

2.2.5 阴虚痢

Manifestations: Red and white pus and blood or sticky fresh blood, burning pain around the naval and abdomen, tenesmus, little intake, irritation and dry mouth; red tongue with little tongue fur; rapid fine pulse.

证候: 痢下赤白脓血,或下鲜血黏稠,脐腹灼痛,里急后重,食少,心烦口干。舌质红绛少苔,或舌光红乏津,脉细数。

Treatment: To nourish yin and cleanse the intestines.

治法: 养阴清肠。

Formulas and Herbs: *Parking Pills* (Zhu Che Wan), usually composed of *Coptidis Rhizoma* (Huang Lian) to cleanse the intestines; *Asini Corii Colla* (E Jiao) and *Angelicae Sinensis Radix* (Dang Gui) to nourish yin and harmonize blood, a little *Zingiberis Rhizoma Preparata* (Pao Jiang) to subtract the bitterness and coolness of *Coptidis Rhizoma* (Huang Lian) as well as resolve stagnation.

方药: 驻车丸。常用:黄连苦寒以清肠;阿胶、当归养阴和血;稍佐炮姜以制黄连苦寒太过,且辛能散滞。

Modification: For body fluid injured by heat with symptoms like thirst, little urine, add *Glehniae Radix* (Sha Shen) and *Dendrobii Caulis* (Shi Hu) to nourish yin and generate fluid; for diarrhea with heavy bleeding, add *Moutan Cortex* (Mu Dan Pi), *Paeoniae Radix Rubra* (Chi Shao), *Ecliptae Herba* (Mo Han Lian), *Sanguisorbiae Radix Preparata* (Di Yu Tan), *Cirsii Japonici Herba* (Da Ji), *Cirsii Herba* (Xiao Ji), *Lonicerae Japonicae Flos Preparata* (Yin Hua Tan) to cool blood and stop bleeding without drying; for deficiency complicated with excess and damp-heated not clear awayed with symptoms like bitter mouth, burning anus, add *Fraxini Cortex* (Qin Pi) and *Purslane* (Ma Chi Xian) to clear away deep heat.

加减: 若热灼津伤,而见口渴、尿少者,可加沙参、石斛养阴生津;若见痢下血多者,可加牡丹皮、赤芍药、墨旱莲、地榆炭、大蓟、小蓟、银花炭等凉血止血而又不失甘润;若虚中夹实,湿热未清,见口苦、肛门灼热者,可加秦皮、马齿苋等清解湿热。

2.2.6 Intermitten Dysentery

2.2.6 休息痢

Manifestations: Dysentery off and on, prolonged without cure, often triggered by improper diet, cold and overstrain, diarrhea with red and white glue-like materials, fullness in the abdomen, little intake, fatigue and drowsiness; pale tongue with greasy tongue fur; soft soft pulse or rapid weak pulse.

证候: 下痢时发时止,迁延不愈,常因饮食不当、受凉、劳累而发,发时大便次数增多,夹有赤白黏冻,腹胀食少,倦怠嗜卧。舌质淡苔腻,脉濡软或虚数。

Treatment: To warm zhong jiao and cleanse the intestines; regulate qi and resolve stagnation.

治法: 温中清肠,调气化滞。

Formulas and Herbs: *Coptidis-Regulating*

方药: 连理汤。常用:人

Decoction (Lian Li Tang), usually compose of *Ginseng Radix et Rhizoma* (Ren Shen), *Atractylodis Macrocephalae Rhizoma* (Bai Zhu), *Zingiberis Rhizoma* (Gan Jiang), *Poria* (Fu Ling), *Glycyrrhizae Radix et Rhizoma* (Gan Cao) to warm the middle and strengthen the spleen; *Coptidis Rhizoma* (Huang Lian) to cleanse the remaining pathogenic damp-heat in the intestines.

参、白术、干姜、茯苓、甘草温中健脾；黄连清除肠中湿热余邪。

Modification: For weak spleen and stomach, middle-qi descending with manifestation like prolonged dysentery and rectocele, fatigue and weakness, qi shortage and laziness to talk, use modified *Center-Supplementing qi-Boosting Decoction* (Bu Zhong Yi Qi Tang); for dysentery with white glue-like materials, which attacks at times of cold, fatigue, little intake pale tongue, white tongue fur with deep pulse due to extreme deficiency of spleen-yang with cold accumulated in the intestines, use *Spleen-Warming Decoction* (Wen Pi Tang) from *Thousand Ducat Prescriptions for Emergencies* (Bei Ji Qian Jin Yao Fang) to warm the middle and dispel cold, resolve retention and stagnation; for prolonged dysentery with deficient and weakening kidney-yang that it is hard to hold anus tight, add *Four Gods Pills* (Si Sheng Wan) to warm the kidney and spleen as well as consolidate the intestines and stop dysentery; for complication of deficiency and excess with manifestations like intermitten dysentery with loose stool, irritation, hunger without appetite and cold limbs, use modified *Black Plum Pills* (Wu Mei Wan).

加减：如久痢脱肛，神疲乏力、少气懒言，属脾胃虚弱、中气下陷，可用补中益气汤加减；若为脾阳虚极，肠中寒积不化，遇寒即发，下痢白冻、倦怠少食、舌淡苔白脉沉者，则可用《千金》温脾汤，温中散寒、消积导滞、攻补两施；若久痢兼见肾阳虚衰，关门不固者，宜加四神丸以温肾暖脾、固肠止痢；若下痢时作、大便稀溏、心中烦热、饥不欲食、四肢不温，证属寒热错杂，可用乌梅丸加减。

Constipation

Constipation is a disease of stool conpressed and blocked in the large intestine, usually caused by the failure of the large intestine to transport, featuring long stool time or long intervals, dry stool, difficult defecation, or frequent sticky stool.

1 Etiology and Pathogenesis

Improper diet, emotional and spiritual disorder, weak constitution, or zang-fu organ injuries cause the failure of the large intestines to tranport and waste retains in the intestines which for long, turns dry and hard, leading to constipation.

1.1 Pathogenic Heat from Food Gathers in the Intestines and Stomach

Weak constitution with excessive yang or over intake of spicy food and over-drinking of alcohol, or over intake of herbs with heat nature will lead to excessive heat in the body. Or remaining heat after fever or dry-heat in the lung and middle moving downward to the intestines can lead to heat accumulated in the intestines and stomach, making damage to body fluid, causing dry and astrigent intestines and diffcult defecation.

1.2 Emotional and Spiritual Disorder; Qi Activities Depressed and Stagnated

Excessive worry, depression, anger, long sitting without moving, intestinal adhesions after operation or refined food will all lead to depression and stagnation of qi activities in the large intestine, which fails to dredge, descend, transport waste

便 秘

便秘主要是因大肠传导功能失常导致大便秘结不通，排便时间或间隔时间延长，或粪质干结，排出艰难，或经常便而不畅为主要临床表现的一种病证。

1 病因病机

便秘的发生主要是由于饮食不节、情志失调、体虚病后、脏腑损伤等因素，导致大肠传导功能失常，糟粕停积于肠，时间过久便质干燥或坚硬所致。

1.1 饮食热邪，肠胃积热

素体阳盛，或过食辛辣醇酒，或过服热药而致热邪内盛；亦有热病之后，余热留恋，或肺中燥热下移大肠，均可导致肠胃积热，耗伤津液，以致肠道干涩燥结，排便艰涩。

1.2 情志失调，气机郁滞

忧思过度、抑郁恼怒、久坐少动、术后肠道黏连或食偏精细等均可导致大肠气机郁滞，通降失常，传导失职，糟粕内停，不得下行。

downward.

1.3 Deficiency of Qi, Blood and Yin Due to Weak Constitution after Illness

Weak constitution with yin deficiency; or qi and blood deficiency due to prolonged illness, postpartum, old age; or yin-fluid injured by over use of perspiring, laxative or drying medicine; or qi, blood, yin and essence exhaustion due to plenty of sweating, intercourse, or overstrain, all can lead to qi defeciency and incapability to transport, yin-blood defeciency and the intestines lacking in moisturizing. Therefore, waste retains and constipation is resulted in.

1.3 体虚病后,气血阴亏

素体阴虚;久病、产后及年老体弱之人,气血亏虚;或过用汗、利、燥热之剂,损伤阴津;或汗出过多,房室、劳役过度,耗伤气血阴精,致气虚而传导无力,阴血亏而肠道失于濡润,糟粕不行,因虚而秘。

1.4 Yang-qi Weakens and Yin-cold Gathers and Stagnates

Favor for cold and raw food, or overuse of bitter cold medicine will hurt yang-qi. Weak constitution due to old age or shortage ofgenuine yang will make it difficult to warm and transfer body fluid to moisturize the intestines. As a result, yin-cold gathers and waste remains in the intestines.

Constipation features the failure of the large intestine to transport, hampered qi activities and waste accumulation inside. It lies in the large intestine but is closely related to the functions ofthe lung, spleen, stomach, liver and kidney. Constipation, by pathological nature, comes into four types: cold, heat, deficiency and excess. Constipation of heat is characterized by dry-heat in the intestines while excess type is featured by qi activity depression and stagnation. Deficiency type features deficiency of qi, blood, yin and yang while cold type is characterized by yin-cold retention. Of the four types, deficiency and excess is the guidance for i-

1.4 阳气虚衰,阴寒凝滞

嗜食寒凉生冷,或过用苦寒药物,伐伤阳气;或年老体弱,真阳不足,均可因温煦无权,不能蒸化津液,温润肠道,而致阴寒内结,糟粕不行,凝积肠道。

便秘的基本病机特点为大肠传导失常,气机不畅,糟粕内停。病位在大肠,同时与肺、脾、胃、肝、肾等脏腑的功能失调息息相关。病性可概括为寒、热、虚、实四个方面:燥热内结于肠胃者,属热秘;气机郁滞者,属实秘;气血阴阳亏虚者,为虚秘;阴寒积滞者,为冷秘或寒秘。四者之中,又以虚实为纲,热秘、气秘、冷秘属实,阴阳气血不足的便秘属虚。而寒、

dentification. Constipation of heat, qi, cold falls into excess type while yin, yang, qi and blood deficiency falls into deficiency type. Meanwhile, the four interchangeable types are often complicated with another.

热、虚、实之间，常又相互兼夹或相互转化。

2　Syndrome Differentiation and Treatment

2　辨证论治

2.1　Key Points of Syndrome Differentiation

2.1　辨治要点

Doctors should inquire carefully about patients' eating habits, life habits andherbsl history to speculate on the possible causes of constipation and decide on different types of constipation. For patients who favor spicy food with heavy dressings, or fired food and drinking, it is more likely to be constipation of heat due to heat gathering in the stomach and intestines. For patients with depression and excessive worry, or who sit for long without moving, or lie for long without moving, or who have had operation in the abdomen, it is constipation of excess type due to depression and stagnation of qi activity. Old people or women after labor are more likely to have constipation of deficiency type due to deficiency of qi, blood, yin and essence. For patients with deficient and weak yang or who favor cold and raw food, it is, more often than not, constipation of cold type. Stool quality and defecation situations are also helpful for pattern identification. Dry and rocky stool, burning anus and thick yellow dirty greasy dry tongue fur reveals dry-heat inside while dry stool, difficult defecation, white moist slippery tongue fur means yin-cold inside. Not very dry stool, yet difficult defecation, distention in the abdomen and hypochondria are usually manifestations of depression and stagnation of qi activity. Howev-

详细询问患者的饮食习惯、生活习惯及其他病史，以推测可能的致秘之因，有助于判别虚实寒热的不同。如平素喜食辛辣厚味、煎炒酒食者多致胃肠积热而成热秘；长期忧郁思虑过度或久坐、久卧少动，或有腹部手术者，多致气机郁滞而为气秘实证；年老体衰，病后产后多为气血阴精亏虚之虚秘；平素阳气虚衰或嗜食寒凉生冷者，其便秘多为冷秘。辨别粪质、排便情况亦有助辨证：如大便干燥坚硬，排便时肛门有热感，苔见黄厚，垢腻而燥者，多为燥热内结；大便干结，排出艰难，苔见白润而滑者为阴寒内结；粪质不甚干结，欲便不出，胁腹作胀者多为气机郁滞；便质干如栗状或如羊屎，舌红少津，无苔或苔少者多为血虚津枯。治疗上应以通下为主，但决不可单纯用泻下药，应针对不同的病因采取相应的治疗方

er, nut-shaped or goat-stool shaped stool, red tongue with little fluid, no tongue fur or little tongue fur are symptoms of blood deficiency and fluid shortage. The treatment should focus on dredging downward. However, it is unwise to use purgative herbs. Instead, different therapeutic methods should be adopted according to different causes. For excess type, dispelling the pathogenic factor is the main method, together with others, such as purging heat, warming and dispersing and dredging to eliminate pathogenic factors and promote defecation. For deficiency type, restoring healthy qi should come first by boosting qi, warming yang, nourishing yin and nurturing blood to strenghten healthy qi and promote defecation. Meanwhile, regualation of qi activity should not be ignored. It is advisable to use herbs that can regulate qi and help qi descend to resolve stagnation.

法:实秘以祛邪为主,给予泻热、温散、通导之法,使邪去便通;虚秘以扶正为先,给予益气温阳、滋阴养血,使正盛便通。同时应重视对气机的调畅,参用理气沉降之品以助行滞。

2.2 Therapeutic Methods for Different Patterns

2.2.1 Constipation Due to Heat

Manifestations: Dry stool, distention or pain in the abdomen, dry mouth with bad smell, dark short urine, fever and red complexion; red tongue with yellow dry tongue fur; rapid rolling pulse.

Treatment: To clear away heat and moisturize the intestines.

Formulas and Herbs: *Cannabis Pills* (Ma Ren Wan), usually composed of *Rhei Radix et Rhizoma* (Da Huang) and *Cannabis Fructus* (Huo Ma Ren) to purge heat and moisturize the intestines to promote defecation; *Armeniacae Semen Amaru* (Ku Xing Ren) to help qi descend and moisturize the intestines, *Paeoniae Radix Alba* (Bai Shao) to nourish yin and harmonize ying; *Aurantii Fructus Immaturus* (Zhi

2.2 分型论治

2.2.1 热秘

证候: 大便干结,腹胀或痛,口干口臭,小便短赤,身热面赤。舌红苔黄燥,脉滑数。

治法: 清热润肠。

方药: 麻仁丸。常用:大黄、火麻仁泻热润肠通便;杏仁降气润肠;白芍药养阴和营;枳实、厚朴行气除满;白蜜以加强润肠通下。

Shi) and *Magnoliae Officinalis Cortex* (Hou Po) to promote qi flow and eliminate fullness; *Mel* (Feng Mi) to help moisturize the intestines and defecation.

Modification: For dry and hard stool, add *Natrii Sulfas* (Mang Xiao) to soften the stool and ease defecation with salt and cool herbs; for dry tongue and mouth and fair exhaustion of body fluid, add *Rehmannia Radix* (Sheng Di Huang), *Scrophulariae Radix* (Xuan Shen) and *Ophiopogonis Radix* (Mai Men Dong) to nourish yin and generate body fluid just as increase water to float the boat; for reddish eye and tendency of irritation without rapid taut pulse due to depressed anger injuring the liver, add *Toillette Pills* (Geng Yi Wan) or *Angelicae Sinensis and Aloe Pills* (Dang Gui Lu Hui Wan) to cleanse the liver and ease stool; for constipation due to heat in the large intestines resulting from lung blocked by phlegm-heat, add *Scutellariae Radix* (Huang Qin), *Trichosanthis Fructus* (Gua Lou) and *Mori Cortex* (Sang Bai Pi) to cleanse the lung, moisturize the intestines and purge heat; for not very remarkable dry and heat, or sticky stool after herbstion, use *Harengula Zunasi Pills* (Qing Lin Wan) to dredge the fu-organs and ease defecation; for constipation with bleeding due to hemorrhage, add *Sophorae Flos* (Huai Hua) and *Sanguisorbiae Radix* (Sheng Di Yu) to cleanse the intestines and stop bleeding.

加减：大便干结而坚硬者，可加芒硝以咸寒软坚而通便；口舌干燥，津液耗伤较盛者，加入生地黄、玄参、麦门冬等以养阴生津，增水行舟；如见目赤易怒、脉弦数者，为郁怒伤肝，加服更衣丸或当归龙荟丸以清肝通便；如因痰热壅肺以致大肠结热便秘者，可加黄芩、瓜蒌、桑白皮等以清肺润肠泄热；若燥热不甚，或药后大便不爽者，可用青麟丸以通腑缓下；如兼痔疮便秘出血，可加槐花、生地榆以清肠止血。

2.2.2 Constipation Due to Qi

Manifestations: Dry and clotted stool, difficult defecation, distention and fullness in the hypochondria and abdomen, ever pain in the abdomen, frequent burping; thin greasy tongue fur; taut pulse.

Treatment: To regulate qi and resolve stagna-

2.2.2 气秘

证候：大便秘结，欲便不得，胁腹胀满，甚则腹中胀痛，嗳气频作。苔薄腻，脉弦。

治法：顺气导滞。

tion.

Formulas and Herbs: *Six Milled Ingredients Decoction* (Liu Mo Tang), usually composed of *Aucklandiae Radix* (Mu Xiang), *Linderae Radix* (Wu Yao) and *Aquilariae Lignum Resinatum* (Chen Xiang) to regulate qi and resolve depression; *Rhei Radix et Rhizoma* (Da Huang), *Aurantii Fructus Immaturus* (Zhi Shi) and *Arecae Semen* (Bing Lang) to break qi blockage and eliminate stagnation.

方药: 六磨汤。常用:木香、乌药、沉香顺气解郁;大黄、枳实、槟榔破气行滞。

Modification: For long depressed qi transforming into fire with symptoms like bitter mouth and dry throat, yellow tongue fur and rapid pulse, add *Gardeniae Fructus* (Zhi Zi) *Gentianae Radix et Rhizoma* (Long Dan) to cleanse and purge liver heat; for disharmony between the liver and the spleen with symtoms like constipation, abdominal fullness, poor appetite and pain around hypochondria, use moderately *Free Wanderer Powder* (Xiao Yao San); for constipation due to qi stagnation and blood stasis after falling to the ground and operation, add *Carthami Flos* (Hong Hua), *Paeoniae Radix Rubra* (Chi Shao) and *Persicae Semen* (Tao Ren) to promote blood circulation and eliminate stasis; for lung failing to disperse, descend and transfer, with such symptoms as constipatin, asthmatic cough, discomfort and oppression in the heart and abdomen, distention and fullness in the chest and around the hypochondria, deep taut pulse, use *Fructus-Perillae-Lowering-Qi Decoction* (Su Zi Jiang Qi Tang) moderately to lower qi and ease defecation.

加减: 如气郁日久化火,见口苦咽干、苔黄脉数者,加山栀、龙胆草以清泻肝热;如肝脾不和,症见便秘、腹胀、纳呆、胁肋作痛等症,可酌用逍遥散加减;若跌仆损伤,腹部术后,便秘不通,属气滞血瘀者,可加红花、赤芍药、桃仁等药活血化瘀;如肺失宣降,传导失司,症见便秘、咳喘、心腹痞闷、胸胁胀满、脉沉弦者,可选用降气通便的苏子降气汤加减。

2.2.3 Constipation Due to Cold

2.2.3 冷秘

Manifestations: Hard stool, inabiltiy to hold

证候: 大便艰涩,腹痛拘

stool at abdominal pain, distention and fullness in the abdomen which resists pressing, some pain under the hypochondria, cold hands and feet, regurgitation and vomiting; white greasy tongue fur; taut tight pulse.

急,胀满拒按,胁下偏痛,手足不温,呃逆呕吐。舌苔白腻,脉弦紧。

Treatment: To warm the interior and dispel cold; promote defecation and stop pain.

治法: 温里散寒,通便止痛。

Formulas and Herbs: *Spleen-Warming Decoction* (Wen Pi Tang) and *Pinellia and Sulfur Pills* (Ban Liu Wan), usually composed of *Aconm Lateralis Radix Praeparata* (Fu Zi) to warm the interior and dispel cold, *Rhei Radix et Rhizoma* (Da Huang) to cleanse retention and stagnation; *Codonopsis Radix* (Dang Shen), *Zingiberis Rhizoma* (Gan Jiang) and *Glycyrrhizae Radix et Rhizoma* (Gan Cao) to warm zhong jiao and boost qi.

方药: 温脾汤合半硫丸。常用:附子温里散寒;大黄荡涤积滞;党参、干姜、甘草温中益气。

Modification: For constipation with abdominal pain, add *Aurantii Fructus Immaturus* (Zhi Shi), *Magnoliae Officinalis Cortex* (Hou Po) and *Aucklandiae Radix* (Mu Xiang) to help purge; for cold and pain in the abdomen, cold hands and feet, add *Alpiniae Officinarum Rhizoma* (Gao Liang Jiang) and *Foeniculi Fructus* (Xiao Hui Xiang) to help dispel cold.

加减: 若便秘腹痛,可加枳实、厚朴、木香助泻下之力;若腹部冷痛,手足不温,加高良姜、小茴香增散寒之功。

2.2.4 Constipation Due to Qi Deficiency

2.2.4 气虚便秘

Manifestations: Stool awareness but feeling powerless in defecation, not very hard stool but difficult to defecate, sweating and short breath, fatigue after stool, waxy pale complexion, general weakness and laziness to talk; pale tender tongue with white tongue fur; weak pulse.

证候: 虽有便意而临厕努挣乏力,大便并不干硬,但难于排出,汗出短气,便后乏力,面色㿠白,肢倦懒言。舌淡嫩,苔白,脉弱。

Treatment: To boost qi and moisturize the intestines.

治法: 益气润肠。

Forumulas and Herbs: *Astragali Radix* Decoc-

方药: 黄芪汤。常用:黄

tion (Huang Qi Tang), usually composed of *Astragali Radix* (Huang Qi) to supplement lung-qi and spleen-qi; *Cannabis Fructus* (Huo Ma Ren) and *Mel* (Feng Mi) to moisturize the intestines to ease defecation; *Citri Reticulatae Pericarpium* (Chen Pi) to regulate qi and harmonize the stomach.

芪补肺脾之气;火麻仁、白蜜润肠通便;陈皮理气和胃。

Modification: For rectocele due to qi deficiency, add *Cimicifugae Rhizoma* (Sheng Ma), *Bupleuri Radix* (Chai Hu), *Platycodi Radix* (Jie Geng) and *Ginseng Radix et Rhizoma* (Ren Shen) to boost qi and reverse descending; for along with blood deficiency with such symptoms as pale color in tongue, lips and nails, add *Angelicae Sinensis Radix* (Dang Gui), *Polygoni Multiflori Radix* (He Shou Wu) and *Rehmannia Radix* (Sheng Di Huang) to nourish the blood, moisturize the intestines and ease defecation; for prolonged qi deficiency, sore and weakness in the waist and knees, it is advisable to invigorate the kidney with *Major Yuan (Primary) Qi-Reinforcing Decoction* (Da Bu Yuan Jian).

加减: 气虚下陷脱肛者,可加升麻、柴胡、桔梗、人参以益气升陷;兼血虚者,其唇舌爪甲色淡,可加当归、生首乌、生地黄等养血润肠通便;气虚日久,肢倦腰酸者,宜兼补肾,可用大补元煎。

2.2.5 Constipation Due to Blood Deficiency

2.2.5 血虚便秘

Manifestations: Dry stool, lusterless face, dizziness and vertigo, palpitation and insomnia; pale tongue and lips; fine pulse.

证候: 大便干结,面色无华,头晕目眩,心悸少寐。唇舌淡,脉细。

Treatment: To nourish blood and moisturize dryness.

治法: 养血润燥。

Formulas and Herbs: *Intestine-Moisturizing Pills* (Run Chang Wan), usually composed of *Angelicae Sinensis Radix* (Dang Gui) and *Rehmannia Radix* (Sheng Di Huang) to supplement blood and nourish yin; *Cannabis Fructus* (Huo Ma Ren) and *Persicae Semen* (Tao Ren) to moisturize the intestine to ease stool; *Aurantii Fructus* (Zhi Qiao) to move the qi downwards.

方药: 润肠丸。常用:当归、生地黄补血养阴;火麻仁、桃仁润肠通便;枳壳导气下行。

Modification: For blood deficiency with heat, along with dry mouth and irritation, peeled tongue fur and fine rapid pulse, add *Polygoni Multiflori Radix* (He Shou Wu), *Polygonati Odorati Rhizoma* (Yu Zhu) and *Anemarrhenae Rhizoma* (Zhi Mu) to generate body fluid and cleanse heat; for dry stool despite recovered body fluid, use *Five Kernels Pills* (Wu Ren Wan) to moisturize the intestines to ease stool; for constipation due to qi and blood deficiency after birth labor, use *Eight Jewel Decoction* (Ba Zhen Tang) with *Polygoni Multiflori Radix* (He Shou Wu), *Persicae Semen* (Tao Ren) and *Mel* (Feng Mi) to boost qi, supplement blood and moisturize the intestines.

加减: 若血虚有热,兼见口干心烦、苔剥、脉细数,可加生首乌、玉竹、知母以生津清热;若津液已复而大便仍干燥,可用五仁丸以润肠通便;如妇人产后,气血虚弱见大便秘结,可用八珍汤加生首乌、桃仁、白蜜等以益气补血润肠。

2. 2. 6 Constipation Due to Yin Deficiency

2. 2. 6 阴虚便秘

Manifestations: Dry stool in shape of goat-stool, dry mouth, dry eyes, emaciation, flushed cheeks, feverish sensations, night sweating, irriation and heat in the five centers, dizziness and vertigo; red tongue with little tongue fur; rapid fine pulse.

证候: 大便干结如羊屎状,口干,目涩,形体消瘦,可见颧红,潮热盗汗,五心烦热,眩晕耳鸣。舌红少苔,脉细数。

Treatment: To nourish yin and moisturize the intestines to ease stool.

治法: 滋阴润肠通便。

Formulas and Herbs: *Humor-Increasing Decoction* (Zeng Ye Tang), usually composed of *Rehmannia Radix* (Sheng Di Huang), *Scrophulariae Radix* (Xuan Shen) and *Ophiopogonis Radix* (Mai Men Dong) to nourish yin and increase body fluid.

方药: 增液汤。常用生地黄、玄参、麦门冬滋阴增液。

Modification: For dry stool like goats', add *Cannabis Fructus* (Huo Ma Ren), *Platycladi Semen* (Bai Zi Ren), and *Trichosanthis Semen* (Gua Lou Zi) to help moisturize the intestines; for shortage of stomach-yin, dry mouth and thirst, use *Stomach-Benefiting Decoction* (Yi Wei Tang); for deficiency

加减: 便秘干结如羊屎状,加火麻仁、柏子仁、瓜蒌仁增润肠之效;若胃阴不足,口干口渴者,可用益胃汤;若肾阴不足,腰膝酸软者,可用六味地黄丸;若阴亏燥结,热

of kidney-yin, sore and weakness in the waist and knees, use *Rehmannia Pills with Six Ingredients* (Liu Wei Di Huang Wan); for yin deficiency and dryness and body fluid damaged by exuberant heat, use *Humor-Increasing Purgative Decoction* (Zeng Ye Cheng Qi Tang) to increase yin (increase the water to float the boat).

盛伤津者,可用增液承气汤增水行舟。

2. 2. 7 Constipation Due to Yang Deficiency

Manifestations: Dry or not dry stool, defecation difficulties, long clear away urine, waxy pale complexion, cold limbs, favor for warmth and dread of cold, cold in the abdomen, sore and weakness in the waist and knees; pale tongue or pale enlarged tongue with white moist slippery tongue fur; deep retard pulse.

Treatment: To warm yang to ease stool.

Formulas and Herbs: *Fluid Nourishing Decoction* (Ji Chuan Jian), usually composed of *Cistanchis Herba* (Rou Cong Rong) and *Achyranthis Bidentatae Radix* (Niu Xi) to warm yang and strengthen the kidney as well as mointurize the intestines and ease stool; *Angelicae Sinensis Radix* (Dang Gui) to nourish blood and moisturize the intestines; *Cimicifugae Rhizoma* (Sheng Ma) and *Alismatis Rhizoma* (Ze Xie) to raise clarity and lower turbidity; *Aurantii Fructus*(Zhi Qiao) to loosen the intestines and move qi downwards.

Modification: For cold accumulation and qi stagnation with severe abdominal pain, add *Cinnamomi Cortex* (Rou Gui) and *Aucklandiae Radix* (Mu Xiang) to warm yang, promote qi flow and stop pain.

2. 2. 7 阳虚便秘

证候: 大便干或不干,排出困难,小便清长,面色㿠白,四肢不温,喜热怕冷,腹中冷,腰膝酸冷,舌淡或淡胖,苔白润而滑,脉沉迟。

治法: 温阳通便。

方药: 济川煎。常用:肉苁蓉、牛膝温阳补肾,润肠通便;当归养血润肠;升麻、泽泻升清降浊;枳壳宽肠下气。

加减: 若寒凝气滞、腹痛较甚,加肉桂、木香温中行气止痛。

Hematemesis

Hematemesis is a disease of spitting red or purple dark blood often with some food remainders, mainly caused by damages of stomach collaterals and blood overspilling into the stomach so that blood moves upward with stomach-qi, which results in hematemesis.

1 Etiology and Pathogenesis

Improper diet, emotional and spiritual extremes, overstrain and fatigue will lead to fire-heat burning inside, forcing blood to move frenetically or blood spill-over the vessels due to qi deficiency. That is the main cause of hemompotysis.

1.1 Improper Diet Leads to Heat Retained in the Stomach

Gluttony, over intake of spicy food with heavy dressings leads to heat accumulated in the stomach or damp-heat, which makes damages to the stomach collaterals, causinghematemesis.

1.2 Emotional, Spiritual Extremes and Liver Depression Transforming Into Fire

Emotional and spiritual satisfaction and long depressed liver-qi transforming into fire override the stomach and injure the stomach collaterals, causing hematemesis.

1.3 Qi Exhaustion Due to Overstrain and Qi fails togather blood

Overstrain or irregualar dietwill damage Middle-qi which fails to gather blood. Then blood over spills into the stomach, which causes hemopotysis.

The pathological position of hemopotysis is in the stomach, but the liver and spleen are also involved. The pathological features come into two

吐 血

吐血主要因胃络损伤，血溢胃内，以致胃气上逆，血随气逆，而致血经呕吐而出，血色红或紫黯，常夹有食物残渣的一类病证。

1 病因病机

吐血的发生主要因饮食不节、情志过极、劳倦过度，导致火热薰灼、迫血妄行，或气虚不摄、血溢脉外而产生本病。

1.1 饮食不节，胃中积热

暴饮暴食，过食辛辣厚味，以致胃中积热，或滋生湿热，热伤胃络，引起吐血。

1.2 情志过极，肝郁化火

情志不遂，肝气郁结，郁久化火，逆乘于胃，胃络损伤，则引起吐血。

1.3 劳倦耗气，气不摄血

劳倦过度，饥饱失常，中气亏虚，气不摄血，血溢胃内而致吐血。

吐血的病位在胃，并与肝、脾密切相关。病机特点可以归结火热薰灼、迫血妄

types of fire-heat forcing blood to move frenetically and blood spilling over the vessels due to qi deficiency. By pathological nature, it comes into two kinds: the deficiency type and the excess type. Hemopotysis due to fire-heat belongs to the excess type with hemopotysis due to qi deficiency, the deficiency type. Although the two types are different in pathogenesis and pathology, there will be some interchanges as it develops.

行，气虚不摄、血溢脉外两大类。病理性质有虚有实，由火热亢盛所致者属于实证，由气虚不摄所致者属于虚证。实证和虚证虽各有其不同的病因病机，但在疾病发展变化的过程中，又常发生实证向虚证的转化。

2 Syndrome Differentiation and Treatment

2 辨证论治

2.1 Key Points of Syndrome Differentiation

Doctors should first locate the pathological organs since some lie in the stomach while some in the liver, which can be distinguished by symptoms. Then doctors should distinguish betweendeficiency from excess. Acute hemopotysis of excess type lasts short with scarlet fresh blood and signs of fever. Meanwhile, continuous hemopotysis of deficiency type is sometimes better and sometimes worse with dark blood. In terms of treatment, treating fire, treating qi and blood should be the fundamental principles. For fire of excess, purge it. For qi-deficiency, boost it with cool herbs and astringent herbs to cease bleeding.

2.1 辨治要点

吐血的辨证首先应辨清脏腑病位，有病在胃及病在肝之别，可根据伴随症状加以辨别。其次分清虚实，出血急骤：病程较短，血色鲜红，且伴有热象者，为实证；吐血缠绵，时轻时重，血色暗淡者，多属虚证。治疗上以治火、治气、治血为基本原则，实火当清热泻火，气虚当补气益气，并配合凉血止血、收敛止血等法。

2.2 Therapeutic Methods for Different Patterns

2.2 分型论治

2.2.1 Hyperpyrexia of Stomach

Manifestations: Spitting red or dark purple blood with food remainders, stool as black as tar, distention and fullness in the stomach and abdomen or even pain, dry mouth with smells or constipation; red tongue with yellow greasy tongue fur; rapid rolling pulse.

2.2.1 胃热壅盛

证候：吐血色红或紫黯，常夹有食物残渣，大便色黑如柏油，脘腹胀闷，甚则作痛，口干口臭，或便秘。舌质红，苔黄腻，脉滑数。

Treatment: To clear away stomach heat and purge fire; resolve stasis and stop bleeding.

治法： 清胃泻火，化瘀止血。

Formulas and Herbs: *Heart-Draining Decoction* (Xie Xin Tang) and *Ten Ashes Powder* (Shi Hui San), usually composed of *Scutellariae Radix* (Huang Qin), *Coptidis Rhizoma* (Huang Lian) and *Rhei Radix et Rhizoma* (Da Huang) to purge fire and clear away the stomach with bitter and cool herbs; *Cirsii Japonici Herba* (Da Ji), *Cirsii Herba* (Xiao Ji), *Platycladi Cacumen Preparata* (Ce Bai Ye), *Rubiae Radix et Rhizoma* (Xi Cao Gen) and *Imperatae Rhizoma* (Bai Mao Gen) to clear away heat, cool blood and stop bleeding; Palm Tree barks (Zong Lü Pi) to astringe and stop bleeding, *Moutan Cortex* (Mu Dan Pi) and *Gardeniae Fructus* (Zhi Zi) to clear away heat and cool blood; *Rhei Radix et Rhizoma* (Da Huang) to dredge fu-organs, purge heat and resolve stasis. The formula features stoping bleeding and resolving stasis.

方药： 泻心汤合十灰散。常用：黄芩、黄连、大黄苦寒泻火清胃；大蓟、小蓟、侧柏叶、茜草根、白茅根清热凉血止血；棕榈皮收敛止血；牡丹皮、栀子清热凉血；大黄通腑泻热散瘀，全方具有止血不留瘀的特点。

Modification: For stomach-qi upward flow, nausea and vomiting, add *Inulae Flos* (Xuan Fu Hua), *Haematitum* (Zhe Shi) and *Bambusae Caulis in Taenias* (Zhu Ru) to harmonize the stomach and lower upward flow; for stomach-yin injured by heat with symptoms like thirst, red and dry tongue and fine rapid pulse, add *Ophiopogonis Radix* (Mai Men Dong), *Dendrobii Caulis* (Shi Hu) and *Trichosanthis Radix* (Tian Hua Fen) to nourish the stomach and generate body fluid.

加减： 胃气上逆而致恶心呕吐者，可加旋覆花、代赭石、竹茹和胃降逆；热伤胃阴而表现口渴、舌红而干、脉象细数者，加麦门冬、石斛、天花粉养胃生津。

2.2.2 Liver-fire Attacks the Stomach

2.2.2 肝火犯胃

Mainfestations: Spitting red or dark purple blood, bitter mouth and pain around the hypochondria, restlessness and irritation, insomnia and dreaminess; dark red tongue; rapid taut pulse.

证候： 吐血色红或紫黯，口苦胁痛，心烦易怒，寐少梦多。舌质红绛，脉弦数。

Treatment: To purge the liver and cleanse the stomach; cool blood and stop bleeding.

治法： 泻肝清胃，凉血止血。

Formulas and Herbs: *Gentian Liver-Draining Decoction* (Long Dan Xie Gan Tang), usually composed of *Gentianae Radix et Rhizoma* (Long Dan), *Bupleuri Radix* (Chai Hu), *Scutellariae Radix* (Huang Qin) and *Gardeniae Fructus* (Zhi Zi) to cleanse the liver and purge fire; *Alismatis Rhizoma* (Ze Xie), *Akebiae Caulis* (Mu Tong), *Plantaginis Semen* (Che Qian Zi) to clear away heat and eliminate dampness; *Rehmannia Radix* (Sheng Di Huang) and *Angelicae Sinensis Radix* (Dang Gui) to nourish yin and nourish blood.

方药： 龙胆泻肝汤。常用：龙胆草、柴胡、黄芩、栀子清肝泻火；泽泻、木通、车前子清热利湿；生地、当归滋阴养血。

Modification: Add *Imperatae Rhizoma* (Bai Mao Gen), *Nelumbinis Rhizomatis Nodus* (Ou Jie) *Ecliptae Herba* (Han Lian Cao), *Rubiae Radix et Rhizoma* (Qian Cao) and *Ten Ashes Powder* (Shi Hui San) to help cool blood and stop bleeding; for severe pain around the hypochondria, add *Curcumae Radix* (Yu Jin), *Cyperi Rhizoma* Praeparata (Zhi Xiang Fu) to regulate qi, activate colleterals and stop pain; for sudden spitting blood in a great amount, it is better to use *Rhinoceros Horn and Rehmannia Decoction*(Xi Jiao Di Huang Tang) and *Notoginseng Radix et Rhizoma* (San Qi) powder to clear away heat, cool blood and stop bleeding.

加减： 可加白茅根、藕节、旱莲草、茜草，或合用十灰散，以加强凉血止血的作用；胁痛甚者，加郁金、制香附等理气活络定痛；若吐血暴发，出血如涌，宜清热凉血止血，选用犀角地黄汤配三七末调服。

2.2.3 Blood Overspilt Due to Qi Deficiency

2.2.3 气虚血溢

Manifestations: Continuous spitting bleeding, better or worse at times, dark pale blood, fatigue and tiredness, palpitation and short of breath, pale complexion; pale tongue; fine weak pulse.

证候： 吐血缠绵不止，时轻时重，血色暗淡，神疲乏力，心悸气短，面色苍白，舌质淡，脉细弱。

Treatment: To strengthen the spleen and nourish the heart; boost qi to gather blood.

治法： 健脾养心，益气摄血。

Formulas and Herbs: *Angelica Splenic Decoction*

方药： 归脾汤。常用：黄

(Gui Pi Tang), usually composed of *Astragali Radix* (Huang Qi), *Angelicae Sinensis Radix* (Dang Gui), *Longan Arillus* (Long Yan Rou) and *Jujubae Fructus* (Da Zao) to boost qi and nourish blood; *Codonopsis Radix* (Dang Shen), *Atractylodis Macrocephalae Rhizoma* (Bai Zhu) and *Zingiberis Rhizoma Recens* (Sheng Jiang) to supplement qi and strengthen the spleen; *Poria* (Fu Ling), *Polygalae Radix* (Yuan Zhi), *Ziziphi Spinosae Semen* (Suan Zao Ren) to nourish the heart-blood and calm the spirits; *Aucklandiae Radix* (Mu Xiang) to promote qi flow without causing stagnation.

芪、当归、龙眼肉、大枣益气养血;党参、白术、生姜补气健脾;茯神、远志、酸枣仁养心血而安神;木香行气,使补而不滞。

Modification: Add moderately *Agrimoniae Herba* (Xian He Cao), *Bletillae Rhizoma* (Bai Ji), *Sepiae Endoconcha* (Hao Piao Xiao) and *Zingiberis Rhizoma Preparatae* (Pao Jiang Tan) to warm the meridians, astringe and stop bleeding; for yang injured by qi, cold and deficiency in the stomach and spleen with such symptoms as cold limbs, aversion to cold, loose stool, change for *Kashiwaba Decoction* (Bai Ye Tang) and *Regulating Zhong jiao Decoction* (Fu Zi Li Zhong Tang) to warm the meridians and stop bleeding; for over bleeding and qi exhaustion together with blood with symptoms like pale complexion, cold limbs, sweating and weak pulse, give *immediately Ginseng Decoction* (Du Shen Tang) to boost qi and stop exhaustion.

加减: 可酌加仙鹤草、白及、乌贼骨、炮姜炭等温经固涩止血;若气损及阳,脾胃虚寒,症见肢冷、畏寒、大便溏薄者,可改用柏叶汤合理中丸温经止血;若出血过多,气随血脱,症见面色苍白、四肢厥冷、汗出、脉微者,应急服独参汤益气固脱。

Hemafecia

便 血

Hemafecia is a disease of blood in stool or stool as black as tar due to injuries of colleterals of the stomach and intestines.

便血是胃肠脉络受损,出现血液随大便而下,或大便呈柏油样为主要临床表现的病证。

1 Etiology and Pathogenesis

Helmafecia is caused by burning heat-fire forcing the blood to move frenetically or by qi not so deficient as togather blood so that blood overspills due to exogenous pathogenic factors, improper diet, emotional and spiritual extremes, fatigue and overstrain.

1.1 Exogenous Pathogenic Factors Injure the Blood and Collaterals

Among the pathogenic factors, pathogenic heat is the most common one as pathogenic heat or damp heat hurts lower collaterals, causing blood in stool.

1.2 Stomach and Spleen Injury Due to Intake of Alcohol and Savoury Food

Improper diet, over drinking and over intake of spicy andsavoury food will bring about damp-heat, which makes damage to collaterals, causing blood in stool.

1.3 Liver Depression Transforming Into Fire Due to Extreme Emotional Changes

Over worry and anger turn depressed liver qi into fire, which attacks the nearby stomach and stomach collaterals. Blood spills over into the stomach and moves downward with stool, causing hemofecia.

1.4 Deficiency of Spleen-qi Due to Overstrain and Prolonged Illness

Overstrain and prolonged illness make damage to the stomach and spleen, the latter of which fails togather blood, and blood spills over into the intestines, causing hemefecia.

Hemecefica lies in the the stomach and intestines but is related with the liver and the spleen.

1 病因病机

便血的发生主要由感受外邪、饮食不节、情志过极、劳倦久病等因素，导致火热薰灼，迫血妄行，或气虚不摄，血溢脉外而产生本病。

1.1 感受外邪，损伤血络

外邪侵袭，其中以感受热邪所致者为多，热邪或湿热损伤下部脉络，则引起便血。

1.2 嗜食醇酒厚味，脾胃受伤

饮食不节，饮酒过多及过食辛辣厚味，滋生湿热，热伤脉络，引起便血。

1.3 情志过极，肝郁化火

忧思恼怒过度，肝气郁结化火，肝火横逆犯胃，热伤胃络，血溢胃内，随大便而下，引起便血。

1.4 劳倦久病，脾气亏虚

劳倦久病，脾胃受损，脾不统血，血溢肠内，而出现便血。

便血病位在胃肠，并与肝、脾相关。基本病机为火

The pathogensis is buring of fire-heat or the failure of the spleen to gather blood. The pathological nature comes into deficiency type and excess type. Damp-heat in the intestines and depressive heat in the liver and stomach belongs to excess type while deficiencyof spleen-qi and spleen-yang belong to deficiency type.

热熏灼，或脾不统血。病理性质有虚有实，实为肠道湿热、肝胃郁热，虚为脾气、脾阳亏虚。

2 Syndrome Differentiation and Treatment

2 辨证论治

2.1 Key Points of Syndrome Differentiation

2.1 辨治要点

Doctors can distinguish deficiency from excess type and identify the pathological zang-fu organs by stool color, symptoms, tongue and pulse. Generally speaking, scarlet blood in stool usually comes from the intestines while black blood in stool often comes from the stomach. Bitter and dry mouth, red tongue with yellow tongue fur andsoft rapid or rapid taut pulse are symptoms of excess type while tiredness, fatigue, pale tongue with fine pulse are symptoms of deficiency type. In terms of treatment, treating fire, qi and blood is the principle. For fire, purge it. For qi deficiency, warm and supplement it together with cooling, astringing, nurturing blood to stop bleeding.

可根据便血颜色、伴随症状、舌脉来辨别虚实和脏腑病位。一般而言：便血色红，其血多来自肠；便血色黑，其血多来自胃。伴口干口苦，舌红苔黄，脉濡数或弦数，多为实证；伴倦怠乏力，舌淡脉细，多为虚证。治疗上以治火、治气、治血为原则，实火宜清，气虚宜补宜温，同时配合凉血止血，收敛止血，养血止血等法。

2.2 Therapeutic Methods for Different Patterns

2.2 分型论治

2.2.1 Damp-heat in the Intestines

2.2.1 肠道湿热

Manifestations: Scarlet blood in stool, unsmooth or loose stool or with abdominal pain, bitter mouth; red tongue with yellow greasy tongue fur; rapid soft pulse.

证候：便血色红，大便不畅或稀溏，或有腹痛，口苦。舌质红，苔黄腻，脉濡数。

Treatment: To purge and resolve damp-heat; cool blood to stop bleeding.

治法：清化湿热，凉血止血。

Formulas and Herbs: *Sanguisorbae Powder* (Di Yu San) and *Sophorae Pills* (Huai Jiao Wan), usu-

方药：地榆散或槐角丸。常用：地榆、槐角、茜草凉血

ally composed of *Sanguisorbiae Radix* (Di Yu), *Sophorae Fructus* (Huai Jiao) and *Rubiae Radix et Rhizoma* (Qian Cao) to cool blood to stop bleeding; *Gardeniae Fructus* (Zhi Zi), *Scutellariae Radix* (Huang Qin) and *Coptidis Rhizoma* (Huang Lian) to clear away heat and dry dampness as well as purge fire to detoxify; *Poria* (Fu Ling) to stop penetrating and resolve dampness; *Saposhnikoviae Radix*(Fang Feng), *Aurantii Fructus*(Zhi Qiao) and *Angelicae Sinensis Radix* (Dang Gui) to disperse wind, regulate qi and promote blood circulation.

止血;栀子、黄芩、黄连清热燥湿,泻火解毒;茯苓淡渗利湿;防风、枳壳、当归疏风理气活血。

Modification: For prolonged hemafecia, deficiency of yin and blood and unclear awayed damp-heat with such symptoms as dizziness and vertigo, lusterless face, *Organ-Cleansing Decoction* (Qing Zang Tang) or Pork Intestines and *Coptidis Pills* (Zang Lian Wan) is used to clear away heat and eliminate dampness as well as supplement and strengthen yin and blood, in which way, both deficiency and excess into account have been considered and healthy qi is strengthened and pathological factors dispelled.

加减:便血日久,阴血已亏,湿热未清,症见头晕目眩、面色少华者,宜予清脏汤或脏连丸清热除湿与补益阴血双管齐下,以虚实兼顾,扶正祛邪。

2.2.2 Depressed Heat in the Liver and Stomach

2.2.2 肝胃郁热

Manifestations: Dark red or black blood in stool, burning pain in the stomach, epigastric upset and regurgitation, irritation and restlessness, bitter and dry mouth; red tongue with yellow tongue fur; taut or rapid pulse.

证候:便血暗红或黑便,胃脘灼痛,嘈杂泛酸,烦躁易怒,口干口苦。舌红苔黄,脉弦或数。

Treatment: To disperse liver and purge heat; harmominze the stomach and cool blood.

治法:疏肝泄热,和胃凉血。

Formulas and Herbs: *Moutan Cortex and Gardeniae- Free Wanderer Powder* (Dan Zhi Xiao Yao San) and *Coptis and evodia Pills* (Zuo Jin Wan), usually composed of *Moutan Cortex* (Mu Dan Pi) and

方药:丹栀逍遥散合左金丸。常用:牡丹皮、山栀清肝泻火;柴胡、薄荷疏肝;当归、白芍药柔肝养肝;白术、

Gardeniae Fructus (Zhi Zi) to cleanse the liver and purge fire, *Bupleuri Radix* (Chai Hu) and *Menthae Haplocalycis Herba* (Bo He) to disperse the liver; *Angelicae Sinensis Radix* (Dang Gui) and *Paeoniae Radix Alba* (Bai Shao Yao) to soften and nourish the liver; *Atractylodis Macrocephalae Rhizoma* (Bai Zhu), *Poria* (Fu Ling), *Glycyrrhizae Radix et Rhizoma* (Gan Cao) and *Zingiberis Rhizoma Preparata* (Wei Jiang) to strengthen the spleen and harmonize the stomach; *Coptidis Rhizoma* (Huang Lian) and *Euodiae Fructus* (Wu Zhu Yu) to purge the liver and harmonize the stomach.

茯苓、甘草、煨姜健脾和胃；黄连、吴茱萸泻肝和胃。

Modification: *Rubiae Radix et Rhizoma* (Xi Cao), *Ecliptae Herba* (Han Lian) and *Platycladi Cacumen Preparata* (Ce Bai Ye) can be added to help cool blood to stop bleeding; for constipation, add *Gentianae Radix et Rhizom* (Long Dan) and *Rhei Radix et Rhizoma* (Da Huang) to purge fire and ease stool.

加减：可加茜草、旱莲草、侧柏叶等凉血止血；若大便秘结者，加龙胆草、大黄以泻火通便。

2.2.3 Deficienct Qi Failing to Control Blood

2.2.3 气虚不摄

Manifestations: Red or dark purple blood in stool, little intake, fatigue, withered yellow complexion, palpipation, insomnia; pale tongue; fine pulse.

证候：便血色红或紫黯，食少，体倦，面色萎黄，心悸，少寐。舌质淡，脉细。

Treatment: To boost qi and control blood.

治法：益气摄血。

Formulas and Herbs: *Angelica Splenic Decoction* (Gui Pi Tang), usually composed of *Codonopsis Radix* (Dang Shen), *Atractylodis Macrocephalae Rhizoma* (Bai Zhu), *Poria* (Fu Ling) and *Glycyrrhizae Radix et Rhizoma* (Gan Cao) to boost qi and strengthen the spleen; *Angelicae Sinensis Radix* (Dang Gui) and *Astragali Radix* (Huang Qi) to boost qi and generate blood; *Ziziphi Spinosae Semen* (Suan Zao Ren), *Polygalae Radix* (Yuan Zhi) and

方药：归脾汤。常用：党参、白术、茯苓、甘草补气健脾；当归、黄芪益气生血；酸枣仁、远志、龙眼肉补心益脾，安神定志；木香理气醒脾。

Longan Arillus (Long Yan Rou) to nourish the heart and strengthen the spleen as well as calm the spirits and the minds; *Aucklandiae Radix* (Mu Xiang) to regulate qi and waken the spleen.

Modification: *Sophorae Flos* (Huai Hua), *Sanguisorbiae Radix* (Di Yu), *Bletillae Rhizoma* (Bai Ji) and *Agrimoniae Herba* (Xian He Cao) can be added moderately to help stop bleeding; for middle-qi descending, lassitude and short breath, and bulging annus, add *Center-Supplementing qi-Boosting Decoction* (Bu Zhong Yi Qi Tang).

加减: 可酌加槐花、地榆、白及、仙鹤草,以增强止血作用;若中气下陷,神疲气短、肛门坠胀,可加补中益气汤。

2.2.4 Deficiency-cold of Spleen and Stomach

2.2.4 脾胃虚寒

Manifestations: Frequent dull pain in the abdomen at ordinary times, favor warmth and pressing, dark purple blood in stool or even tar-black, lusterless face, lassitude and laziness to talk, loose stool; pale tongue; fine weak pulse.

证候: 平素腹部隐痛,喜温喜按,便血紫黯,甚则色黑如柏油样,面色不华,神倦懒言,大便溏薄。舌质淡,脉细弱。

Treatment: To strengthen the spleen and warm zhong jiao; nourish blood and stop bleeding.

治法: 健脾温中,养血止血。

Formulas and Herbs: *Baked Yellow Earth Decoction* (Huang Tu Tang), usually composed of baked yellow earth from Cshinese traditional cooking ranges to warm the middle-Jiao and stop bleeding, *Atractylodis Macrocephalae Rhizoma* (Bai Zhu), *Aconm Lateralis Radix Praeparata* (Fu Zi), *Glycyrrhizae Radix et Rhizoma* (Gan Cao) to warm zhong jiao and strengthen the spleen; *Rehmannia Radix* (Di Huang) and *Asini Corii Colla* (E Jiao) to nourish blood and stop bleeding; *Scutellariae Radix* (Huang Qin) which is cool, bitter, hard for counteracting assistance.

方药: 黄土汤。常用:灶心土温中止血;白术、附子、甘草温中健脾;地黄、阿胶养血止血;黄芩苦寒坚阴,起反佐作用。

Modificiation: For remarkable yang deficiency, dread of cold and cold limbs, add *Cervi Cornu Degelatinatum* (Lu Jiao Shuang), *Zingiberis Rhizoma*

加减: 若阳虚较甚,畏寒肢冷者,加鹿角霜、炮姜、艾叶等温阳止血;下血日久,气

(Pao Jiang) and *Folium Artemistae Argyi* (Ai Ye) to warm yang and stop bleeding; for prolonged bleeding, causing qi deficiency and descending, and bulging annus, add *Center-Supplementing qi-Boosting Decoction* (Bu Zhong Yi Qi Tang) to boost qi and raise yang.

虚下陷,肛门下坠者,可合用补中益气汤以益气升阳。

Chapter 4 Liver System Diseases

第4章 肝系病证

Hypochondriac Pain

胁 痛

Hypochondriac pain is a disease featured by pain on one or two sides of the hypochondria due to blockade or slack of the liver collaterals.

胁痛主要因肝络不通或不荣而导致一侧或两侧胁肋部疼痛为主要表现的病证。

1 Etiology and Pathogenesis

1 病因病机

Hypochondriac pain is caused by disharmoncy of seven emtions, improper diet, falling and injury or weak constitution due to prolonged illness. All these factors will cause liver-qi to be depressed, which when not dispersed in time, stagnates and blocks the spleen-earth and finally generate dampness. Or when qi is depressed for long, qi stagnates and affects blood circulation, causing blood stasis and water fluid retention, which in turn, damages the liver and kidney and makes blood fail to nourish the collaterals. Finally, hypochondriac pain is resulted.

胁痛的发生主要是由于七情失和、饮食不节、跌仆损伤、久病体虚等因素，导致肝气郁结，疏泄不及，肝郁气滞，脾土壅滞，湿自内生；或气郁日久，气滞及血，瘀血停积；或肝肾亏损，血不荣络等，发为胁痛。

1.1 Depressed Liver-qi Due to Injury of the Seven Emotions

1.1 七情所伤，肝气郁结

When emtions and minds are depressed, the liver is not well dispersed in time. Meanwhile, when outrage makes qi flows reversely, the liver is over-dispersed. Under both of those circumstances, the liver will fail to

情志抑郁则疏泄不及，暴怒气逆则疏泄太过，均可导致肝脏功能失调，肝失条达，疏泄不利，气阻络痹而致

function properly and be dispersed, blocking the collaterals which leads to hypochondriac pain.

胁痛。

1.2 Blood Stasis Obstructing Collaterals Due to Trauma and Sprain

Overstrain damages the liver collaterals and hinders blood circulation. Injury and sprain also will hurt liver collaterals and cause blood statis, resulting unsmooth movement of qi and blood, which will block the collaterals on both sides and causehypochondriac pain.

1.2 外伤闪搓，瘀血阻络

强力负重，肝络受损，血行不畅；外伤闪挫损伤胁络，瘀血停留，导致气血运行不畅，阻塞胁络，不通则痛，而致胁痛。

1.3 Pathogenic Damp-heat Accumulating in the Liver and Gallbladder

Pathogenic damp-heat comes into exogenous type and endogenous type. When exogenous damp-heat gathers in the liver and gallbladder, the liver and gallbladder fail to disperse, causing hypochondriac pain. When overintake of sweat, greasy food and alcohol damages the spleen and stomach, the spleen and stomach fails to function properly and dampness is generated. Then phlegm-damp blocks the qi activities which is depressed and turns into heat. Damp-heat then attacks the liver and gallbladder, causing disharmony between the liver and gallbladder. When the liver fails to disperse, hypochondriac pain is resulted in.

1.3 湿热之邪，蕴结肝胆

湿热之邪，有内外之分：外感湿热，蕴于肝胆，肝胆失于疏泄条达，可致胁痛；饮食不节，或进食肥甘美酒，或过食生冷，伤及脾胃，健运失司，湿自内生，痰湿中阻，气机不利，郁而化热，湿热侵犯肝胆，使肝络失和，胆失疏泄，而致胁痛。

1.4 Dystrophy of the Liver Collaterals Due to Prolonged Illness, Overstrain and Excessive Intercourse

Prolongedillness, overstrain or excessive intercourse will exhaust and damage the essence and blood, causing the colleterals lacking in nurturing and side stiches then.

1.4 久病劳欲，肝络失养

久病耗伤，劳欲过度，精血亏损，络脉失养，致使不荣则痛。

Hypochondriac pain lies primarily in the live and gallbladder but is also related to the spleen, the

胁痛主要病位在肝胆，且与脾、胃、肾相关。本病以

stomach and kidney. Pain due to blockade by qi stagnation, blood stasis and damp-heat is of excess type while pain due to dystrophy because of blood and essence deficiency is of deficiency type. The excess type is the majority. The pathological change is quite complicated. Generally speaking, hypochondriac pain for the first time is of excess type while prolonged hypochondriac pain is of deficiency type. However, when excess type is prolonged and depressed liver-qi transforms into fire, liver-yin will be damaged and blood stasis remains. As a result, not enough new blood can be produced which leads to the shortage of blood and essence and excess type turns into deficiency type. On the other hand, as deficiency of the liver and kidney, and shortage of essence and blood render it more likely to generate heat or blood stasis, deficiency type, together with emotional disorder and improper diet, will be complicated with excess type or they are interchanged. Hypochondriac pain also sees the transformation of qi and blood. That is, qi stagnation will affect blood while blood stasis will blocks qi. But in a nutshell, it is no more than qi, blood or both.

气滞、血瘀、湿热所致不通则痛者属实，以精血不足所致不荣则痛者属虚，而以实证为多见。病机转化较为复杂，一般初病多实证，久病多虚证。实证日久，因肝郁化火，耗伤肝阴，或瘀血不去，新血不生，精血虚少，即可由实转虚；而肝肾亏虚，精血不足的虚证，又易于化热或产生瘀血，或因情志、饮食因素可产生虚中夹实，或本虚标实的变化。胁痛还有气血的转化，即可气滞及血，又可血瘀阻气，但不外乎病在气，或病在血，或气血同病。

2 Syndrome Differentiation and Treatment

2.1 Key Points of Syndrome Differentiation

Doctors should be able to distguish qi, blood, deficiency and excess by the nature, position of pain and accompanying symptoms. Distending pain is the main characteristics and changes its position randomly. Hypochondriac pain due to qi stagnation changes with emotions. Stabbing pain in fixed positions which gets worse at night and is caused by falling and sprain is due to injured collaterals and blood

2 辨证论治

2.1 辨治要点

胁痛的辨证可从疼痛的性质、部位、伴随症状等方面进行气血虚实的辨别：胁痛以胀痛为主，走窜不定，每因情志变化而增减，病属气滞；胁肋呈刺痛，部位固定，入夜痛甚，因跌仆闪挫所致，为胁络受损，瘀血停着；胁痛如

stasis. Twisting pain reaching the back with fever, bitter mouth, or jaundice, or spitting roundworms is due to steaming damp-heat or sandstones or roundworms blocking the gallbladder. Dull pain on the hypochondria, restlessness, dry mouth, dizziness, vertigo and red tongue with little tongue fur is due to yin and blood deficiency. The treatment abides by dispersing the liver and harmonizing the collaterals to stop pain. For excess type, it is advisable to dispel the pathogenic factors and dredge, including dispersing the liver, regulating qi, promoting blood circulation, resolving dampness and puring fu-organs. For deficiency type, soften the liver and strengthen healthy qi, by means of nourishing yin to soften the liver, and nourishing the liver collaterals. At the same time, herbs for qi regulation can be added moderately to disperse and dredge qi activities to improve herbsl effects. However, remember qi-regulating herbs with the nature of aroma and dryness shall not be applied in case of hurting yin.

绞，痛彻肩背，伴发热口苦，胸闷恶心，或见黄疸，或呕吐蛔虫，多为湿热交蒸，或砂石或蛔虫阻滞胆道；胁肋隐痛，心烦口干，伴头晕目眩，舌红少苔，病属阴血亏损。治疗上以疏肝和络止痛为基本治则：实证以祛邪疏通为要，分别采用疏肝、理气、活血、清热、利湿、泻腑等法；虚证以柔肝扶正为主，采用滋阴柔肝，滋养肝络之法。同时亦可适量加入理气之品，以疏通气机，提高疗效。但理气药不宜香燥，以免更伤其阴。

2.2 Therapeutic Methods of Different Patterns

2.2.1 Depressed Liver and Qi Stagnation

Manifestations: Distenting pain on hypochondria which changes positions randomly, even stretching to shoulders and backs, aggravation or relief with changes of emotions and minds, oppression in the chest, sighs, burping, poor appetite, distention and fullness in the stomach and abdomen; white thin tongue fur; taut pulse.

Treatment: To disperse the liver and regulate qi.

Formulas and Herbs: *Bupleurum-Dispersing-Liver Powder* (Chai Hu Shu Gan San), usually composed of *Bupleuri Radix* (Chai Hu), *Cyperi*

2.2 分型论治

2.2.1 肝郁气滞

证候：胁肋胀痛，走窜不定，甚则连及胸肩背，随情志变化而加重或减轻，胸闷，善太息，嗳气频作，伴有纳呆，脘腹胀满。舌苔薄白，脉弦。

治法：疏肝理气。

方药：柴胡疏肝散。常用：柴胡、香附、枳壳疏肝理气解郁；川芎活血行气；白芍

Rhizoma (Xiang Fu) and *Aurantii Fructus* (Zhi Qiao) to disperse the liver, regulate qi and resolve depression; *Chuanxiong Rhizoma* (Chuan Xiong) to promote blood circulation and qi flow; *Paeoniae Radix Alba* (Bai Shao Yao) and *Glycyrrhizae Radix et Rhizoma* (Gan Cao) to relieve and stop pain.

药、甘草缓急止痛。

Modification: For remarkable hypochondriac pain, add *Citri Reticulatae Pericarpium Viride* (Qing Pi), *Citri Reticulatae Pericarpium* (Chen Pi), *Curcumae Radix* (Yu Jin), *Aucklandiae Radix* (Mu Xiang), *Corydalis Rhizoma* (Yan Hu Suo) and *Toosendan Fructus* (Chuan Lian Zi) to help regulate qi and stop pain; for long depressed liver-qi turning into fire with such symptoms as dragging pain on hypochondria, irriataion and restlessness, bitter and dry mouth, yellow urine and constipation, red tongue with yellow tongue fur and rapid taut pulse, add *Moutan Cortex* (Mu Dan Pi), *Gardeniae Fructus* (Zhi Zi) and *Gentianae Radix et Rhizom* (Long Dan) to cleanse the liver and purge fire, regulate qi and stop pain, or add *Golden Bell Powder* (Jin Ling Zi San) and *Coptis and evodia Pills* (Zuo Jin Wan) to cleanse the live and regulate qi, promote blood circulation and stop pain; for depressed qi turning into fire, buring the liver-yin with symptoms like dull pain on hypochondria, dizziness and dim eyesight, dry mouth, red tongue and fine taut pulse, add *Lycii Fructus* (Gou Qi Zi), *Polygoni Multiflori Radix* Praeparata (Zhi Shou Wu), *Ecliptae Herba* (Han Lian Cao) and *Chrysanthemi Flos* (Ju Hua) to nourish yin and cleanse the liver; for living qi attacking the stomach, causing disharmony between the liver and stomach, poor appetite, burping, nausea and vomiting, add

加减：胁痛重者，加青皮、陈皮、郁金、木香、延胡索、川楝子以增强理气止痛之功；若肝气郁结，久而化火，症见胁肋掣痛、心烦急躁、口干口苦、溺黄便秘、舌红苔黄、脉弦数，可加牡丹皮、山栀、龙胆草等清肝泻火、理气止痛，或加金铃子散、左金丸以清肝理气、活血止痛；若气郁化火，灼伤肝阴，症见胁肋隐痛、头晕眼花、口干舌红、脉弦细、可加枸杞子、制首乌、旱莲草、菊花以滋阴清肝；若肝气横逆犯胃，导致肝胃不和，纳呆嗳气、恶心欲呕者，加半夏、竹茹以和胃止呕。

Pinelliae Rhizoma (Ban Xia) and *Bambusae Caulis in Taenias* (Zhu Ru) to harmonize the stomach and stop vomiting.

2. 2. 2　Liver-blood Stasis and Blockade

Manifestations: Stabbing pain on hypochondria in fixed positions which gets worse at night or soot-black complexion, dark red blood streads and red moles in palm, lumps under the hypochondria; dark purple tongue or sometimes with stasis spots; deep taut uneven pulse.

Treatment: To promote blood circulation and remove blood stasis; dredge collaterals and stop pain.

Formulas and Herbs: *Subphrenic Stasis-Expelling Decoction* (Ge Xia Zhu Yu Tang), usually composed of *Persicae Semen* (Tao Ren) and *Carthami Flos* (Hong Hua) to resolve stasis and break clots, *Angelicae Sinensis Radix* (Dang Gui), *Toosendan Fructus* (Chuan Lian Zi), *Paeoniae Radix Rubra* (Chi Shao) to resolve stasis and break clots; *Cyperi Rhizoma* (Xiang Fu), *Aurantii Fructus*(Zhi Qiao), *Linderae Radix* (Wu Yao), *Corydalis Rhizoma* (Yan Hu Suo, Yuan Hu) and *Faeces Trogopterorum* (Wu Ling Zhi) to regulate qi, dredge collaterals and stop pain.

Modification: For remarkable blood stasis with hard painful lumps under the hypochondria and healthy qi not injured, add *Trionycis Carapax* (Bie Jia), *Sparganii Rhizoma* (San Leng), *Curcumae Rhizoma* (E Zhu) and *Eupolyphaga Steleophaga* (Zhe Chong) to eliminate stasis and lumps, or use Rhei and *Eupolyphaga Steleophaga Pills* (Da Huang Zhe Chong Wan) and *Trionycis Carapax* Pills (Bie Jia Jian Wan) to soften and loosen lumps; for blood

2. 2. 2　肝血瘀阻

证候: 胁肋刺痛,痛处不移,入夜尤甚,或见面色黧黑,手掌赤痕,赤缕红痣,胁下积块,舌质紫暗或有瘀点瘀斑,脉沉弦涩。

治法: 活血化瘀,通络止痛。

方药: 膈下逐瘀汤。常用:桃仁、红花化瘀散结;当归、川楝子、赤芍药养血活血,行瘀散结;香附、枳壳、乌药、延胡索、五灵脂理气通络止痛。

加减: 瘀血较重,胁下有癥块坚硬疼痛而正气未虚者,加鳖甲、三棱、莪术、地鳖虫等破瘀消坚,或合用大黄䗪虫丸、鳖甲煎丸以软坚散结;因跌仆闪挫而致瘀血内停,胁肋疼痛者,可用复元活血汤,同时吞服三七粉或云南白药等。

stasis and fluid retention due to falling and sprain with pain on hypochondria, use Vitality-Restoring Blood-Activating Decoction (Fu Yuan Huo Xue Tang) and swallow Notoginseng Powder (San Qi Fen) or Yunnan White Medicine (Yun Nan Bai Yao).

2. 2. 3 Damp-heat in the Liver and Gallbladder

Manifestations: Distenting pain or buring pain, or sharp pain on hypochondria, bitter and dry mouth, oppression in the chest, poor appetite, discomfort in the stomach, distention in the abdomen, or yellow eyes and skin, yellow-dark urine; yellow greasy tongur fur; rapid taut rolling pulse.

Treatment: To clear away and dispel damp-heat in the liver and gallbladder.

Formulas and Herbs: *Gentian Liver-Draining Decoction* (Long Dan Xie Gan Tang), usually composed of *Gentianae Radix et Rhizom* (Long Dan) to purge damp-heat in the liver and gallbladder; *Scutellariae Radix* (Huang Qin) and *Gardeniae Fructus* (Zhi Zi) to clear away heat and purge fire; *Bupleuri Radix* (Chai Hu), *Angelicae Sinensis Radix* (Dang Gui) and *Rehmannia Radix* (Sheng Di Huang) to disperse the liver, activate blood and cool blood; *Alismatis Rhizoma* (Ze Xie), *Akebiae Caulis* (Mu Tong) and *Plantaginis Semen* (Che Qian Zi) to clear away heat and resolve dampness through urine.

Modification: For heat predominance, constipation or loose but sticky stool, abdominal distention, add *Rhei Radix et Rhizoma* (Da Huang) and *Natrii Sulfas* (Mang Xiao) to purge heat and help urination; for dampness predominance, discomfort and distention in the abdomen and stomach, poor appetite and fatigue, add *Atractylodis Macrocephalae*

2. 2. 3 肝胆湿热

证候: 胁肋胀痛、灼痛,或剧痛,口干口苦,胸闷纳差,脘痞腹胀,或目黄身黄,小便黄赤。舌苔黄腻,脉弦滑数。

治法: 清利肝胆湿热。

方药: 龙胆泻肝汤。常用:龙胆草清泻肝胆湿热;黄芩、山栀清热泻火;柴胡、当归、生地黄疏肝、活血、凉血;泽泻、木通、车前子清热利湿,使湿热从小便而解。

加减: 若热重于湿,大便秘结或溏垢不爽、腹胀者,可加大黄、芒硝以泄热通便;如湿重于热,脘腹痞胀、纳呆乏力者,可加白术、茯苓、薏苡仁以健脾化湿;如发热黄疸、口渴便秘,加茵陈蒿汤以清

Rhizoma (Bai Zhu), *Poria* (Fu Ling) and *Coicis Semen* (Yi Yi Ren) to strengthen the spleen and dry dampness; for fever, jaundice, thirst and constipation, add *Artemisia, Poria and Artemisiae Chinghao Decoction* (Yin Chen Hao Tang) to clear away heat, resolve dampness and dispel yellowness; for sandstone blocking the gallbladder, remarkable hypochondriac pain reaching shoulders and back, add *Lysimachiae Herba* (Jin Qian Cao), *Lygodii Spora* (Hai Jin Sha) and *Aucklandiae Radix* (Mu Xiang) to dredge the gallbladder and eliminate sandstone; for roundworms finding way into gallbladder, twisting pain on sides, turing round and sleeplessness, use *Roundworm-Calming Mume Pills* (Wu Mei An Hui Wan) to calm the worms.

热利湿退黄；若因砂石阻于胆道，胁痛剧烈、牵引肩背者，加金钱草、海金砂、木香等利胆排石；若因蛔虫钻胆，胁痛如绞、辗转不安者，可用乌梅安蛔丸以安蛔。

2. 2. 4 Deficiency of Liver-yin

Manifestations: Dull continuous pain on hypochondria which gets worse at work, dry mouth and throat, vertigo and dry eyes, restlessness and irritation in five centers, feverish sensation in the afternoon; red tongue with little tongue fur; fine rapid taut pulse.

Treatment: To nourish yin and soften the liver; nourish blood and dredge collaterals.

Formulas and Herbs: *An Ever Effective Decoction for Nourishing Liver and Kidney* (Yi Guan Jian), usually composed of *Rehmannia Radix* (Sheng Di Huang) and *Lycii Fructus* (Gou Qi Zi) to nourish and nourish the liver and kidney; *Glehniae Radix* (Sha Shen), *Ophiopogonis Radix* (Mai Men Dong) and *Angelicae Sinensis Radix* (Dang Gui) to nourish yin and soften the liver; *Toosendan Fructus* (Chuan Lian Zi) to disperse the liver, regulate qi, harmonize collaterals and stop pain.

2. 2. 4 肝阴不足

证候：胁肋隐痛，其痛悠悠，绵绵不休，遇劳则重，口干咽燥，眩晕目涩，五心烦热，午后潮热，舌红少苔，脉弦细数。

治法：滋阴柔肝，养血通络。

方药：一贯煎。常用：生地黄、枸杞子滋养肝肾；沙参、麦门冬、当归养阴柔肝；川楝子疏肝理气、和络止痛。

Modification: Dizziness and vertigo, dim eyes, remarkable yin deficiency of liver and kidney, add *Ligustri Lucidi Fructus* (Nü Zhen Zi), *Ecliptae Herba* (Han Lian Cao), *Paeoniae Radix Alba* (Bai Shao Yao), *Polygonati Rhizoma* (Huang Jing) and *Chrysanthemi Flos* (Ju Hua) to nourish and nourish the liver and kidney, relieve vertigo and improve eyesight; for thirst and plenty of drink, slippery red tongue with no tongue, add *Trichosanthis Radix* (Tian Hua Fen), *Polygonati Odorati Rhizoma* (Yu Zhu), *Dendrobii Caulis* (Shi Hu) to nourish yin and generate fluid; for lassitude and fatigue, add *Ginseng Radix et Rhizoma* (Ren Shen) or *Pseudostellariae Radix* (Tai Zi Shen) to boost qi and nourish yin.

加减：头晕目眩、视物昏花，肝肾阴虚明显者，加女贞子、旱莲草、白芍药、黄精、菊花以滋补肝肾、止眩明目；口渴多饮、舌光红无苔者，加天花粉、玉竹、石斛以养阴生津；神疲乏力者，加人参或太子参以益气养阴。

Jaundice

黄 疸

Jaundice is a disease featuring yellow eyes, yellow skins and yellow urine, in particular, yellow eyes and pupils, caused by the liver and gallbladder's failure to disperse so that the bile deviates from the usual way into blood and is reflected on the skin.

黄疸主要因肝胆疏泄失常，胆汁不循常道，渗入血液，溢于肌肤，而导致的以目黄、身黄、尿黄为主症的一种病证。其中尤以目睛黄染为主要特征。

1 Etiology and Pathogenesis

1 病因病机

Jaundice is mainly caused by epidemic pathogenic factors, improper diet and zang-fu organ disorders. Pathogenic dampnessencumbers the spleen and stomach, blocks the liver and gallbladder, which fail to disperse properly and bile erupts, leading to jaundice.

黄疸的病因主要有感受时邪疫毒、饮食所伤及脏腑功能失调等，导致湿邪困阻脾胃，壅塞肝胆，疏泄失常，胆汁泛溢而发病。

1.1 Invasion of Damp-heat Due to Affection of Epidemic Pathogenic

1.1 感受邪毒，湿热内侵

Epidemic pathogenic factors, after invading into the body via mouth or skin, gather in zhong jiao,

感受时邪疫毒，自口而入，或从表入里，蕴结于中

disenabling the stomach of transferring and transporting. Then damp-heat steams the liver and gallbladder, disenabling the liver of dispersing. The bile spills over and reveals itself through skin, the eyes upwards and bladder downwards. The eyes and urine turn yellow and that is jaundice. In case of severe epidemic pathogenic affection, it sets on rapidly, deadly and is contagious in which the yin-blood will be greatly damaged by exuberant heat. That is called acute jaundice.

焦，致脾胃运化失常，湿热交蒸于肝胆，肝失疏泄，胆液外溢，浸淫肌肤，上侵于目，下注膀胱，使身目小便俱黄，发为黄疸。若疫毒重者，其病势暴急凶险，具有传染性，表现为热毒炽盛、迅速伤及营血的严重现象，称为急黄。

1.2 Damp-heat In Spleen and Stomach Due to Improper Diet

1.2 饮食所伤，脾胃湿热

Improper diet, including irregular hunger and gluttony and over-drinking will make damages to the spleen and stomach, disenabling the spleen and stomach of transferring and transporting, which leads to turbidity produced inside and depression transforming into heat, scorching the liver and gallbladder. Thebile overspills and penetrates into skin which turns on yellow.

饮食所伤，饥饱失常或嗜酒过度，皆能损伤脾胃，以致运化功能失职，湿浊内生，郁而化热，熏蒸肝胆，胆汁外溢，浸淫肌肤而发黄。

1.3 Yang Deficiency Due to Weak Constitution and Deficieny-cold of the Spleen and Stomach

1.3 素体阳虚，脾胃虚寒

Innate weakness of the spleen and stomach or spleen-yang injured due to prolonged illness causes the spleen and stomach to fail to transfer and transport, resulting in the damge of qi and blood, which causes the transformation of cold into dampness. When it lasts for long, the liver lacks in nurturing and fail to disperse and purge, leading to bile overspilling.

素体脾胃虚弱，或久病脾阳受损，导致脾胃运化失司，气血亏损，湿从寒化，久之肝失所养，疏泄失职而致胆汁外溢发黄。

1.4 Stasis and Blockade of Vessels and Collaterals Due to Prolonged Illness

1.4 久病迁延，脉络瘀阻

Retention which cannot be eliminated due to prolonged illness will cause stasis and blockade in

久病迁延不愈，积聚日久不消，脉络瘀阻，或因砂

vessels and collaterals. Or sandstones and worms obstruct the gallbladder, preventing the liver and gallbladder from functioning properly. When the gallbladder is blocked, the bile spills over, leading to jaundice.

石、虫体阻滞胆道，肝胆疏泄不畅，胆道淤滞，胆汁外溢，发为黄疸。

Pathogenic dampness is the key to jaundice. Malfunction of the spleen, stomach, liver, and gallbladder is the cause. Besides, it is more often than not that liver and gallbladder are affected by the dysfunction of the spleen and stomach. Jaundice can be put into different types according to yin, yang, defiency and excess by its pathological nature. Generally speaking, exuberant yang and heat, fairly high stomach-fire, damp-heat accumulated inside are likely to be jaundice of yang type. Damp-heat along with epidemic pathogenic factors is acute jaundice. Excess yin and cold and weak spleen-yang tend to be jaundice of yin type. All of the three types are interchangeable. For example, if jaundice of yang is not treated in time and prolonged, or has been treated with cold and bitter herbs that may hurt the spleen-yang, jaundice of yang type would grow into yin type. When damp-heat turns into pathogenic factors and grows serious, it will soon get worse and change to acute jaundice.

黄疸病机关键在于湿邪，主要责之于脾胃肝胆功能失调，且往往由脾胃涉及肝胆。黄疸的病理性质有阴阳虚实之分。一般而言：阳盛热甚，胃火偏旺之人，湿热内蕴，多为阳黄；湿热夹毒，热毒炽盛发为急黄；阴盛寒甚，脾阳不振之人，寒湿阻遏，多为阴黄。阳黄、阴黄、急黄三者可相互转化，如阳黄失治，迁延日久，或过用苦寒之品，致脾阳受伐，则可转为阴黄；若阳黄因湿热化毒，病邪深重，致黄疸迅速加深，病情迅速加重，而转化为急黄危候。

2 Syndrome Differentiation and Treatment

2 辨证论治

2.1 Key Points of Syndrome Differentiation

2.1 辨治要点

Jaundice can be identifiedby the guidance of yin and yang and in terms of pathogenesis, clinical history, stages, complexion, stool and urine, tongue and pulse and diet. Jaundice of yang type is caused by damp-heat which starts quickly but lasts short. The color looks fresh like orange. Other symptoms

黄疸的辨证应以阴阳为纲，围绕病因、病史、病程、肤色、二便、舌脉，结合饮食等情况来进行：阳黄以湿热为患，一般起病急，病程短，黄色鲜明如橘色，常伴口干发

are dry mouth and fever, short and dark urine, dry stool, yellow greasy tongue fur and rapid taut pulse. All these are symptoms of damp-heat in the liver and gallbladder. On the contrary, jaundice of yin type takes on gradually and unconsciously which lasts long. The color is dull and dark yellow or smoky. Usually, there are other symptoms such as poor appetite, distention in the stomach, loose stool, lassitude and physical cold, tastelessness and no thirst, pale tongue with white greasy tongue fur, slippery soft pulse or deep retarded pulse. All these features spleen-yang deficiency and damp-cold blockade. Clinically, jaundice can be further distinguished according to the severity of dampness and heat along with the predominance of yin or yang in the human body. In terms of treatment, the principle should be to dissolve dampness and promote urination. Dissolving dampness can effectively expel yellowness. For damp-heat, clear away heat and dissslove dampness and dredge fu-organ if necessary to purge damp-heat. For cold-dampness, invigorate the spleen and dissolve dampness by warming. For promoting urination, eliminate dampness with bland drugs to dispel yellowness. For acute jaundice and pathogenic factors invading into heart-ying, clear away heat to detoxify and cool ying to open into orifices. For jaundice of yin type due to spleen deficiency and dampness stagnation, invigorate the spleen and nourish blood to eliminate dampness and dispel yellowness.

热，小便短赤，大便秘结，舌苔黄腻，脉弦数等肝胆湿热之证；阴黄多以寒湿为主，起病隐匿或缓慢，病程长，黄色晦暗，或如烟薰，常伴纳少、脘胀、大便不实、神疲形寒、口淡不渴、舌淡苔白腻、脉濡滑或沉迟等脾阳不足、寒湿阻遏之证。阳黄由于感受湿与热邪的程度不同，患者机体阴阳偏盛不同，故临床有湿与热邪孰轻孰重之分，治疗上以化湿邪、利小便为原则。化湿可以退黄，湿热当清热化湿，必要时应通利腑气，以使湿热下泄，寒湿当健脾温化；利小便主要是通过淡渗利湿以退黄。至于急黄热毒炽盛，邪入心营者，当以清热解毒，凉营开窍为主。阴黄脾虚湿滞者，治以健脾养血，利湿退黄。

2.2 Therapeutic Methods for Different Patterns

2.2 分型论治

2.2.1 Jaundice of Yang Type with Predomination of Heat

2.2.1 阳黄热重于湿

Manifestations: Eyes turning yellow and yellow

证候：白睛发黄，迅速至

all over in a short time, bright yellow, quite severe jaundice, fever, thirst, irritation, nausea, vomiting, poor appetite, short and dark yellow urine, dry stool; red tongue with yellow greasy or yellow coarse tongue fur; rapid taut pulse or slippery rapid pulse.

全身发黄，黄疸较重，色泽鲜明，发热口渴，心中懊侬，恶心，呕吐，纳呆，小便赤黄、短少，大便秘结。舌红苔黄腻或黄糙，脉弦数或滑数。

Treatment: To clear away heat and eliminate dampness along with dredging fu-organs.

治法：清热利湿，佐以通腑。

Formulas and Herbs: *Artemisia, Poria and Artemisiae Chinghao Decoction* (Yin Chen Hao Tang), usually composed of *Artemisiae Scopariae Herba* (Yin Chen) to clear away heat, eliminate dampness and dispel yellowness, *Gardeniae Fructus* (Zhi Zi) to purge damp-heat in the three jiaos and *Rhei Radix et Rhizoma* (Da Huang) to purge heat and dredge downward.

方药：茵陈蒿汤。常用：茵陈清热利湿退黄；栀子清泄三焦湿热；大黄清热通下。

Modification: Add moderately *Isatidis Radix* (Ban Lan Gen), *Forsythiae Fructus* (Lian Qiao), *Isatisdis Folium* (Da Qing Ye), *Polygoni Cuspidati Rhizoma et Radix* (Hu Zhang) and *Herba Hyperici Japonici* (Tian Ji Huang) to clear away heat and detoxify and *Plantaginis Semen* (Che Qian Zi), *Polyporus* (Zhu Ling) and *Alismatis Rhizoma* (Ze Xie) to injuce pathogenic dampness; for distention in the abdomen and sharp pain around hypochondria, add *Bupleuri Radix* (Chai Hu), *Curcumae Radix* (Yu Jin) and *Toosendan Fructus* (Chuan Lian Zi) to diperse the liver and regulate qi; for nausea and feeling to vomit, add *Citri Reticulatae Pericarpium* (Chen Pi), *Bambusae Caulis in Taenias* (Zhu Ru) and *Pinelliae Rhizoma* (Ban Xia) to lower the upward flow and stop vomiting; for irritation and spontaneous external bleeding, add *Moutan Cortex* (Mu Dan Pi) and *Paeoniae Radix Rubra* (Chi Shao)

加减：可酌加板蓝根、连翘、大青叶、虎杖、田基黄等以清热解毒，车前子、猪苓、泽泻等以渗利湿邪；如腹胀胁痛较甚可加柴胡、郁金、川楝子等疏肝理气；如恶心欲吐可加陈皮、竹如、半夏以降逆止呕；如心烦、衄血者，可加牡丹皮、赤芍药以凉血止血；如因虫体阻止胆道，突然出现黄疸、胁痛时发时止、痛而有钻顶感，宜加乌梅丸以安蛔止痛。

to cool blood and stop bleeding; for worms blocking the gallbladder, and sudden jaundice with coming-and-going penetrating pain around the hypochondria, add *Black Plum Pills* (Wu Mei Wan) to calm roundworms to stop pain.

2. 2. 2　Jaundice of Yang Type with Predonimation of Dampness

Manifestations: Yellow skin and eyes but not as evident as jaundice of yang type proodimated by heat, recessive heat, general heaviness, favor lying, fatigue, discomfort and oppression in the chest and abdomen, poor appetite, vomiting, nausea, aversion to greasy food, slimy sensation in the mouth, inhibited urination, grimy sloppy stool; thick yellowish greasy tongue fur; slow soft pulse or slippery taut pulse.

Treatment: To eliminate dampness and dissolve turbidity along with clear awaying away heat.

Formulas and Herbs: *Artemisia and Poria Five Powder* (Yin Chen Wu Ling San) or *Sweet Dew Toxin-Dispersing Elixir* (Gan Lu Xiao Du Dan), usually composed *Artemisiae Scopariae Herba* (Yin Chen) is used to clear away heat, eliminate dampness and dispel yellowness; *Polyporus* (Zhu Ling), *Poria* (Fu Ling) and *Alismatis Rhizoma* (Ze Xie) to eliminate dampness with bland herbs; *Atractylodis Macrocephalae Rhizoma* (Bai Zhu) to strengthen the spleen and dry dampness; *Talcum* (Hua Shi) and *Akebiae Caulis* (Mu Tong) to clear away heat and eliminate dampness through urination;, *Scutellariae Radix* (Huang Qin) and *Forsythiae Fructus* (Lian Qiao) to clear away heat, dry dampness and detoxify; *Acori Tatarinowii Rhizoma* (Shi Chang Pu), Semen Amomi Rotundus (Bai Kou Ren), *Pogostemonis Herba*

2. 2. 2　阳黄湿重于热

证候: 身目发黄,但不如前者鲜明,身热不扬,头重身困,嗜卧乏力,胸脘痞闷,纳呆呕恶,厌食油腻,口黏不渴,小便不利,大便溏垢。舌苔厚腻微黄,脉濡缓或弦滑。

治法: 利湿化浊,佐以清热。

方药: 茵陈五苓散或甘露消毒丹。常用:茵陈清热利湿退黄;配以猪苓、茯苓、泽泻淡渗利湿;白术健脾燥湿;滑石、木通清热利湿,引湿热之邪从小便而出;黄芩、连翘清热燥湿解毒;石菖蒲、白蔻仁、藿香、薄荷芳香化浊,行气悦脾,宣利气机而化湿浊。

(Huo Xiang) and *Menthae Haplocalycis Herba* (Bo He) to dissolve turbidity with aromatizing to promote qi flow, disperse qi and dissolve turbidity.

Modification: For dampness encumbering the spleen and stomach, oppression and distention in the stomach, sweet in the mouth, add *Magnoliae Officinalis Cortex* (Hou Pu) and *Atractylodis Rhizoma* (Cang Zhu); for poor appetite or no appetite, add *Stir-fried Hordei Fructus Germinatus* (Chao Mai Ya) and *Galli Gigerii Endothelium Corneum* (Ji Nei Jin) to awaken the spleen and resolve food retention; for onset stage of jaundice of yang type with exterior symptoms, use *Ephedrae, Forsythiae and Phaseoli Decoction* (Ma Huang Lian Qiao Chi Xiao Dou Tang) to relieve exterior symptoms, clear away heat and resolve dampness; for lingering fever due to unpurged damp-heat, add *Gardenia and Phellodendron Decoction* (Zhi Zi Bai Pi Tang) to help purge heat and resolve dampness; for exburant heat in Yangming meridian consumes body fluid, resulting in constipation, use *Rhubarb and Niter Decoction* (Da Huang Xiao Shi Tang) to purge heat and expel excess, in order to preserve yin.

加减：若湿困脾胃，胃脘闷胀、口中甜者，可加厚朴、苍术；纳呆或无食欲者加炒麦芽、鸡内金以醒脾消食；阳黄初起见表证者，宜用麻黄连翘赤小豆汤以解表清热利湿；如热留未退，乃因湿热未得透泄，可加用栀子柏皮汤，增强泻热利湿作用；病程中如见阳明热盛，灼伤津液，积滞成实，大便不通者，宜用大黄硝石汤泻热去实、急下存阴。

2.2.3 Acute Jaundice

Manifestations: Sudden attack, yellowness turning into golden in a short period of time, excessive heat, irritation, thirst, frequent burping, little urine, constipation, distention in abdomen, hypochondriac pain, restlessness, unconsciousness and delirium, vomiting or blood stool, ecchymosis; scartlet tongue with dry yellow tongue fur; rapid taut pulse or large surging pulse.

Treatment: To clear away heat and detoxify; cool blood and open into orifices.

2.2.3 急黄

证候：起病急骤，黄疸迅速加深，其色如金，壮热烦渴，呕吐频作，尿少便结，腹胀，胁痛，烦躁不安，或神昏谵语，或呕血便血，皮下瘀斑。舌质红绛，苔黄而干燥，脉弦数或洪大。

治法：清热解毒，凉血开窍。

Formulas and Herbs: *Thousand-Gold Rhinoceros Horn Powder* (Qian Jin Xi Jiao San), usually composed of *Cornu Rhinoceri Asiatici* (Xi Jiao) [which can be substituted for *Bubali Cornu* (Shui Niu Jiao)] to clear away heat and detoxify; *Coptidis Rhizoma* (Huang Lian), *Gardeniae Fructus* (Zhi Zi) and *Cimicifugae Rhizoma* (Sheng Ma) to clear away heat, detoxify and cool ying; *Artemisiae Scopariae Herba* (Yin Chen) to clear away heat, eliminate dampness and dispel yellowness.

方药: 千金犀角散。常用:犀角(可用水牛角代之)清热解毒凉血;黄连、栀子、升麻清热解毒凉营;茵陈清热利湿退黄。

Modification: For excessive heat and constipation, add *Rhei Radix et Rhizoma* (Da Huang) and *Natrii Sulfas* (Mang Xiao), or *Five-Ingredient Toxin-Dispersing Beverage* (Wu Wei Xiao Du Yin) to clear away heat and detoxify; for irritation and restlessness, spiritual disturbance, add *Peaceful Palace Bovine Bezoar Pills* (An Gong Niu Huang Wan) or *Crown Jewel Elixir* (Zhi Bao Dan) to cool and open into orifices; for external bleeding or ecchymosis, add *Sanguisorbiae Radix Preparata* (Di Yu Tan) and *Platycladi Cacumen Preparata* (Bai Ye Tan) to cool blood and stop bleeding; for little and short urine and difficult urination, or abdominal dropsy, add *Imperatae Rhizoma* (Bai Mao Gen), *Plantaginis Herba* (Che Qian Cao), *Plantaginis Semen* (Che Qian Zi), *Polyporus* (Zhu Ling) and *Arecae Pericarpium* (Da Fu Pi) to clear away heat and induce urination.

加减: 热毒炽盛,大便秘结者,可加大黄、芒硝,或加用五味消毒饮以清解热毒;如出现躁扰不宁、心神昏乱,可配服安宫牛黄丸或至宝丹以凉开清窍;如衄血、便血或者肌肤瘀斑重者,可加用地榆炭、柏叶炭等凉血止血之品;如小便短少不利,或出现腹水者,可加用白茅根、车前草、车前子、猪苓、大腹皮等清热利尿之品。

2.2.4 Jaundice of Yin Type

Manifestations: Yellow skin and eyes, dark dull yellowness or smoky yellowness, discomfort in the stomach, little intake, lassitude, aversion to cold, distention in abdomen, loose stool; pale tongue with white greasy tongue fur; slow soft pulse or deep re-

2.2.4 阴黄

证候: 身目俱黄,黄色晦暗不泽,或如烟熏,痞满食少,神疲畏寒,腹胀便溏,口淡不渴。舌淡苔白腻,脉濡缓或沉迟。

tarded pulse.

Treatment: To warm the middle and dissolve dampness; strengthen the spleen and harmonize the stomach.

治法: 温中化湿,健脾和胃。

Formulas and Herbs: *Artemisia, Atractylodis and Aconiti Decoction* (Yin Chen Zhu Fu Tang), usually composed of *Artemisiae Scopariae Herba* (Yin Chen) to expel dampness, induce the gallbladder and dispel yellowness; *Aconm Lateralis Radix Praeparata* (Fu Zi) and *Zingiberis Rhizoma* (Gan Jiang) to warm the middle and expel cold; *Atractylodis Macrocephalae Rhizoma* (Bai Zhu) and *Glycyrrhizae Radix et Rhizoma* (Gan Cao) to strengthen the spleen and harmonize the stomach.

方药: 茵陈术附汤。常用:茵陈除湿利胆退黄;附子、干姜温中散寒;白术、甘草健脾和胃。

Modification: For distention in abdomen and thick tongue fur, delete *Glycyrrhizae Radix et Rhizoma* (Gan Cao) and add *Atractylodis Rhizoma* (Cang Zhu) and *Magnoliae Officinalis Cortex* (Hou Po) to dry dampness and remove distention; for distention due to lumps under the hypochondria in fixed spots, dark yellow complexion, dizziness, fatigue, dark red tongue fur, fine taut pulse, which are the characteristics of deficiency of qi and blood, pathogenic turbidity blocking the vessels and collaterals, use *Niter and Alum Powder* (Xiao Shi Fan Shi San) to remove turbidity and stasis, and soften the hard lumps; for prolonged jaundice, qi stagnation and blood stasis, lingering turbidity, lumps under hypochondria with sharp pain which refuse to be pressed, use *Decocted Turtle Shell Pills* (Bie Jia Jian Wan) to promote blood circulation and remove stasis and *Free Wanderer Powder* (Xiao Yao San) can be used along to disperse the liver and strengthen the spleen; for remarkable weak spleen and stom-

加减: 若腹胀苔厚者,可去甘草加苍术、厚朴以燥湿消胀;如胁下积块胀痛、固定不移,肤色暗黄,头晕乏力,舌质暗红,脉弦细,乃属气血两虚、浊邪瘀阻脉络,可用硝石矾石散以化浊祛瘀软坚;如因黄疸日久,气滞血瘀,湿浊残留,结于胁下,并见胁下积块、刺痛拒按,宜服鳖甲煎丸,活血化瘀,并可配服逍遥散以疏肝扶脾;如脾胃虚弱明显者,可配服香砂六君子汤以健脾和胃。

ach, add *Aucklandia, Amomum and Six Nobles Decoction* (Xiang Sha Liu Jun Zi Tang) to strengthen the spleen and harmonize the stomach.

Tympanites

Tympanites is a disease characteriszing abdominal distention, or even prominent green-blue abdominal veins, protruding navel and greenish yellow or soot black complextion due to retention of qi, blood, fluid and water, casued by malfunction of the liver, spleen, and kidney.

1 Etiology and Pathogenesis

Tympanites is mainly caused by malfunction of the liver, spleen and kidney due to emotional and spiritual injuries, over-drinkig and overstrain, schistosome infection, jaundice and accumulation that has not been resolved in time, leading to qi stagnation, blood stasis, water-damp intertangled in the abdomen.

1.1 Liver and Spleen Injuries Due to Emotional and Spiritual Factors, Drink and Diet

Emotional and Spiritual depression causes liver-qi to be depressed and then qi stagnation and blood stasis. When depressed live-qi interferes with the spleen or when over worry injuries the spleen, the spleen will lose itscontrolance of transportation and therefore, water and grain cannot be turned into essence but water-damp instead. When water-damp gathers in zhong jiao along with qi stagnation and blood stasis affecting one another for long, it will cause discomfort and blockade in zhong jiao, resulting in tympanites.

鼓　胀

鼓胀主要是因肝脾肾功能失调,气、血、水内停而导致的以腹部胀大,甚则腹壁青筋显露,脐心突起,面色苍黄或黧黑为主症的一种的病证。

1　病因病机

鼓胀的发生主要是由于情志所伤、酒食不节、劳欲过度、感染血吸虫及黄疸、积聚失治等因素,导致肝脾肾三脏功能失调,气滞、瘀血、水湿互结于腹中而发病。

1.1　情志酒食,损伤肝脾

情志抑郁,肝气郁结,致气滞血瘀;肝气郁结,横逆犯脾,或思虑伤脾,均能使脾运不健,水谷不化精微而成水湿,水湿停聚中焦,与气滞、瘀血蕴结日久不化,痞塞中焦,便成鼓胀。

Favor for alcohol and sweat greasy food, improper diet oraccumulation of cold food will damage the spleen and the stomach and disenable them as controlance of transference and transportation, leading to damp-turbidity. Or when the liver is injured by alcohol toxin, liver-qi will be depressed which leads to qi stagnation and blood stasis. All of qi, blood and water finally block in the abdomen, resulting in tympanites.

嗜酒肥甘，饮食不节，或寒食积滞，损伤脾胃，运化失职，湿浊内生；或因酒毒伤肝，肝郁气滞血瘀，终致气、血、水三者交阻腹中，变成鼓胀。

1.2 Spleen and Kidney Deficiency Due to Overstrain

1.2 劳欲过度，脾肾两虚

The kidney stores essence and is thecongenital foundation and the spleen controls the transportation and transference and is the foundation of acquired constitution. These two are the source of life. Overstrain will damage the spleen and kidney. When the spleen is damaged, it fails to transport and transfer and therefore water-damp is produced inside. When the kidney is hurt, it fails to transform qi and breaks down qi activities and then dampness accumulates and water is produced. All these will lead to tympanites.

肾藏精为先天之本，脾主运化为后天之源，两者为生命之根本。劳欲过度伤及脾肾，脾伤则不能运化水谷，水湿内生；肾损则气化不行，湿聚水生而成鼓胀。

1.3 Stagnation of Liver Vessels Dueto Water-toxin Affection

1.3 水毒久病，肝脉瘀阻

Damage of Schistosoma infection to the liver and spleen causes the accumulation of water-toxin, stagnation of qi activity, stasis of vessels and collaterals, the dysfuction of qi ascending and descending, and the mixture of clarity and turdity, which all finally results in tympanites. Besides, when jaundice is prolonged, damp-turbidity goes so intense that the middle-qi is hurt and exhausted, qi and blood of the liver and spleen fail to move smoothly and vessels and collaterals are blocked. Or

感染血吸虫，内伤肝脾，水毒内结，气机郁滞，脉络瘀阻，升降失常，清浊相混，逐渐而形成鼓胀。另外，黄疸日久，湿浊壅甚，中气亏耗，肝脾气血运行不畅，脉络瘀阻；或因积聚日久，气血瘀滞，水湿内聚，而为鼓胀。

when there is retention for long, qi and blood will be stagnated and water-damp is produced, causing tympanites.

Tympanites lies in the liver, spleen and kidney. The main pathological factors are qi stagnation, blood stasis and water-damp which interact one with another and interchange. During the onset stage, qi stagnation and damp-blockage are the main factors. Later, it is more likely due to malfunctions of zang-fu organs because of which, qi, blood and water block in the abdomen and fail to be transferred. The deficient will go even more deficient and the excessive, more execesive and it takes on the signs of tangled stasis and heat, yin-deficiency of the liver and kidney, yang-deficiency of the spleen and kidney. The pathological features are primary deficiency and the secondary excess as well as complication of the primary and secondary symptoms.

鼓胀的病位在肝、脾、肾，病理因素主要有气滞、瘀血、水湿，三者相互壅结，相互转化：初期多以气滞湿阻或湿热壅结为主；后期则多因脏腑功能失调，气血水壅滞腹中而不化，虚者愈虚，实者愈实，呈现瘀热互结，肝肾阴虚，脾肾阳虚之象。主要病机特点是本虚标实、虚实夹杂。

2 Syndrome Differentiation and Treatment

2.1 Key Points of Syndrome Differentiation

Doctors should identifytympanites in light of the primary symptoms and the secondary symptoms, defiency and excess. For the secondary excess, doctors should distinguish predominance of qi stagnation, water-damp and blood stasis. For the primary deficiency, distinguish the predominance of yin deficiency and yang deficiency and main pathological organ, the liver, spleen or kidney. The treatment should follow the principle of simultaneous supplementating and attacking therapy. For the secondary excess, it is advisable to promote qi flow, active blood circulation, dispel dampness, and eliminate dampness. Or use temporarily attacking and dispel-

2 辨证论治

2.1 辨治要点

鼓胀辨证当分清标本虚实：标实当辨气滞、水湿、瘀血的偏盛；本虚当辨阴虚与阳虚之不同，并分肝、脾、肾之侧重。治疗原则为攻补兼施：标实为主者，当根据气、血、水的偏盛，分别采用行气、活血、祛湿利水或暂用攻逐之法，同时配以疏肝健脾；本虚为主者，当根据阴阳的不同，分别采取温补脾肾或滋养肝肾法，同时配合行气活血利水；本虚标实错杂，治

ling methods along with other methods to disperse the liver and strengthen the spleen. For the primary deficiency, according to the difference between yin and yang, adopt methods of warming and supplementing the spleen and kidney or nourishing and nurturing the liver and kidney respectively, along with methods of promoting qi flow, activating blood and inducing diuresis. For complication of both the primary and secondary symptoms, attack and supplement simultaneously. Supplement deficiency without neglecting the excess and purge excess without neglecting deficiency.

当攻补兼施，补虚不忘实，泻实不忘虚。

2.2　Different Types of Tympanites

2.2　分型论治

2.2.1　Qi Stagnation and Damp Blockage

2.2.1　气滞湿阻

Manifestations: Abdominal distention that doesn't feel hard when pressed, distention and fullness or pain in hypochondria, decreasing intake, distention after diet, burping and discomfort, little and short urination; white greasy tongue fur; taut pulse.

证候： 腹胀大按之不坚，胁下胀满或疼痛，饮食减少，食后作胀，嗳气不适，小便短少。舌苔白腻，脉弦。

Treatment: To disperse the liver and regulate qi; eliminate dampness and remove fullness.

治法： 疏肝理气，行湿散满。

Formulas and Herbs: *Bupleurum-Dispersing-Liver Powder* (Chai Hu Shu Gan San) and *Poria Stomach Decoction* (Wei Ling Tang), usually composed of *Bupleuri Radix* (Chai Hu), *Aurantii Fructus* (Zhi Qiao), *Paeoniae Radix Alba* (Bai Shao Yao) and *Cyperi Rhizoma* (Xiang Fu) to diperse the liver and regulate qi; *Chuanxiong Rhizoma* (Chuan Xiong) to promote qi flow and activate blood circulation; *Glycyrrhizae Radix et Rhizoma* (Gan Cao) to harmonize zhong jiao, *Atractylodis Macrocephalae Rhizoma* (Bai Zhu), *Poria* (Fu Ling), *Polyporus* (Zhu Ling) and *Alismatis Rhizoma* (Ze Xie) to strength-

方药： 柴胡疏肝散合胃苓汤。常用：柴胡、枳壳、白芍药、香附疏肝理气；川芎行气活血；甘草和中；白术、茯苓、猪苓、泽泻健脾利湿；桂枝辛温通阳；苍术、陈皮、厚朴行湿散满。

en the spleen and eliminate dampness; *Cinnamomi Ramulus* (Gui Zhi) to free yang with warmth and acridity, *Atractylodis Rhizoma* (Cang Zhu), *Citri Reticulatae Pericarpium* (Chen Pi) and *Magnoliae Officinalis Cortex* (Hou Pu) to eliminate dampness and remove fullness.

Modification: For yellowish greasy tongue fur, dry and bitter mouth, taut pulse and depressed qi transforming into fire, add *Moutan Cortex* (Mu Dan Pi) and *Gardeniae Fructus* (Zhi Zi); for dizziness, insomnia, red tongue, fine rapid taut pulse and depressed qi transforming into heat that injuries yin, add *Polygoni Multiflori Radix* Praeparata (Zhi Shou Wu), *Lycii Fructus* (Gou Qi Zi) and *Ligustri Lucidi Fructus* (Nü Zhen Zi) to nourish and nourish yin; for stabbing pain in hypochondria, dark complexion, purple tongue, taut uneven pulse, which are areh symptoms of qi stagnation and blood stasis, add *Corydalis Rhizoma* (Yan Hu Suo, Yuan Hu), *Curcumae Rhizoma* (E Zhu) and *Salviae Miltiorrhizae Radix et Rhizoma Radix* (Dan Shen) to active blood and remove stasis.

加减： 如苔腻微黄、口干而苦、脉弦数，气郁化火者，可加丹皮、栀子；如头晕、不寐、舌质红、脉弦细数，气郁化热伤阴者，可加制首乌、枸杞子、女贞子等养血滋阴之品；如胁下刺痛不移、面色晦暗、舌紫、脉弦涩，气滞血瘀者，可加延胡索、莪术、丹参等活血化瘀之品。

2.2.2 Cold-damp Emcumbering the Spleen

2.2.2 寒湿困脾

Manifestations: Distention and fullness in the abdomen which feels like a bag containing full water when pressed, slight swollen face, edema of lower limbs, discomfort and distention in the stomach which is slightly relieved when warmed, general heaviness, fatigue and tiredness, fear of cold and laziness to move, little short urine, loose thin stool; white greasy tongue fur; slow pulse.

证候： 腹大胀满，按之如囊裹水，甚则颜面微肿，下肢浮肿，脘腹痞胀，得热稍舒，周身困重，精神困倦，怯寒懒动，小便短少，大便溏薄，舌苔白腻，脉缓。

Treatment: To warm yang and strengthen the spleen; regulate qi and eliminate dampness.

治法： 温阳健脾，行气利水。

Formulas and Herbs: *Spleen-Firming Decoction*

方药： 实脾饮。常用：附

(Shi Pi Yin), usually composed of *Aconm Lateralis Radix Praeparata* (Fu Zi), *Zingiberis Rhizoma* (Gan Jiang), *Atractylodis Macrocephalae Rhizoma* (Bai Zhu) and *Glycyrrhizae Radix et Rhizoma* (Gan Cao) to boost spleen-yang; *Chaenomelis Fructus* (Mu Gua), *Arecae Pericarpium* (Da Fu Pi) and *Poria* (Fu Ling) to regulate qi and eliminate dampness; *Aucklandiae Radix* (Mu Xiang), *Tsaoko Fructus* (Cao Guo) and *Jujubae Fructus* (Da Zao) to regulate qi, strengthen the spleen and dry dampness.

子、干姜、白术、甘草振奋脾阳;木瓜、大腹皮、茯苓行气利水;厚朴、木香、草果、大枣以理气健脾燥湿。

Modification: For serious water-damp, add *Cinnamomi Cortex* (Rou Gui), *Polyporus* (Zhu Ling), *Alismatis Rhizoma* (Ze Xie) to help the bladder to transform qi and induce urination; for qi deficiency and short breath, add moderately *Astragali Radix* (Huang Qi) and *Codonopsis Radix* (Dang Shen) to supplement qi of the lung and spleen; for distention and pain around hypochondria and in the abdomen, add *Curcumae Radix* (Yu Jin), *Citri Reticulatae Pericarpium Viride* (Qing Pi) and *Amomi Fructus* (Sha Ren) to regulate qi and relieve the middle.

加减:如水湿过重,可加肉桂、猪苓、泽泻以助膀胱气化而利小便;气虚息短者,可酌加黄芪、党参以补肺脾之气;如胁腹胀痛,可加郁金、青皮、砂仁等理气宽中。

2.2.3 Accumulation of Dampness-heat

2.2.3 湿热蕴结

Manifestations: Large, hard and full abdomen, bulging feeling in the stomach and abdomen, feverish sensation, irritation, bitter mouth, hot urine, constipation or loose stool, or yellow complexion, eyes and skin; red tongue tip and sides, yellow greasy or yellow greasy grayish black tongue fur; taut rapid pulse.

证候:腹大坚满,脘腹撑急,烦热口苦,渴不欲饮,小便赤涩,大便秘结或溏垢,或有面目肌肤发黄。舌尖边红,苔黄腻或兼灰黑,脉象弦数。

Treatment: To clear away heat and eliminate dampness; eliminate retention of fluid by purgation.

治法:清热利湿,攻下逐水。

Formulas and Herbs: *Center Fullness Separating and Dispersing Pill* (Zhong Man Fen Xiao Wan) and *Artemisia, Poria and Artemisiae Chinghao Decoction* (Yin Chen Hao Tang), usually composed of *Scutellariae Radix* (Huang Qin), *Coptidis Rhizoma* (Huang Lian), *Anemarrhenae Rhizoma* (Zhi Mu), *Artemisiae Scopariae Herba* (Yin Chen), *Rhei Radix et Rhizoma* (Da Huang) and *Gardeniae Fructus* (Zhi Zi) to clear away heat and dissolve dampness; *Magnoliae Officinalis Cortex* (Hou Pu), *Aurantii Fructus* (Zhi Qiao), *Pinelliae Rhizoma* (Ban Xia) and *Citri Reticulatae Pericarpium* (Chen Pi) to regulate qi and dry dampness; *Poria* (Fu Ling), *Polyporus* (Zhu Ling) and *Alismatis Rhizoma* (Ze Xie) to eliminate dampness with bland herbs.

方药：中满分消丸合茵陈蒿汤。常用：黄芩、黄连、知母、茵陈、大黄、栀子等清热化湿；厚朴、枳壳、半夏、陈皮等理气燥湿；茯苓、猪苓、泽泻等淡渗利湿。

Modification: For hot urination, add old *Fructus Lagenariae Depressae* (Chen Hu Lu), *Talcum* (Hua Shi) and *Cricket Powder* (Xi Shuai Fen) (swallowed seperately) to activate metabolism of fluid by promoting defecation and urination; for acute abdominal distention, use for time being, *Boats and Carts Pills* (Zhou Che Wan) and Ten Jujubes Decoction (Shi Zao Tang) to drastically expel water; for heat forcing blood to overspill, casuing bleeding in teeth and nose, purple plague and bleeding, use *Rhinoceros Horn and Rehmannia Decoction* (Xi Jiao Di Huang Tang) with *Notoginseng Radix et Rhizoma* (San Qi), *Sanguisorbiae Radix* (Sheng Di Yu) and *Agrimoniae Herba* (Xian He Cao) to clear away heat, cool blood and stop bleeding.

加减：小便赤涩不利者，加陈葫芦、滑石、蟋蟀粉（另吞服）以行水利窍；腹部胀急较甚，可暂用舟车丸、十枣汤峻下逐水；若伴有热迫血溢而齿衄、鼻衄、紫斑、出血诸症，可用犀角地黄汤加参三七、生地榆、仙鹤草等清热凉血止血。

2.2.4 Blood Stasis in the Liver and Spleen

Manifestations: Large, hard and full abdomen, expanding vessels and collaterals, stabbing pain around hypochondria and in the abdomen, soot-black

2.2.4 肝脾血瘀

证候：腹大坚满，脉络怒张，胁腹刺痛，面色黧黑，面颈胸臂有血痣，呈丝纹状，手

complexion, blood moles on the neck, in the chest and on the arms in the shape of thread, reddish mark in the palms, purple and dark lips, thirst but no desire for drink, black stool; dark purple tongue with stasis spots; fine uneven pulse.

掌赤痕,唇色紫褐,口渴不欲饮,大便色黑。舌质紫暗或有瘀斑,脉细涩。

Treatment: To activate blood and resolve stasis; promote qi flow and eliminate dampness.

治法: 活血化瘀,行气利水。

Formulas and Herbs: *Construction-Regulating Decoction* (Tiao Ying Yin), usually composed of *Angelicae Sinensis Radix* (Dang Gui), *Chuanxiong Rhizoma* (Chuan Xiong) and *Paeoniae Radix Rubra* (Chi Shao) to active blood and resolve stasis; *Curcumae Rhizoma* (E Zhu), *Corydalis Rhizoma* (Yan Hu Suo) and *Rhei Radix et Rhizoma* (Da Huang) to disperse qi and break blood; *Dianthi Herba* (Qu Mai), *Arecae Semen* (Bing Lang), *Descurainiae Semen Lepidii Semen* (Ting Li Zi), *Poria* (Fu Ling) and *Mori Cortex* (Sang Bai Pi) to promote qi flow and eliminate dampness.

方药: 调营饮。常用:当归、川芎、赤芍药等活血化瘀;莪术、延胡索、大黄以散气破血;瞿麦、槟榔、葶苈子、赤茯苓、桑白皮等以行气利水。

Modification: For black stool, add *Notoginseng Radix et Rhizoma* (San Qi), and *Platycladi Cacumen Preparata* (Ce Bai Ye) to resolve stasis and stop bleeding; for severe water fullness, powerful rapid taut pulse with fairly good constitution, use for time being, *Boats and Carts Pills* (Zhou Che Wan) to precipitate to expel water; for evident lumps under hypochondria, use *Decocted Turtle Shell Pills* (Bie Jia Jian Wan).

加减: 如大便色黑,可加参三七、侧柏叶等化瘀止血;如水胀满过甚、脉弦数有力、体质尚好,可暂用舟车丸攻逐水气;若胁下积块明显,可加用鳖甲煎丸。

2.2.5 Yang Deficiency of the Spleen and Kidney

2.2.5 脾肾阳虚

Manifestations: Large, distended abdomen in discomfort which get relieved in the moring and get worse in the evening, withering yellow complexion or waxy pale complexion, oppression in the stomach, poor appetite, lassitude, fear of cold, cold

证候: 腹大胀满不舒,朝宽暮急,面色苍黄,或呈㿠白,脘闷纳呆,神倦怯寒,肢冷,或下肢浮肿,小便短少不利,舌质胖淡紫,苔滑腻,脉沉细

limbs or lower limbs edema, oliguresis and unsuccessful urination; enlarged light purple tongue fur with slippery greasy tongue fur; deep fine powerless pulse.

无力。

Treatment: To warm and supplement the spleen and kidney; transform qi and promote water flow.

治法: 温补脾肾,化气行水。

Formulas and Herbs: *Aconiti Praeparata-Regulating Zhong jiao Decoction* (Fu Zi Li Zhong Tang) and *Poria Five Powder* (Wu Ling San) and *Spleen-qi Pills for Succoring the Sick* (Ji Sheng Shen Qi Wan), usually composed of *Aconm Lateralis Radix Praeparata* (Fu Zi), *Zingiberis Rhizoma* (Gan Jiang) to warm and transfer zhong jiao and expel pathogenic cold, *Codonopsis Radix* (Dang Shen), *Atractylodis Macrocephalae Rhizoma* (Bai Zhu) and *Glycyrrhizae Radix et Rhizoma* (Gan Cao) to boost qi, strengthen the spleen and expel pathogenic dampness; *Polyporus* (Zhu Ling), *Poria* (Fu Ling) and *Alismatis Rhizoma* (Ze Xie) to eliminate diuresis with bland herbs; *Cinnamomi Ramulus* (Gui Zhi) to free yang with warmth and acridity; *Rehmanniae Radix Praeparata* (Shu Di Huang), *Corni Fructus* (Shan Zhu Yu), *Dioscoreae Rhizoma* (Shan Yao) and *Moutan Cortex* (Mu Dan Pi) to nourish the kidney and store essence; *Achyranthis Bidentatae Radix* (Niu Xi), *Plantaginis Semen* (Che Qian Zi) to eliminate dampness and remove edema.

方药: 附子理中丸合五苓散、济生肾气丸。常用:附子、干姜温运中焦,驱散寒邪;党参、白术、甘草补气健脾,祛除湿邪;猪苓、茯苓、泽泻淡渗利湿;桂枝辛温通阳;熟地黄、山茱萸、山药、牡丹皮滋肾填精;牛膝、车前子利水退肿。

Modification: For poor appetite and abdominal fullness which gets worse after diet, add *Dioscoreae Rhizoma* (Shan Yao), *Coicis Semen* (Yi Yi Ren), *Lablab Semen Album* (Bai Bian Dou), *Galli Gigerii Endothelium Corneum* (Ji Nei Jin), *Aucklandiae Radix* (Mu Xiang), *Hordei Fructus Germinatus* (Mai Ya) and *Setariae Fructus Germinatus* (Gu Ya)

加减: 若纳呆腹满、食后尤甚,可加山药、薏苡仁、白扁豆、鸡内金、木香、谷麦芽等健脾理气消食;若畏寒神疲、面色青灰、脉弱无力,酌加淫羊藿、巴戟天、仙茅等温阳;若腹筋暴露者酌加桃仁、

to strengthen the spleen, regulate qi and remove food retention; for aversion to cold, lassitude, greenish gray complexion and weak pulse, add moderately *Epimedii Folium* (Yin Yang Huo), *Morindae Officinalis Radix* (Ba Ji Tian) and *Curculiginis Rhizoma* (Xian Mao) to warm yang; for prominent green-blue veins, add moderately *Persicae Semen* (Tao Ren), *Paeoniae Radix Rubra* (Chi Shao Yao), *Sparganii Rhizoma* (San Leng) and *Curcumae Rhizoma* (E Zhu) to activate blood.

赤芍药、三棱、莪术等活血。

2.2.6 Yin Deficiency of the Liver and Kidney

Manifestations: Large and distended full abdomen, or prominent veins on the abdomen, dull stagnant facial complexion, purple lips, dry mouth, insomnia, bleeding in the teeth and nose, oliguresis; scarlet tongue fur with little fluid; fine rapid taut pulse.

Treatment: To nourish the liver and kidney; activate blood and remove stasis.

Formulas and Herbs: *Rehmannia Pills with Six Ingredients* (Liu Wei Di Huang Wan) or *An Ever Effective Decoction for Nourishing Liver and Kidney* (Yi Guan Jian) and modified *Infradiaphragmatic Stasis-Expelling Decoction* (Ge Xia Zhu Yu Tang), usually composed of *Rehmanniae Radix Praeparata* (Shu Di Huang), *Corni Fructus* (Shan Zhu Yu) and *Dioscoreae Rhizoma* (Shan Yao) to nourish the liver and kidney; *Poria* (Fu Ling), *Alismatis Rhizoma* (Ze Xie) and *Moutan Cortex* (Mu Dan Pi) to eliminate dampness with bland herbs; *Rehmannia Radix* (Sheng Di Huang), *Glehniae Radix* (Bei Sha Shen), *Ophiopogonis Radix* (Mai Men Dong) and *Lycii Fructus* (Gou Qi Zi) to nourish the liver and kidney; *Angelicae Sinensis Radix* (Dang Gui) and

2.2.6 肝肾阴虚

证候: 腹大胀满,或见青筋暴露,面色晦滞,唇紫,口燥,心烦,不寐,牙宣出血,鼻衄,小便短少。舌质红绛少津,脉弦细数。

治法: 滋养肝肾,活血化瘀。

方药: 六味地黄丸或一贯煎合膈下逐瘀汤加减。常用:熟地黄、山茱萸、山药滋养肝肾;茯苓、泽泻、牡丹皮淡渗利湿;生地黄、沙参、麦门冬、枸杞滋养肝肾;当归、川楝子和血疏肝;五灵脂、赤芍药、桃仁、红花活血化瘀;川芎、乌药、延胡索、香附、枳壳行气活血;甘草调和诸药。

Toosendan Fructus (Chuan Lian Zi) to harmonize blood and disperse the liver; *Faeces Trogopterorum* (Wu Ling Zhi), *Paeoniae Radix Rubra* (Chi Shao Yao), *Persicae Semen* (Tao Ren) and *Carthami Flos* (Hong Hua) to activate blood circulation and remove stasis; *Chuanxiong Rhizoma* (Chuan Xiong), *Linderae Radix* (Wu Yao), *Corydalis Rhizoma* (Yan Hu Suo, Yuan Hu), *Cyperi Rhizoma* (Xiang Fu) and *Aurantii Fructus*(Zhi Qiao) to promote qi follow and activate blood circulation; *Glycyrrhizae Radix et Rhizoma* (Gan Cao) to harmonize all the other herbs.

Modification: For yin deficiency and interior heat, dry mouth, scarlet tongue fur with little fluid, add *Scrophulariae Radix* (Xuan Shen), *Dendrobii Caulis* (Shi Hu) and *Ophiopogonis Radix* (Mai Men Dong) to clear away heat and generate fluid; for serious abdominal distention, add *Raphani Semen* (Lai Fu Zi) and *Arecae Pericarpium* (Da Fu Pi) to promote qi flow and remove distention; for other accompanying symptoms such as feverish sensations, irritation, insomnia, add *Stellariae Radix* (Yin Chai Hu), *Lycii Cortex* (Di Gu Pi), Stir-fried *Gardeniae Fructus* (Chao Zhi Zi), *Polygoni Multiflori Caulis* (Ye Jiao Teng); for oliguresis, add *Polyporus* (Zhu Ling), *Talcum* (Hua Shi), *Imperatae Rhizoma* (Bai Mao Gen), or add a little *Cinnamomi Cortex* (Rou Gui) to give counteracting assistance; for yin deficiency and floating yang with symptoms like tinnitus and dark red cheeks, add *Testudinis Carapax et Plastrum* (Gui Jia), *Trionycis Carapax* (Bie Jia) and *Ostreae Concha* (Mu Li) to nourish yin and subdue yang.

加减：如阴虚内热口干、舌绛少津，加玄参、石斛、麦门冬以清热生津；如腹胀甚，加莱菔子、大腹皮以行气消胀；如兼有潮热、烦躁、不寐，加银柴胡、地骨皮、炒栀子、夜交藤；如小便短少，加猪苓、滑石、白茅根，或少加肉桂心反佐；如阴虚阳浮，症见耳鸣、面赤颧红，加龟甲、鳖甲、牡蛎等以滋阴潜阳。

Headache

头 痛

Headache is a disease of pain in the head due to meridians and vessels convulsion or lackof nourishing in the head caused by six climatic pathogenic factors and internal injuries.

头痛是指因外感六淫、内伤诸因引起头部经脉绌急或失养，以头部疼痛为主要表现的病证。

1 Etiology and Pathogenesis

1 病因病机

The causes of headache comes into two categories: exogenous and endogenous factos.

引起头痛的病因不外乎外感、内伤两大类。

1.1 Six Climatic Pathogenic Factors and Vessels Convulsion

1.1 外感六淫，绌急经脉

Careless living allows pathogenic factors such as wind, cold, damp and heat to invade, attackthe head and blocks meridians and collaterals, leading to headache.

起居不慎，感受风、寒、湿、热之邪，上犯清空，阻遏清阳，邪壅经络，发为头痛。

1.2 Hyperactivity of Liver Yang Due to Emotional and Spiritual Disorder

1.2 情志失调，肝阳上亢

Depressed anger makes damage to the liver and when depressed qi turns into firewhich inflames up along the meridians to interfere with the head, leading to headache.

郁怒伤肝，气郁化火，火性炎上，循经上扰清空而致头痛。

1.3 Eating Unclean Food and Spleen Injury Due to Overstrain

1.3 饮食不洁，劳倦伤脾

Favor for alcohol, greasy and sweet food makes the spleen to fail to transport, resulting in phlegm due to accumulation of dampness. The turbid phlegm blocks clear yang, leading to headache.

嗜酒肥甘，脾失健运，聚湿生痰，痰浊阻遏清阳，发为头痛。

1.4 Consitutional Weakness and Deficiency of Kidney Essence

1.4 禀赋不足，肾精亏虚

Congenital deficiency and too much sexual life orprolonged illness damaging and exhausting the kidney essence leads to head marrow deficiency, resulting in headache.

先天亏虚，房劳过度；或久病及肾，肾精久亏，脑髓空虚而致头痛。

1.5 Falling Injuries and Vessels and Collaterals Stasis

Falling or external injuries or prolonged illness affects the colleterals causes qi stagnation and blood stasis, which blocks the vessels and collaterals, causing headache.

In a word, headache lies in thehead and is grouped into exogenous and endogenous types. The pathologenesis of exogenous headache is exogenous pathogenic factors interferering the head and blocks the meridians and collaterals. Endogenous headache is relate to the liver, spleen and kidney. Headache related to the liver is due to wind-yang disturbing the head. Headache related to the spleen is due to turbid phlegm blinding the orifices or due to lack of nourishment of head collaterals resulting from qi and blood deficiency. Meanwhile, headache related to the kidney is due to the lack of nourishment resulting from marrow sea deficiency. Falling and other external injuries, when prolonged, will affect and block the collaterals.

2 Syndrome Differentiation and Treatment

2.1 Key Points of Syndrome Differentiation

Doctors should first identify exogenous headache from endogenous headache. Exogenous headache takes on suddenly and usually has accompanying symptoms of pathogenic factorstightening the exterior. Doctors should tell the differences among wind, cold, damp and heat. For headache due to wind-cold, it is sharp pain and stretches to the nape and back. For headache due to wind-heat, it is splitting bulging pain. For headache due to wind-damp, it is head heaviness as if swathed. Endoge-

1.5 跌仆损伤,瘀阻脉络

外伤跌仆或久病入络,气滞血瘀,脉络瘀阻,不通则痛。

总之,头痛病位在脑。病因有外感与内伤两大类。外感头痛的病机为外邪上扰清空,邪壅经脉,络脉不通。内伤者,与肝、脾、肾有关,因于肝者为风阳上扰清空;因于脾者,为痰浊上蒙清窍;或为气血亏虚,脑脉失养;因于肾者,髓海空虚,脑失濡养。跌仆外伤,久病入络,瘀血阻络。

2 辨证论治

2.1 辨治要点

头痛首辨外感与内伤。外感头痛起病较急,常伴有外邪束表的症状,应区别风、寒、湿、热之不同:因于风寒者,头痛剧烈而连项背;因于风热者,头胀痛如裂;因于风湿者,头痛如裹。内伤者头痛反复发作,时轻时重,应分辨气虚、血虚、肾虚、肝阳、痰浊、瘀血之异。因于虚者,头

nous headache comes and goes with varying intensity. Doctors should tell the differences among qi deficiency, blood deficiency, kidney deficiency, liver yang, turbid phlegm and blood stasis. For headache due to deficiency, it is dull and continuous pain or empty pain. For headache due to phlegm-damp, it is sagging heaviness or distention in the head. For headache due to liver-fire, it is throbbing pain. For headache due to liver-yang, it is distending pain in the head. For that due to blood stasis, it is sharp pain in fixed spots. Doctors also have to distinguish meridians and collaterals by the positions of pain. Pain in the back of head stretching to the nape is related to taiyang while pain in the forehead and eyebrows is related to yangming. Pain on the two sides of the head stretching to the ears is related to shaoyang while pain on the top of head stretching to eyes is related to jue yin.

隐痛绵绵，或空痛；因于痰湿者，头重坠或胀；因于肝火者，头痛呈跳痛；因于肝阳者，头痛而胀；因于瘀血者，头痛剧烈而部位固定。还根据头痛部位辨病变经络，大抵太阳头痛，在头后部，下连于项；阳明头痛，在前额部及眉棱骨等处；少阳头痛，在头之两侧，并连及于耳；厥阴头痛则在巅顶部位，或连目系。

Exogenous headache belongs to excess type and should be treated mainly by dispersing wind along with dispelling cold, clear awaying away heat and eliminate dampness. Endogenous headache pertains to deficiency type or complication of deficiency and excess. It is advisable to nourish yin and blood, and tonifying kidney and replenishing essence. For excess headache, try to calm the liver, resolve phlegm and remove stasis. For headache with complication of deficiency and excess, both deficiency and excess should be treated simultaneously and use herbs ingeniously to Clear Spirit to reach the upper orifices and use meridian guiding herbs to strengthen herbal effect. For example, *Notopterygii Rhizoma et Radix* (Qiang Huo), *Viticis Fructus* (Man Jing Zi) and *Chuanxiong Rhizoma* (Chuan Xiong) can be chan-

外感头痛属实证，治疗主以疏风，兼以散寒、清热、祛湿；内伤头痛多属虚证或虚实夹杂证，虚者以滋阴养血，益肾填精为主。实证当平肝、化痰、行瘀；虚实夹杂者，酌情兼顾并治用药宜清灵以达上窍。头痛用药还可根据头痛部位选用引经药以增强药效，如太阳头痛选用羌活、蔓荆子、川芎，阳明头痛选用葛根、白芷、知母，少阳头痛选用柴胡、黄芩、川芎，厥阴头痛选用吴茱萸、藁本。对于缠绵不愈，部位固定的头部刺痛，可酌情加入

nel conductors for headache of taiyang while *Puerariae Lobatae Radix* (Ge Gen), *Angelicae Dahuricae Radix*(Bai Zhi) and *Anemarrhenae Rhizoma* (Zhi Mu) for head of yangming, *Bupleuri Radix* (Chai Hu), *Scutellariae Radix* (Huang Qin) and *Chuanxiong Rhizoma* (Chuan Xiong) for shaoyang, *Euodiae Fructus* (Wu Zhu Yu) and *Imperatae Rhizoma* (Gao Ben) for jueyin. For continuous sharp pain in fixed positions that cannot be cured, add moderately some insect materia such as *Scorpio* (Quan Xie), *Scolopendra* (Wu Gong), *Bombyx Batryticatus* (Jiang Can) and *Pheretima* (Di Long) to eliminate stasis and dredge collaterals, relieve convulsion and stop pain.

全蝎、蜈蚣、僵蚕、地龙等虫类药祛瘀通络，解痉止痛。

2.2 Therapeutic Methods for Different Pattern

2.2 分型论治

2.2.1 Exogenous Headache

2.2.1 外感头痛

2.2.1.1 Headache Due to Wind-cold

2.2.1.1 风寒头痛

Manifesations: Intermittent headache stretching to the nape and back, aversion to cold and wind, aggravation by wind, no thirst; white thin tongue fur; floating pulse.

证候：头痛时作，痛连项背，恶寒畏风，遇风尤剧，口不渴。苔薄白，脉浮。

Treatment: To disperse wind-cold.

治法：疏散风寒。

Formulas and Herbs: *Tea-Blended Chuanxiong Powder* (Chuan Xiong Cha Tiao San), usually composed of acrid and warm herbs such as *Chuanxiong Rhizoma* (Chuan Xiong), *Schizonepetae Herba* (Jing Jie), *Saposhnikoviae Radix*(Fang Feng), *Notopterygii Rhizoma et Radix* (Qiang Huo), *Angelicae Dahuricae Radix*(Bai Zhi) and *Asari Radix et Rhizoma* (Xi Xin) to disperse wind-cold to stop pain.

方药：川芎茶调散。常用川芎、荆芥、防风、羌活、白芷、细辛等辛温药疏散风寒止痛。

Modification: If pathogenic cold has attacked jueyin with such symptoms as pain on the head top, hiccup and drooling and foam at the mouth and even

加减：若寒邪侵犯厥阴经，症见巅顶头痛、干呕、吐涎沫，甚则四肢厥冷，脉弦，

cold of the limbs and taut pulse, use *Euodiae Decoction* (Wu Zhu Yu Tang) from which, delete *Ginseng Radix et Rhizoma* (Ren Shen) and *Jujubae Fructus* (Da Zao) and to which, add *Pinelliae Rhizoma* (Ban Xia), *Imperatae Rhizoma* (Gao Ben) and *Chuanxiong Rhizoma* (Chuan Xiong) to warm and disperse to lower reversal flow; when pathogenic cold restrains shaoyang meridian with such symptoms as headache, cold back, cold feet and deep fine pulse, use *Ephedra, Aconite, and Asarum Decoction* (Ma Huang Fu Zi Xi Xin Tang) and *Angelicae Dahuricae Radix* (Bai Zhi), *Chuanxiong Rhizoma* (Chuan Xiong) to warm shaoyin and disperse pathogenic cold.

用吴茱萸汤去人参、大枣，加半夏、藁本、川芎之类温散降逆；若寒邪克于少阴经脉，症见头痛、背冷、足寒、脉沉细，可用麻黄附子细辛汤加白芷、川芎以温散少阴寒邪。

2.2.1.2 Head Due to Wind-heat

2.2.1.2 风热头痛

Manifestations: Distending pain in the head, even splitting pain, fever or aversion to wind, red cheeks and reddish eyes, thirst for drink, constipation and yellow urine; red tongue with yellow tongue fur; rapid floating pulse.

证候：头痛且胀，甚则头痛如裂，发热或恶风，面红目赤，口渴欲饮，便秘溲黄。舌质红，苔黄，脉浮数。

Treatment: To disperse wind and clear away heat.

治法：疏风清热。

Formulas and Herbs: *Chuanxiong, Dahurian Angelica, and Gypsum Fibrosum Decoction* (Xiong Zhi Shi Gao Tang), usually composed of *Chuanxiong Rhizoma* (Chuan Xiong) to promote blood circulation and dredge orifices; *Chrysanthemi Flos* (Ju Hua) and *Gypsum Fibrosum Fibrosum* (Shi Gao) to disperse wind and clear away heat; *Angelicae Dahuricae Radix* (Bai Zhi), *Imperatae Rhizoma* (Gao Ben) and *Notopterygii Rhizoma et Radix* (Qiang Huo) to disperse wind and dredge orifices to stop pain.

方药：芎芷石膏汤。常用：川芎活血通窍，菊花、石膏疏风清热；白芷、藁本、羌活散风通窍而止头痛。

Modification: For heavy heat, delete *Imperatae*

加减：若热甚去羌活、藁

Rhizoma (Gao Ben) and *Notopterygii Rhizoma et Radix* (Qiang Huo), add *Scutellariae Radix* (Huang Qin), *Menthae Haplocalycis Herba* (Bo He) and *Gardeniae Fructus* (Zhi Zi) to clear away heat with their acrid-cool nature; for constipation and sores in the mouth and nose, add *Coptis Upper-Body-Clear awaying Pills* (Huang Lian Shang Qing Wan) to subdue fire with bitter cool herbs and dredge fu-organs and purge heat; for thundering pain, lumps on the head and face or hot swollen head and face, called "Thunder Head Wind", which is usually caused by pathogenic wind and damp-toxin surging upward, it is better to use *Clear awaying and Vibrating Decoction* (Qing Zheng Tang) and *Universal Salvation Detoxifying Cool Decoction* (Pu Ji Xiao Du Yin) to dispel wind, dry dampness, clear away heat and detoxify.

本，改用黄芩、薄荷、栀子辛凉清解；若大便秘结、口鼻生疮，加黄连上清丸苦寒降火、通腑泄热；若头痛如雷鸣、头面起核或肿痛红热，名“雷头风”，多为风邪湿毒上冲所致，宜用清震汤合普济消毒饮以祛风燥湿、清热解毒。

2.2.1.3　Headache Due to Wind-damp

Manifestations: Headache as if swathed, general heaviness, poor appetite, oppression in the chest, inhibited urination; white greasy tongue fur; soft pulse.

Treatment: To dispel wind and overcome dampness.

Formulas and Herbs: *Notopterygium Dampness-Overcoming Decoction* (Qiang Huo Sheng Shi Tang), usually composed of *Notopterygii Rhizoma et Radix* (Qiang Huo), *Angelicae Pubescentis Radix* (Du Huo), *Saposhnikoviae Radix* (Fang Feng), *Viticis Fructus* (Man Jing Zi) and *Imperatae Rhizoma* (Gao Ben) to dispel wind and overcome dampness with its warm and acrid nature; *Chuanxiong Rhizoma* (Chuan Xiong) to dredge orifice, activate blood flow and stop pain with its warm and acrid

2.2.1.3　风湿头痛

证候： 头痛如裹，肢体困重，纳呆胸闷，小便不利。苔白腻，脉濡。

治法： 祛风胜湿。

方药： 羌活胜湿汤。常用：羌活、独活、防风、蔓荆子、藁本辛温祛风胜湿；川芎辛温通窍、活血止痛。

nature.

Modification: For damp-turbid blocks in the middle, oppression in the chest, poor appetite and loose stool, add *Stomach-Calming Powder* (Ping Wei San); for oliguresis, add *Coicis Semen* (Yi Yi Ren) and *Lophatheri Herba* (Dan Zhu Ye) to eliminate dampness with bland herbs; for at the turn of spring and summer, headache along with fever and little sweating, or slight aversion to cold, inhibited sweating, thirst, oppression in the chest, dry hiccup and no intake, use *Coptidis and Elsholtziae Decoction* (Huang Lian Xiang Ru Yin) with *Pogostemonis Herba* (Huo Xiang), *Eupatorii Herba* (Pei Lan), *Nelumbinis Folium* (He Ye) and *Bambusae Caulis in Taenias* (Zhu Ru) to clear away summer heat and dissolve dampness.

加减：若湿浊中阻，胸闷纳呆、便溏，加平胃散；小便短少，加薏苡仁、淡竹叶淡渗利湿；暑夏之际，头痛兼见身热汗少或微恶寒、汗出不畅、口渴胸闷、干呕不食，用黄连香薷饮加藿香、佩兰、荷叶、竹茹等清暑化湿。

2.2.2 Endogenous Headache

2.2.2.1 Headache Due to Liver Yang

Manifestations: Headache and vertigo, irritation, unpeaceful sleep, or hypochondriac pain, red face and bitter mouth; yellow thin tongue fur; powerful taut pulse.

Treatment: To calm the liver and subdue yang.

Formulas and Herbs: *Gastrodia and Uncaria Decoction* (Tian Ma Gou Teng Yin), usually composed of *Gastrodiae Rhizoma* (Tian Ma), *Uncariae Ramulus cum Uncis* (Gou Teng) and *Haliotidis Concha* (Shi Jue Ming) to calm the liver and subdue yang, *Scutellariae Radix* (Huang Qin) and *Gardeniae Fructus* (Zhi Zi) to clear away liver-fire; *Achyranthis Bidentatae Radix* (Niu Xi), *Eucommiae Cortex* (Du Zhong) and *Taxilli Herba* (Sang Ji Sheng) to nourish the heart and calm and spirits; *Os Draconis* (Long Gu) and *Ostreae Concha* (Mu Li) to settle

2.2.2 内伤头痛

2.2.2.1 肝阳头痛

证候：头痛而眩，心烦易怒，夜眠不宁，或兼胁痛，面红口苦。苔薄黄，脉弦有力。

治法：平肝潜阳。

方药：天麻钩藤饮。常用：天麻、钩藤、石决明平肝潜阳，黄芩、栀子清肝火；牛膝、杜仲、桑寄生补肝肾；夜交藤、茯神养心安神；龙骨、牡蛎重镇潜阳。

and subdue yang.

Modification: If depressed liver-qi tranforms into fire with symptoms like heavy headache, reddish eyes, bitter mouth, irritation, constipation and yellow urine, add *Prunellae Spica* (Xia Ku Cao), *Gentianae Radix et Rhizoma* (Long Dan) and *Rhei Radix et Rhizoma* (Da Huang); for deficiency of the liver and kidney and water failing to moisten wood, with such symptoms as dizziness, sore eyes, dim sight which worsens at work, soreness in the waist and knees, add *Lycium, Chrysanthemun and Rehmannia Pills* (Qi Ju Di Huang Wan).

加减：若肝郁化火，而症见头痛剧烈、目赤口苦、急躁、便秘溲黄者，加夏枯草、龙胆草、大黄。若兼肝肾亏虚、水不涵木，症见头晕目涩、视物不明，遇劳加重，腰膝酸软者，可加杞菊地黄丸。

2.2.2.2　Headache Due to Kidney Deficiency

2.2.2.2　肾虚头痛

Manifesatations: Empty pain in the head, vertigo, soreness in the waist, lassitude and fatigue, spermatorrhea and vaginal discharge, tinnitus and little sleep; red tongue with little tongue fur, weak fine pulse.

证候：头痛且空，每兼眩晕，腰痛酸软，神疲乏力，遗精带下，耳鸣少寐。舌红少苔，脉细无力。

Treatment: To nourish yin and strengthen the kidney.

治法：养阴补肾。

Formulas and Herbs: *Major Yuan (Primary) Qi-Reinforcing Decoction* (Da Bu Yuan Jian), usually composed of *Rehmanniae Radix Praeparata* (Shu Di Huang), *Corni Fructus* (Shan Zhu Yu), *Dioscoreae Rhizoma* (Shan Yao) and *Lycii Fructus* (Gou Qi Zi) to nourish and supplement kidney-yin and liver-yin; *Ginseng Radix et Rhizoma* (Ren Shen) and *Angelicae Sinensis Radix* (Dang Gui) to supplement qi and blood; *Eucommiae Cortex* (Du Zhong) to strengthen the kidney and strenghten the waist.

方药：大补元煎。常用：熟地黄、山茱萸、山药、枸杞子滋补肝肾之阴；人参、当归气血双补；杜仲益肾强腰。

Modification: For kidney-yang deficiency, with symptoms like headache, aversion to cold, waxy pale complexion, cool limbs, pale tongue and deep fine slow pulse, use *Vital Gate Pills* (You Gui Wan)

加减：若肾阳不足，症见头痛而畏寒、面色㿠白、四肢不温、舌淡、脉沉细而缓，可用右归丸温补肾阳、填补精

to warm and supplement kidney-yang, and replenish essence and blood; for kidney-yin deficiency and deficiency-fire inflaming upward with symptoms such as headache, dizziness, hot head and face, dark red cheeks and sweating at times, use *Anemarrhena, Phellodendron, and Rehmannia Pills* (Zhi Bai Di Huang Wan) to nourish yin and purge fire.

血；若属肾阴亏虚，虚火上炎，症见头痛而晕、头面烘热、面颊红赤、时伴汗出者，用知柏地黄丸滋阴泄火。

2.2.2.3 Headache Due to Blood Deficiency

2.2.2.3 血虚头痛

Manifeastations: Headache, dizziness, palpitation, lassitude, fatigue, waxy pale complexion; pale tongue with white thin tongue fur; fine weak pulse.

证候：头痛而晕，心悸不宁，神疲乏力，面色㿠白。舌质淡，苔薄白，脉细弱。

Treatment: To nourish and regulate blood.

治法：养血调血。

Formulas and Herbs: Supplemented *Four Agents Decoction* (Jia Wei Si Wu Tang), usually composed of *Angelicae Sinensis Radix* (Dang Gui), *Paeoniae Radix Alba* (Bai Shao Yao), *Rehmannia Radix* (Sheng Di Huang) and *Chuanxiong Rhizoma* (Chuan Xiong) to nourish and regulate blood; *Chrysanthemi Flos* (Ju Hua), *Viticis Fructus* (Man Jing Zi) to calm the liver and dispel wind to clear the head and eyes.

方药：加味四物汤。常用：当归、白芍药、生地黄、川芎养血调血；菊花、蔓荆子平肝祛风清头目。

Modification: For accompanying qi deficiency with symptoms like sweating, short breath and aversion to cold, add *Astragali Radix* (Huang Qi), *Codonopsis Radix* (Dang Shen) and *Asari Radix et Rhizoma* (Xi Xin); for liver-blood deficiency, yin failing to astringe yang and liver-yang interfering upward with symptoms like headache, tinnitus, soreness in the waist and knees, feverish sensations in five centers, add *Four Agents Decoction* (Si Wu Tang), from which, delete *Chuanxiong Rhizoma* (Chuan Xiong) and to which, add *Haliotidis Concha* (Shi Jue Ming), *Ostreae Concha* (Mu Li), *Ligustri Lucidi Fructus* (Nü Zhen Zi) and *Uncariae*

加减：若兼有气虚，症见汗出气短、畏风怕冷，加黄芪、党参、细辛；若肝血不足，阴不敛阳，肝阳上扰，症见头痛、耳鸣、腰膝酸软、五心烦热者，加味四物汤去川芎，加石决明、牡蛎、女贞子、钩藤。

Ramulus cum Uncis (Gou Teng).

2.2.2.4　Headache Due to Phlegm-Turbidity

2.2.2.4　痰浊头痛

Manifestations: Headache and clouding, fullness and oppression in the chest and stomach, vomiting, nausea, phlegm and drooling; white greasy tongue fur; rolling pulse or taut pulse.

证候: 头痛昏蒙,胸脘满闷,呕恶痰涎。苔白腻,脉滑或弦滑。

Treatment: To resolve phlegm and lower reversal flow.

治法: 化痰降逆。

Formulas and Herbs: *Pinellia, White Atractyodest, and Gastrodia Decoction* (Ban Xia Bai Zhu Tian Ma Tang), usually composed of *Pinelliae Rhizoma* (Ban Xia), *Atractylodis Macrocephalae Rhizoma* (Bai Zhu), *Poria* (Fu Ling), *Citri Reticulatae Pericarpium* (Chen Pi) and *Zingiberis Rhizoma Recens* (Sheng Jiang) to strengthen the spleen and resolve phlegm; *Gastrodiae Rhizoma* (Tian Ma) to calm the liver and stop wind.

方药: 半夏白术天麻汤。常用:半夏、白术、茯苓、陈皮、生姜健脾化痰;天麻平肝息风。

Modification: For phlegm-turbidity which has been depressed for long and has turned into heat, with symptoms like bitter mouth, inhibited stool, yellow greasy tongue fur and rolling rapid pulse, add *Coptis-Warming-Gallbladder Decoction* (Huang Lian Wen Dan Tang) to clear away heat, dry dampness, regulate qi and resolve phlegm; for oppression in the chest and considerable vomiting and nausea, add *Magnoliae Officinalis Cortex* (Hou Po) and *Aurantii Fructus* (Zhi Qiao) to harmonize zhong jiao and lower reversal flow.

加减: 若痰浊郁久化热,症见口苦、大便不畅、苔黄腻、脉滑数,合黄连温胆汤清热燥湿、理气化痰;若胸闷、呕恶明显,加厚朴、枳壳和中降逆。

2.2.2.5　Headache Due to Blood Stasis

2.2.2.5　瘀血头痛

Manifestations: Prolonged headache, stabbing pain in fixed positions, or having herbsl history of external injury in the head; purple tongue with white thin tongue fur; fine uneven pulse.

证候: 头痛经久不愈,痛处固定不移,痛如锥刺,或有头部外伤史。舌质紫,苔薄白,脉细涩。

Treatment: To activate blood ciruculation to re-

治法: 活血化瘀。

move stasis.

Formulas and Herbs: *Orifice-Dredging and Blood-Activating Decoction* (Tong Qiao Huo Xue Tang), usually composed of *Persicae Semen* (Tao Ren), *Carthami Flos* (Hong Hua), *Chuanxiong Rhizoma* (Chuan Xiong) and *Paeoniae Radix Rubra* (Chi Shao) to activate blood circulation and remove stasis; *Moschus* (She Xiang), *Zingiberis Rhizoma Recens* (Sheng Jiang) and *Bulbus Allii Fistulosi* (Cong Bai) to warm and dredge vessels and collaterals; moderate *Curcumae Radix* (Yu Jin), *Acori Tatarinowii Rhizoma* (Shi Chang Pu), *Asari Radix et Rhizoma* (Xi Xin) and *Angelicae Dahuricae Radix* (Bai Zhi) to regulate qi and disperse orifices as well as warm the meridians and stop pain.

方药：通窍活血汤。常用：桃仁、红花、川芎、赤芍药活血化瘀；麝香、生姜、葱白温通脉络；酌加郁金、石菖蒲、细辛、白芷理气宣窍，温经止痛。

Modification: For heavey headache, add *Scorpio* (Quan Xie), *Scolopendra* (Wu Gong) and *Eupolyphaga Steleophaga* (Zhe Chong) to track wind, dredge colleterals and stop pain; for accompanying qi and blood deficiency, add *Astragali Radix* (Huang Qi) and *Angelicae Sinensis Radix* (Dang Gui).

加减：若头痛甚，可加全蝎、蜈蚣、地鳖虫搜风剔络止痛；兼气血不足者，可加黄芪、当归。

Vertigo

Vertigo is a disease featuring dizziness and dim eyesight due toupper orifices lacking in nourishing and head marrow deficiency caused by yin deficiency and stirring wind. Slight vertigo is relieved after eye being closed while patients of serious vertigo when on vehicles or boat, feel stopless rotation and cannot stand along with nausea, vomiting, sweating, pale complexion and even faint.

眩 晕

眩晕是由阴虚风动、痰浊及瘀血等引起的清窍失养、脑髓不充，临证以头晕、眼花为主症的一类病证。轻者闭目即止；重者如坐车船，旋转不定，不能站立，或伴恶心、呕吐、汗出、面色苍白等症，甚则突然昏倒。

1 Etiology and Pathogenesis

Vertigo is related to emotions and spirits, diet, constitution, old age, falling and injury. Its pathological nature comes into two types: deficiency and excess. The former refers to head lacking in nourishing while the latter, pathogenic factors interfering with upper orifices.

1 病因病机

眩晕的发生与情志、饮食、体虚年高、跌仆损伤等有关，病性有虚有实。虚者脑失所养，实者有邪扰清窍。

1.1 Hyperactivity Liver-yang Due to Emotional and Spiritual Dissatisfaction

Worry, depression and anger will cause liver-qi to transform into fire. Weak constitution with yang exuberance andhyperactivity of liver-yang interfere with the head, resulting in vertigo.

1.1 情志不遂，肝阳上亢

忧郁恼怒，气郁化火，或素体阳盛，肝阳偏亢，上扰清空，发为眩晕。

1.2 Consumption Due to Prolonged Illness and Qi and Blood Deficiency

Weak constitution after prolonged illness or qi and blood deficiency after bleedingwill make the spleen and stomach weak, clear away yang restrained and the head lacking in nurturing, leading to vertigo.

1.2 久病耗伤，气血亏虚

久病体虚，或失血之后，气血亏虚，脾胃虚弱，清阳不展，脑失所养，发为眩晕。

1.3 Kidney Essence Deficiency Due to Old Age and Overstrain

Prolonged ilnness makes damage to the kidney. The kidney will go deficient when one gets old. When kidney essence is exhausted, head marrow is no more produced, leading to vertigo.

1.3 年高久劳，肾精不足

久病伤肾，或年老肾亏，肾精亏耗，不能生髓充脑，发为眩晕。

1.4 ImproperDiet and Phlegm-turbidity Blocking the Middle

Favor for alcohol, greasy and sweet food or worry or overstrain will make the spleen fail to transport. Dampness gathers and phlegm is generated. Phlegm-turbidity blocks the middle and clear away yang cannot ascend and turbid-yin is unable to

1.4 饮食不节，痰浊中阻

嗜酒肥甘，或思虑劳倦，脾失健运，聚湿生痰，痰浊中阻，清阳不升，浊阴不降，蒙蔽清窍，发为眩晕。

descend. The upper orifices are blocked and vertigo is resulted in.

1.5 Falling and Injury Causing Stasis blocking Vessels and Collaterals

Blood stasis due to falling or external injury in thehead remains and blocks collaterals in the head. Therefore, qi and blood cannot move upward to the head and eyes, leading to vertigo.

In a word, vertigo lies in the head orifices but is related tothe malfunctions of the liver, spleen, and kidney. The fundamental pathological change is between deficiency and excess. Marrow sea deficiency, or qi and blood deficiency and upper orifices lacking in nurturing is of deficiency type while wind, fire, phlegm and stasis interfering with the head is of excess type. Different symptoms can be complicated and interchanged.

2 Syndrome Differentiation and Treatment

2.1 Key Points of Syndrome Differentiation

Doctors should identify vertigo by related zang-fu organs and distinguish deficiency from excess and the primary symptoms from the secondary symptoms. By clinical symptoms, doctors should tell differences betweenhyperactivity of liver-yang, dysfunction of the spleen, phlegm-damp blocking the middle resulting in deficiency of qi and blood, deficiency of kidney essence. Moreover, doctors should distinguish deficiency from excess and the primary symptoms from the secondary symptoms by the disease duration and constitution. Generally speaking, newly developed vertigo for good constitution is of excess type while proloned vertigo for poor constitution is of deficiency type or complicated type.

1.5 跌仆损伤,瘀阻脉络

跌仆坠损,头颅外伤,血瘀停留,脑络痹阻,气血不能上荣于头目,故眩晕时作。

总之,眩晕的病位在头窍,与肝、脾、肾功能失调相关。眩晕的基本病理变化不外虚实两端。虚者为髓海不足,或气血亏虚,清窍失养;实者为风、火、痰、瘀扰乱清空。各证候之间可相互兼夹或转化。

2 辨证论治

2.1 辨治要点

眩晕之证应辨相关脏腑和标本虚实。临证根据伴随症状不同辨别肝阳上亢、脾失健运、痰湿中阻或气血亏虚、肾精不足之异。根据新发久发、体质状况辨别虚实:一般新发、体壮者多实;久发、体虚者多虚,或为虚实夹杂。

The treatment should follow the principle of supplementing deficiency and purging excess and regulating yin and yang. For deficiency type, it is to nourish the liver and kidney, to boost qi andnourish blood, and to regulate and supplement the spleen and kidney. For excess type, it is to cleanse the liver and purge fire, to dry dampness and resolve phlegm, and to activate blood circulation and dredge orifices.

眩晕的治疗原则是补虚泻实，调整阴阳：虚者当滋养肝肾、益气养血、调补脾肾；实者当清肝泻火、燥湿化痰、活血通窍。

2.2 Therapeutic Methods for Different Types of Vertigo

2.2 分型论治

2.2.1 Hyperactivity of Liver-yang

2.2.1 肝阳上亢

Manifestations: Vertigo, distention and pain in the head which gets worse at times of vexation or anger, red cheeks, tinnitus, irritation, bitter mouth; red tongue with yellow tongue fur; taut pulse or rapid pulse.

证候： 眩晕，头胀且痛，每因烦劳或恼怒而加剧，面红，耳鸣，急躁易怒，口苦。舌红苔黄，脉弦或数。

Treatment: To calm the liver and subdue yang; nourish the liver and kidney.

治法： 平肝潜阳，滋养肝肾。

Formulas and Herbs: *Gastrodia and Uncaria Decoction* (Tian Ma Gou Teng Yin), usually composed of *Gastrodiae Rhizoma* (Tian Ma), *Uncariae Ramulus cum Uncis* (Gou Teng) and *Haliotidis Concha* (Shi Jue Ming) to calm the liver and subdue yang; *Scutellariae Radix* (Huang Qin) and *Gardeniae Fructus* (Zhi Zi) to clear away liver-fire; *Achyranthis Bidentatae Radix* (Niu Xi), *Eucommiae Cortex* (Du Zhong) and *Taxilli Herba* (Sang Ji Sheng) to supplement the liver and kidney; *Polygoni Multiflori Caulis* (Ye Jiao Teng) and *Poria cum Ligno Hospite* (Fu Shen) to enrich the heart and calm the spirits; *Leonuri Herba* (Yi Mu Cao) to activate blood circulation and induce diuresis.

方药： 天麻钩藤饮。常用：天麻、钩藤、石决明平肝潜阳，黄芩、栀子清肝火；牛膝、杜仲、桑寄生补肝肾；夜交藤、茯神养心安神；益母草活血利水。

Modification: For liver-fire upward inflamma-

加减： 若肝火上炎，目赤

tion, reddish eyes and bitter mouth, add *Gentianae Radix et Rhizoma* (Long Dan Cao), *Chrysanthemi Flos* (Ju Hua) and *Moutan Cortex* (Mu Dan Pi) to cleanse the liver and purge heat; for stirring yang tending to transform into wind, heavy vertigo, numb and trembling hands and feet, add *Os Draconis* (Long Gu), *Ostreae Concha* (Mu Li) and *Margaritifera Concha* (Zhen Zhu Mu) to calm the liver and stop wind and add *Cornu Antelopis* (Ling Yang Jiao) to clear away heat and stop wind; for accompanying yin-deficiency of the liver and kidney, soreness in the waist and knees, dry eyes and tinnitus, fine rapid taut pulse, red tongue with little or no tongue fur, use *Great Wind-Stabilizing Pills* (Da Ding Feng Zhu) to nourish yin and subdue yang.

口苦者，可加龙胆草、菊花、牡丹皮清肝泻热；若有阳动化风之势，眩晕剧烈、手足麻木或震颤者，可加龙骨、牡蛎、珍珠母镇肝息风，羚羊角清热息风；若兼肝肾阴虚，腰膝酸软、目涩耳鸣、脉弦细数、舌红少苔或无苔，可用大定风珠育阴潜阳。

2.2.2 Qi and Blood Deficiency

Manifestations: Vertigo which gets worse at movement and attacks at overstrain, waxy-pale complexion, lusterless lips and nails, hoarse hair, palpiation, insomnia, spiritual fatigue, laziness to talk and less intake; pale tongue; fine weak pulse.

Treatment: To supplement and nourish qi and blood; regulate and nourish the heart and spleen.

Formulas and Herbs: *Angelica Splenic Decoction* (Gui Pi Tang), usually composed of *Codonopsis Radix* (Dang Shen), *Atractylodis Macrocephalae Rhizoma* (Bai Zhu) and *Astragali Radix* (Huang Qi) to boost qi and strengthen the spleen, *Angelicae Sinensis Radix* (Dang Gui), *Rehmanniae Radix Praeparata* (Shu Di Huang), *Longan Arillus* (Long Yan Rou) and *Jujubae Fructus* (Da Zao) to supplement blood, produce blood and nourish the heart, *Poria* (Fu Ling) and *Polygalae Radix* (Yuan Zhi) and *Ziziphi Spinosae Semen* (Zao Ren) to calm the spirits.

2.2.2 气血亏虚

证候：眩晕动则加剧，劳累易发，面色㿠白，唇甲不华，发色不泽，心悸少寐，神疲懒言，饮食减少。舌质淡，脉细弱。

治法：补养气血，调养心脾。

方药：归脾汤。常用：党参、白术、黄芪益气健脾；当归、熟地黄、龙眼肉、大枣补血生血养心；茯苓、远志、枣仁宁心安神。

Modification: For middle-qi deficiency, clear away yang restrained, short breath and fatigue, little intake and lassitude, loose stool and bulging annus, use *Center-Supplementing qi-Boosting Decoction* (Bu Zhong Yi Qi Tang) to supplement the middle and boost qi as well rasie clarity and lower turbidity; for blood deficiency, add *Asini Corii Colla* (E Jiao), *Placenta Hominis* (Zi He Che), *Codonopsis Radix* (Dang Shen) and *Astragali Radix* (Huang Qi) in great amounts to supplement qi and blood, for heart spirit deprived of nourishment, palpitation and forgetfulness, add *Platycladi Semen* (Bai Zi Ren), *Albiziae Cortex* (He Huan Pi) and *Polygoni Multiflori Caulis* (Ye Jiao Teng) to nourish the heart and calm the spirits.

加减：若中气不足，清阳不升，气短乏力、纳少神疲、便溏下坠、脉象无力者，可合用补中益气汤补中益气、升清降浊；血虚甚者，可加阿胶、紫河车粉，重用党参、黄芪以补气血；若心神失养，心悸少寐健忘者加柏子仁、合欢皮、夜交藤养心安神。

2.2.3 Deficiency of Kidney Essence

2.2.3 肾精不足

Manifestations: vertigo for long, spiritual listlessness, tinnitus, insomnia and dreaminess, forgetfulness, soreness in the waist and knees. In case of predominance of yin-deficiency, it sees symptoms like feverish sensations in five minds, red tongue and fine rapid taut pulse. In case of predominance of yang-deficiency, it sees symptoms like physical cold, cold limbs, pale tongue and fine weak powerless pulse.

证候：眩晕日久，精神委靡，耳鸣，少寐多梦，健忘，腰膝酸软。偏于阴虚者，五心烦热，舌质红，脉弦细数。偏于阳虚者，形寒肢冷，舌质淡，脉沉细无力。

Treatment: To supplement the kidney and nourish yin for yin deficiency type and supplement the kidney and assist yang for yang deficiency.

治法：偏阴虚者，治以补肾滋阴；偏阳虚者，补肾助阳。

Formulas and Herbs: *Kidney Pills* (Zuo Gui Wan) to supplement the kidney and nourish yin and *Vital Gate Pills* (You Gui Wan) to supplement the kidney and assist yang. *Kidney Pills* (Zuo Gui Wan) is usually composed of *Rehmanniae Radix Praeparata* (Shu Di Huang), *Corni Fructus* (Shan Zhu Yu),

方药：补肾滋阴宜左归丸；补肾助阳宜右归丸。左归丸中熟地黄、山茱萸、菟丝子、牛膝、龟甲胶补益肾阴，鹿角胶填精补髓。右归丸中熟地黄、山茱萸、杜仲补肾，

Cuscutae Semen (Tu Si Zi), *Achyranthis Bidentatae Radix* (Niu Xi) and *Testudinis Carapacis et Plastri Colla* (Gui Jia Jiao) to supplement and Boost kidney yin. Similarly, *Vital Gate Pills* (You Gui Wan) is usually composed of *Rehmanniae Radix Praeparata* (Shu Di Huang), *Corni Fructus* (Shan Zhu Yu), and *Eucommiae Cortex* (Du Zhong) to supplement the kidney, while *Aconm Lateralis Radix Praeparata* (Fu Zi), *Cinnamomi Cortex* (Rou Gui) and *Cervi Cornus Colla* (Lu Jiao Jiao) to boost fire to assist yang.

附子、肉桂、鹿角胶益火助阳。

Modification: For serious vertigo, yin deficiency and floating yang, add *Os Draconis* (Long Gu), *Ostreae Concha* (Mu Li) and *Margaritifera Concha* (Zhen Zhu Mu) to subdue yang; for yin deficiency and heat inside, add *Anemarrhenae Rhizoma* (Zhi Mu), *Phellodendri Chinensis Cortex* (Huang Bo), *Moutan Cortex* (Mu Dan Pi) and *Lycii Cortex* (Di Gu Pi) to nourish yin and clear away heat.

加减: 若眩晕较甚,阴虚阳浮,可加龙骨、牡蛎、珍珠母以潜浮阳;若阴虚内热,可加知母、黄柏、牡丹皮、地骨皮等滋阴清热。

2. 2. 4 Phlegm-turbidity Blocking the Middle

2. 2. 4 痰浊中阻

Manifestations: Vertigo, heavy head as if clouded, or vertigo while watching, oppression in the chest and nausea, little intake and sleepliness; white greasy tongue fur; rolling soft pulse.

证候: 眩晕,头重如蒙,或伴视物眩晕,胸闷恶心,食少多寐。舌苔白腻,脉濡滑。

Treatment: To dry dampness and dispel phlegm; strengthen the spleen and harmonize the stomach.

治法: 燥湿祛痰,健脾和胃。

Formulas and Herbs: *Pinellia, White Atractyodest, and Gastrodia Decoction* (Ban Xia Bai Zhu Tian Ma Tang), usually composed of *Pinelliae Rhizoma* (Ban Xia) and *Citri Reticulatae Pericarpium* (Chen Pi) to strengthen the spleen, dry dampness and eliminate phlegm; *Atractylodis Macrocephalae Rhizoma* (Bai Zhu), *Coicis Semen* (Yi Yi Ren) and *Poria*

方药: 半夏白术天麻汤。常用:半夏、陈皮健脾燥湿化痰;白术、薏苡仁、茯苓健脾化湿;天麻化痰息风,止头眩。

(Fu Ling) to strengthen the spleen and dry dampness; *Gastrodiae Rhizoma* (Tian Ma) to resolve phlegm, stop wind and stop vertigo.

Modification: For frequent vomiting, add *Haematitum* (Zhe Shi), *Bambusae Caulis in Taenias* (Zhu Ru) and *Zingiberis Rhizoma Recens* (Sheng Jiang) to suppress the reserval flow to stop vomiting; for oppression in the stomach and no intake, add *Amomi Fructus Rotundus* (Bai Dou Kou) and *Amomi Fructus* (Sha Ren) to harmonize the stomach with their aroma; for depressed phlegm transforming to fire, distention and pain in the eyes and head, irritation, bitter mouth, thirst without desire for drink, yellow greasy tongue fur, rolling taut pulse, use *Coptis Gallbladder-Warming Decoction* (Huang Lian Wen Dan Tang) to clear away and dissolve phlegm-heat.

加减: 若呕吐频作者,加代赭石、竹茹、生姜镇逆止呕;若脘闷不食,加白豆蔻、砂仁芳香和胃;若痰郁化火,头目胀痛、心烦口苦、渴不欲饮、苔黄腻、脉弦滑者,宜用黄连温胆汤清化痰热。

2. 2. 5　Blood Stasis Blocking Orifices

Manifestations: Vertigo, headache, forgetfulness, insomnia, palpitation, dark purple lips and complexion, coarse skin and nails; stasis spots on the tongue; taut uneven pulse or fine uneven pulse.

Treatment: To remove stasis and generate new blood; dredge orifices and acitivate collaterals.

Formalas and Herbs: *Orifice-Dredging and Blood-Activating Decoction* (Tong Qiao Huo Xue Tang), usually composed of *Chuanxiong Rhizoma* (Chuan Xiong), *Paeoniae Radix Rubra* (Chi Shao Yao), *Persicae Semen* (Tao Ren) and *Carthami Flos* (Hong Hua) to activate blood circulation to remove stasis and dispel stasis to dredge collaterals; old Spring Oinion to break clots and dredge yang, Rice Wine (Huang Jiu) to assist blood flow; *Jujubae Fructus* (Da Zao) to boost qi.

2. 2. 5　瘀血阻窍

证候: 眩晕,头痛,健忘,失眠,心悸,面唇紫暗,肌肤甲错。舌有瘀点或瘀斑,脉弦涩或细涩。

治法: 祛瘀生新,通窍活络。

方药: 通窍活血汤。常用:川芎、赤芍药、桃仁、红花活血化瘀、祛瘀通络;老葱散结通阳,黄酒以助血行,大枣甘温益气。

Modification: For accompanying qi deficiency, lassitude and fatigue, add *Astragali Radix* (Huang Qi) and *Codonopsis Radix* (Dang Shen) to boost qi and promote blood circulation; for accompanying aversion to cold and cold limbs, add *Aconm Lateralis Radix Praeparata* (Fu Zi) and *Cinnamomi Ramulus* (Gui Zhi) to warm collaterals and activate blood; for newly falling injuries, add Lignum Sappan (Su Mu) and Resina Draconis (Xue Jie) to activate blood and eliminate stasis.

加减：若兼气虚，神疲乏力，加黄芪、党参益气行血；若兼有畏寒肢冷，加附子、桂枝温经活血；若新近跌仆坠损，可加苏木、血竭等活血祛瘀。

Stroke

中 风

Stroke is a diseasecharacterized by sudden fall, unconsciousness, facial distortion, barylalia, hemiparalysis or only manifested in deviated and paralyzed face without falling.

中风是以猝然昏仆，不省人事，伴口眼歪斜，言语不利，半身不遂或不经昏仆而仅以㖞僻不遂为主症的一类疾病。

1 Etiology and Pathogenesis

Stroke is caused by the functional disorder of the heart, live and kidney. Accumulated interal injuries, improper diet, emotional and spiritual disorder and exogenous pathogenic attacks will casue yin and yan disorder, qi and blood blockade, skin and collaterals deprived of nourishment or will lead to yinexhaustion downward and surging of liver-yang. When yang transforms into wind movement, blood moves reversely with qi which, along with phlegm and fire, will dash through meridians and collaterals and blind the upper orifices, leading to dangerous disease of upper excess and lower deficiency, poor mutual maintenance between yin and yang.

1 病因病机

中风的发生主要在于患者心、肝、肾三脏功能失调，因内伤积损、饮食不节、情志失调、外邪侵袭等诱因，致机体阴阳失调，气血运行受阻，肌肤筋脉失于濡养，或阴亏于下，肝阳暴张，阳化风动，血随气逆，挟痰挟火，横窜经遂，蒙蔽清窍，而成上实下虚，阴阳互不维系的危重证候。

1.1 Weakening Healthy Qi and Accumulated Internal Injury

Stroke can be caused by weak constitution due to aging, manifested by yin deficiency of the liver and kidney and the hyperactivity of liver-yang, or by innate consumption of yin, deficiency of blood and excessive yang and fire, together with inappropriate recuperation, which will result in the consumption of yin downward, surging of liver-yang, yang transforming into wind movement, and qi and blood reversal flow that blinds the spiritual orifices.

1.1 正气虚衰、内伤积损

年老体衰，肝肾阴虚，肝阳上亢，或素体阴亏血虚，阳盛火旺，复因将息失宜，致阴亏于下，肝阳鸱张，阳化动风，气血上逆，上蒙神窍，突发中风。

1.2 Improper Diet Generating Phlegm Turbidity

Favor for greasy, sweet, savoury, spice, roasted food, irregular hunger or gluttony, or overdrinking will disenable the spleen and then dampess gathers and transforms into phlegm, which blocks the meridians and collaterals, blind the upper orifices. When phlegm is depressed for long and transforms into heat, phlegm-heat will generate wind. Wind, fire, phlegm and heat become frenetical, dash through meridians and collaterals and blind the spiritual orifices, leading to stroke.

1.2 饮食不节、痰浊内生

嗜食肥甘厚味、辛香炙煿之物，或饥饱失宜，或饮酒过度，脾失健运，聚湿成痰，阻滞经络，蒙蔽清窍；日久痰郁化热，痰热生风，风火痰热内盛，横窜经络，上阻清窍，中风乃成。

1.3 Excess among the Five Emotions Transforming into Fire and Generating Wind

Excessamong the fiveemotions causes excessive heart-fire. Wind and fire stimulates each other and force the blood move reversely with qi to interfere with the original spirit. Or innate yin deficiency makes water unable to moisten wood, which when triggered by emotional and spiritual injury will bring about excessive hyperactivity of liver-yang and reverse flow of qi and blood, resulting in unconsciousness and stroke.

1.3 五志过极、化火生风

五志过极，心火暴盛，风火相煽，血随气逆，上扰元神；或素体阴虚，水不涵木，复因情志所伤，肝阳暴亢，气血上逆，心神昏冒而发为中风。

1.4 Attack of the Middle by Exogeneous Wind Due to Deficiency of Qi and Blood

Weak constitution due to aging or qi exhaustion due to overstrain or congenital defects or weakness due to prolonged illness, will lead to deficiency of qi and blood. Pathogenic wind then takes the advantage to find its way into meridians and collaterals to block qi and blood flow, and sinews, muscles, collaterals deprived of nourishment and moist. Or physical excess and qi deficiency, innate excess of phlegm-dampness and exogenous wind triggering phlegm and drooling will block the meridians and collaterals, leading to deviated and paralyzed face.

Stroke lies in thehead but is closely related to the heart, liver, spleen and kidney. Pathologically, it is disorder of yin and yang, reversal flow of qi and blood that attacks the head. To be specific, the six extremes—wind (liver-wind, exogenous wind), fire (heart-fire, liver-fire), phlegm (wind-phlegm, damp-phlegm), qi (reverse qi), blood (blood stasis) and deficiency (yin deficiency, qi deficiency)—will interchange and interact under some circumstances, causing stroke. Its pathological nature is primary deficiency (yin-deficiency of the liver and kidney, weakening and decreasing qi and blood) and secondary excess (wind and fire stimualating each other, phlegm-dampness blockade, reversal flow of qi and blood). For slight stroke, phlegm-dampness dashes through meridians and collaterals, which is also called meridian and collateral stroke. For severe stroke, liver yang and liver wind, along with phlegm and fire move upward and block the upper orifices, which is called organ stroke. The change of the severity of the disease is more likely in the

1.4 气血不足、外风入中

年老体衰，或过劳耗气，或禀赋不足，或久病体虚，皆可致气血不足，脉络空虚，风邪乘虚入中经络，气血痹阻，筋肉筋脉失于濡养；或形盛气虚，痰湿素盛，外风引动痰涎，闭阻经络，而致㖞僻不遂。

中风的病位在脑、与心、肝、脾、肾关系密切。基本病机为阴阳失调、气血逆乱，上犯于脑，细分之，有风（肝风、外风）、火（心火、肝火）、痰（风痰、湿痰）、气（气逆）、血（血瘀）、虚（阴虚、气虚）六端，在一定条件下，可互相作用、影响，突然发病。病性为本虚（肝肾阴虚，气血衰少）标实（风火相煽、痰湿壅盛、气血逆乱），上盛下虚。轻者风痰横窜经络而为中经络，重者肝阳肝风夹痰夹火上闭清窍而为中脏腑。轻重转化往往发生在疾病初发阶段，且变化迅速，与预后密切相关。

onset stage, which happens very rapidly and closely related to prognosis.

2　Syndrome Differentiation and Treatment

2.1　Key Points of Syndrome Differentiation

Doctor should first identify meridian and collateral stoke from organ stroke. The state of consciousness is the critical difference between the two types. Sudden fall and consciousness loss is organ stroke which is quite serious and deep-rooted. In constrast, meridian and collateral stroke is shallow and light without consciousness change. Moreover, organ stroke should be distinguished to be block pattern or depletion pattern. By block pattern, it refers to pathogenic factors blocked inside and is featured by sudden stroke and tend to be excess type. Meanwhile, depletion pattern refers to healthy qi depleted outside and is more likely to be transformed from worsened block pattern. Depletion pattern is mostly caused by deficiency and it is very dangerous and has very poor prognosis. Furthermore, block pattern can be subdivided into yang block and yin block. Besides, doctors should also identify disease stages, including acute stage, convalescent stage, and sequela stage. Acute stage means two weeks period after stroke attack and can be one month in case of organ stroke. Half a year after the acute stage is the convalescent stage and sequela stage refers to half a year after stroke attack. Finally, doctor should identify the developmental tendency of the disease. If it is firstly organ stroke, it can be seen that consciousness is gained gradually, that paralysis gets no worse or even relieved, which indicates the change from organ stroke to meridian

2　辨证论治

2.1　辨治要点

中风首辨中经络与中脏腑:有无神志改变是两者根本区别,即出现突然昏仆,不醒人事为中脏腑,病位较深,病情较重;中经络者,病位较浅,病情较轻,一般无神志改变。其次中脏腑当辨闭证与脱证:闭证乃邪闭于内,多见于中风暴起,病性多实;脱证为正脱于外,多由闭证恶化转变而来,以虚为主,病势笃危,预后凶险。而闭证又当根据有无热象,辨阳闭与阴闭。再者须辨病期,分为急性期、恢复期、后遗症期:急性期为发病后 2 周内,中脏腑可至 1 个月;恢复期为急性期后半年内;后遗症期为发病半年以上。最后辨病势顺逆:先中脏腑,如神志渐转清,不遂未加重或有恢复者,即病渐转化为中经络,病势为顺,预后多好;若属中脏腑重症,如神昏偏瘫症在急性期,仍属顺境;若见呃逆频繁或突然神昏,四肢抽搐不已,或背腹骤然灼热而四肢发凉至手足厥逆,或见戴阳证及呕血证,均属病势逆转。治

and collateral stroke. It is called favorable tendency and a good prognosis can be expected. If it is serious organ stroke such as consciousness loss and paralysis during acute stage, it is still considered to be favorable. If there is frequent hiccup and sudden loss of consciousness, limb convulsions, or sudden burning heat in the back and abdomen while the limbs are icy cold, or occurring yang-floating pattern and hemoptysis, it is considered ill-favored tendency. Doctors should identify the stages, take both the primary and secondary symptoms into account and abide by the principle of nourishing the liver and kidney, subduing yang and extinguishing wind, resolving and expelling phlegm according to the pathology. For meridian and collateral stroke, it should be to calm thc liver and stop wind, resolve stasis and dredge collaterals. For block pattern of organ stroke, it should be to stop wind and clear away fire, resolve phlegm and open into orifices, dredge fu-organs and purge heat. For depletion pattern, it should be to rescue yin, restore yang and prevent depletion. If it is block patter inside and depletion pattern outside, then arouse the spirits and open into orifices as well as to strengthen healthy qi and prevent depletion. During convalescent stage and sequela stage, it is advisable to supplement and strengthen the liver and kidney as well as boost qi and nourish blood. In addition, when stasis-heat blocks inside and obstructs fu-qi, then pathogenic heat interferes upward and the head fails to function. At such time, it is urgent to ensure disinhibited stool to purge phlegm heat and then consciousness can be regained.

当分清阶段,兼顾标本,根据病机,滋补肝肾、潜阳息风、豁痰祛瘀主要治则:中经络者,治以平肝息风、化瘀通络;中脏腑闭证,治以息风清火、豁痰开窍、通腑泻热。脱证,治以救阴回阳固脱;若为内闭外脱,则醒神开窍与扶正固脱兼顾。恢复期与后遗症期,应结合补益肝肾、益气养血。另当瘀热内阻、腑气不通、邪热上扰、神机失用之时,当及时通下,使大便通畅,痰热下泄,神识可清。

2.2 Therapeutic Methods for Different Patterns

2.2.1 Meridian and Collateral Stroke

2.2.1.1 Pathogenic Wind Attack Due to Empty Vessels and Collaterals

Manifestations: Ususally numbness of skin, sudden facial distortion, barylalia, drooling at the mouth or even hemiparalysis or accompanying aversion to cold, innate fever, taut torso and soreness in the joints; white thin tongue fur; rapid floating pulse.

Treatment: To dispel wind and resolve phlegm; nourish blood and dredge collaterals.

Formulas and Herbs: *Major Gentianae Macrophyllae Decoction (Da Qin Jiao Tang) and Pinellia, White Atractyodest, and Gastrodia Decoction* (Ban Xia Bai Zhu Tian Ma Tang), usually composed of *Gentianae Macrophyllae Radix* (Qin Jiao), *Notopterygii Rhizoma et Radix* (Qiang Huo), *Saposhnikoviae Radix* (Fang Feng), *Angelicae Dahuricae Radix* (Bai Zhi) and *Asari Radix et Rhizoma* (Xi Xin) to dispel wind and eliminate pathogens, *Rehmanniae Radix Praeparata* (Shu Di Huang), *Angelicae Sinensis Radix* (Dang Gui), *Chuanxiong Rhizoma* (Chuan Xiong) and *Paeoniae Radix Rubra* (Chi Shao) to nourish blood and activate blood circulation; *Pinelliae Rhizoma* (Ban Xia) and *Citri Reticulatae Pericarpium* (Chen Pi) to dry dampness and resolve phlegm; *Gastrodiae Rhizoma* (Tian Ma) to stop wind and dredge collaterals; *Atractylodis Macrocephalae Rhizoma* (Bai Zhu) and *Poria* (Fu Ling) to strengthen the spleen and eliminate dampness; *Gypsum Fibrosum Fibrosum* (Shi Gao), *Scutellariae Radix* (Huang Qin) and *Rehmannia Radix* (Sheng Di Huang) to clear away heat.

2.2 分型论治

2.2.1 中经络

2.2.1.1 脉络空虚,风邪为中

证候: 平素肌肤不仁,肌肤麻木,突然口眼歪斜,语言不利,口角流涎,甚则半身不遂,或兼见恶寒、平素经常发热、肢体拘急、关节酸痛等。苔薄白,脉浮数。

治法: 祛风化痰,养血通络。

方药: 大秦艽汤合半夏白术天麻汤化裁。常用:秦艽、羌活、防风、白芷、细辛祛风散邪;熟地黄、当归、川芎、赤芍药养血活血;半夏、陈皮燥湿化痰;天麻息风通络;白术、茯苓健脾祛湿;石膏、黄芩、生地黄清热。

Modification: For no interior heat, delete *Gypsum Fibrosum Fibrosum* (Shi Gao), *Scutellariae Radix* (Huang Qin) and *Rehmannia Radix* (Sheng Di Huang) and add *Typhonii Rhizoma* (Bai Fu zi) and *Scorpio* (Quan Xie) to dispel wind-phlegm and dredge collaterals; for wind-heat exterior symptoms, delete *Notopterygii Rhizoma et Radix* (Qiang Huo), *Saposhnikoviae Radix* (Fang Feng) and *Angelicae Sinensis Radix* (Dang Gui) and add *Angelicae Sinensis Radix* (Dang Gui), *Chrysanthemi Flos* (Ju Hua) and *Menthae Haplocalycis Herba* (Bo He) to disperse wind and clear away heat; for vomiting and excessive phlegm, delete *Rehmannia Radix* (Di Huang) and add *Arisaematis Rhizoma* (Nan Xing) to dispel phlegm and dry dampness; for numb feet and hands and coarse skin, add Poria-Pathfinder Pills (Zhi Mi Fu Ling Wan) to induce and dredge collaterals; for weak constitution due to aging, add *Astragali Radix* (Huang Qi) to boost qi and strengthen healthy qi.

加减：若无内热，可去生石膏、黄芩、生地黄，加白附子、全蝎祛风痰，通经络；若有风热表证，可去羌活、防风、当归等辛温之品，加桑叶、菊花、薄荷疏风清热；若呕逆痰盛，苔腻脉滑，可去地黄，加南星、橘红祛痰燥湿；若手足麻木、肌肤不仁，加指迷茯苓丸通利经络；年老体衰者，加黄芪益气扶正。

2.2.1.2 Wind-yang Interfering Upward Due to Yin Deficiency of the Liver and Kidney

2.2.1.2 肝肾阴虚，风阳上扰

Manifestations: Usually dizziness and headache, tinnitus and vertigo, insomnia and dreaminess, sudden deviated mouth and eyes, stiff tongue and barylalia, heaviness of hands and feet or even hemiparalysis; red tongue or with greasy tongue fur; rapid fine taut pulse or rolling taut pulse.

证候：平素头晕头痛，耳鸣目眩，少寐多梦，突然发生口眼歪斜、舌强语蹇、手足重滞，甚则半身不遂等症。舌质红或苔腻，脉弦细数或弦滑。

Treatment: To nourish yin and subdue yang; dispel wind and dredge collaterals.

治法：滋阴潜阳，祛风通络。

Formulas and Herbs: Modified *Liver-Sedating and Wind-Eliminating Decoction* (Zhen Gan Xi Feng Tang), usually composed of *Paeoniae Radix Alba* (Bai Shao Yao), *Scrophulariae Radix* (Xuan

方药：镇肝熄风汤加减。常用：白芍药、玄参、天门冬滋阴柔肝息风；龙骨、牡蛎、龟版、代赭石镇肝潜阳；重用

Shen) and *Asparagi Radix* (Tian Dong) to nourish yin, soften the liver and stop wind; *Os Draconis* (Long Gu), *Ostreae Concha* (Mu Li), *Testudinis Carapax et Plastrum* (Gui Jia) and *Haematitum* (Zhe Shi) to calm the liver and subdue yang; *Achyranthis Bidentatae Radix* (Niu Xi) in great amount to induce blood downward, *Gastrodiae Rhizoma* (Tian Ma), *Uncariae Ramulus cum Uncis* (Gou Teng) and *Chrysanthemi Flos* (Ju Hua) to strengthen the effect of soothing the liver and stopping wind.

牛膝引血下行；加天麻、钩藤、菊花增强平肝息风之力。

Modification: For serious phlegm-heat, add *Arisaema cum Bile* (Dan Xing), *Succus Bambosae* (Zhu Li) and *Fritillariae Cirrhosae Bulbus* (Bei Mu) to clear away phlegm-heat; for irritation in the heart, add *Gardeniae Fructus* (Zhi Zi) and *Scutellariae Radix* (Huang Qin) to clear away heat and remove irritation; for heavy headache, add *Cornu Antelopis* (Ling Yang Jiao), *Haliotidis Concha* (Shi Jue Ming) and *Prunellae Spica* (Xia Ku Cao) to clear away and stop wind-yang; for insomnia and dreaminess, add *Margaritifera Concha* (Zhen Zhu Mu), *Dens Draconis* (Long Chi), *Polygoni Multiflori Caulis* (Ye Jiao Teng) and *Poria cum Ligno Hospite* (Fu Shen) to calm the spirits.

加减：若痰热较重，加胆星、竹沥、川贝清化痰热；若心中烦热，加栀子，黄芩清热除烦；若头痛较重，加羚羊角、石决明、夏枯草清息风阳；若失眠多梦，加珍珠母、龙齿、夜交藤、伏神镇静安神。

2.2.2　Organ Stroke

2.2.2　中脏腑

2.2.2.1　Yang Blockage

2.2.2.1　阳闭

Manifestations: Sudden fall with unconsciousness, teeth clenched, mouth firmly closed, firm fist, difficult defecation and urination, serious limb convulsion, dark red face, fever, rough and foul breath, irritation and restlessness; yellow greasy tongue fur; rolling taut pulse.

证候：突然昏仆，不省人事，牙关紧闭，口噤不开，两手握固，大小便闭，肢体强痉，伴面赤身热，气粗口臭，躁扰不宁。苔黄腻，脉弦滑。

Treatment: To cleanse the liver and stop wind;

治法：清肝息风，辛凉开

open orifices with acrid and cool herbs.

窍。

Formulas and Herbs: *Crown Jewel Elixir* on Imperial Formula (Zhi Bao Dan), *Peaceful Palace Bovine Bezoar Pills* (An Gong Niu Huang Wan) and modificed *Cornu Antelopis Decoction* (Ling Yang Jiao Tang) via mouth or nose. *Cornu Antelopis* (Ling Yang Jiao) can be used to cleanse the liver and stop wind. *Chrysanthemi Flos* (Ju Hua), *Prunellae Spica* (Xia Ku Cao) and *Cicadae Periostracum* (Chan tuei) to stop wind and subdue fire, *Testudinis Carapax et Plastrum* (Gui Jia), *Paeoniae Radix Alba* (Bai Shao Yao) and *Haliotidis Concha* (Shi Jue Ming) to nourish yin and subdue yang, *Rehmannia Radix* (Sheng Di Huang) and *Moutan Cortex* (Mu Dan Pi) to cool blood and clear away heat.

方药：先灌服或鼻饲局方至宝丹、安宫牛黄丸，并用羚羊角汤加减。常用：羚羊角清肝息风；菊花、夏枯草、蝉蜕息风降火；龟版、白芍药、石决明育阴潜阳；生地黄、牡丹皮凉血清热。

Modification: For convulsion, add *Scorpio* (Quan Xie), *Scolopendra* (Wu Gong) and *Bombyx Batryticatus* (Jiang Chan) to stop wind and relieve convulsion; for plenty of phlegm, add *Succus Bambosae* (Zhu Li), *Bambusae Concretio Siliceae* (Tian Zhu Huang) and *Arisaema cum Bile* (Dan Nan Xing) to clear away phlegm-heat; for plenty of phlegm and hypnody, add *Acori Tatarinowii Rhizoma* (Shi Chang Pu) and *Curcumae Radix* (Yu Jin) to dissolve phlegm and open orifices.

加减：若有抽搐，加全蝎、蜈蚣、僵蚕息风止痉；若痰多，加竹沥、天竺黄、胆南星清化痰热；若昏睡，加石菖蒲、郁金豁痰透窍。

2.2.2.2 Yin Blockage

2.2.2.2 阴闭

Manifestations: Sudden fall with unconsciousness, teeth clenched, mouth firmly closed, firm fist, difficult defecation and urination, serious limb convulsion, pale complexion, dark lips, favor for lying down without irritation, excessive phlegm and drool, cool limbs; white tongue fur; deep rolling slow pulse.

证候：突然昏仆，不省人事，牙关紧闭，口噤不开，两手握固，大小便闭，肢体强痉，伴面白唇暗，静卧不烦，痰涎壅盛，四肢不温。苔白，脉沉滑缓。

Treatment: To dissolve phlegm and stop wind;

治法：豁痰息风，辛温开

open orifices with warm and acrid herbs.

Formulas and Herbs: Immediately take *Styrax Pills* (Su He Xiang Wan) via mouth or nose, along with modified *Phlegm-Cleansing Decoction* (Di Tan Tang), usually composed of *Pinelliae Rhizoma* (Ban Xia), *Citri Exocarpium Rubrum* (Ju Hong), *Poria* (Fu Ling) and *Bambusae Caulis in Taenias* (Zhu Ru) to dry dampness and dissolve phlegm, *Acori Tatarinowii Rhizoma* (Shi Chang Pu) and *Arisaema cum Bile* (Dan Nan Xing) to open into orifices and dissolve phlegm, *Aurantii Fructus Immaturus* (Zhi Shi) to lower reversal flow.

Modification: Add *Gastrodiae Rhizoma* (Tian Ma) and *Uncariae Ramulus cum Uncis* (Gou Teng) to strengthen the effect of soothing the liver and stopping wind.

2.2.2.3　Prostration Pattern

Manifestations: Sudden fall with unconsciousness, closed eyes and open mouth, snore and weak breath, loose fist and cold limbs, sweating, incontinence of defecation and urination, flaccid paralysis; flaccid tongue; weak fine pulse or weak disappearing pulse.

Treatment: To boot qi and restore yang; rescue yin and stop prostration.

Formulas and Herbs: *Cirsium Japonicum, Ginseng and Aconite Decoction* (Shen Fu Tang), in great amount together with *Pulse Engendering Powder* (Sheng Mai San), usually composed of *Ginseng Radix et Rhizoma* (Ren Shen), *Ophiopogonis Radix* (Mai Men Dong) and *Schisandrae Chinensis Fructus* (Wu Wei Zi) to greatly supplement qi and yin; *Aconm Lateralis Radix Praeparata* (Fu Zi) to restore yang and stop prostration.

Modification: For endless sweating, add

窍。

方药：急用苏合香丸灌服或鼻饲，并用涤痰汤加减。常用：半夏、橘红、茯苓、竹茹燥湿化痰；石菖蒲、胆南星开窍豁痰；枳实降气。

加减：可加天麻、钩藤以增平肝息风之力。

2.2.2.3　脱证

证候：突然昏仆，不省人事，目合口开，鼻鼾息微，手撒肢冷，汗多，大小便自遗，肢体软瘫，舌痿，脉细弱或脉微欲绝。

治法：益气回阳，救阴固脱。

方药：大剂参附汤合生脉散。常用人参、麦门冬、五味子大补气阴，附子回阳救逆。

加减：若汗出不止，加黄

Astragali Radix (Huang Qi), *Os Draconis* (Long Gu), *Ostreae Concha* (Mu Li) and *Corni Fructus* (Shan Zhu Yu) to astringe sweat and stop prostration.

芪、龙骨、牡蛎、山茱萸敛汗固脱。

2.2.3 Sequela Disease

2.2.3 后遗症

2.2.3.1 Hemiparalysis

2.2.3.1 半身不遂

(1) Qi Deficiency and Blood Stasis Block Collaterals

(1) 气虚血瘀,脉络瘀阻

Manifestations: Hemiparalysis, limp limbs, edema in the affected part, aphasia, deviated eyes and mouth, sallow yellow complexion or dark lusterless complexion; white thin tongue fur, pale purple tongue or deviated tongue; fine uneven weak pulse.

证候: 半身不遂,肢软无力,伴患侧手足浮肿,语言謇涩、口眼歪斜,面色萎黄或暗淡无华。苔薄白,舌淡紫,或舌体不正,脉细涩无力。

Treatment: To boost qi and activate blood flow; dredge and activate collaterals.

治法: 补气活血,通经活络。

Formulas and Herbs: *Enriching-yang and Transforming-Five Decoction* (Bu Yang Huai Wu Tang), usually composed of *Astragali Radix* (Huang Qi) in great amount to boost qi; *Persicae Semen* (Tao Ren), *Carthami Flos* (Hong Hua), *Angelicae Sinensis Radix* (Dang Gui), *Paeoniae Radix Rubra* (Chi Shao) and *Pheretima* (Di Long) to nourish blood and activate blood flow to remove stasis.

方药: 补阳化五汤加减。常重用黄芪补气,桃仁、红花、当归、赤芍药、地龙养血活血化瘀。

Modification: Add *Scorpio* (Quan Xie), *Zaocys* (Wu Shao She), *Cyathulae Radix* (Chuan Niu Xi), *Mori Ramulus* (Sang Zhi), *Eupolyphaga Steleophaga* (Zhe Chong) and *Dipsaci Radix* (Chuan Duan) to help to activate and dredge collaterals; for urinary incontinence, add *Mantidis Ootheca* (Sang Piao Xiao), *Corni Fructus* (Shan Zhu Yu), *Cinnamomi Cortex* (Rou Gui), *Alpiniae Oxyphyllae Fructus* (Yi Zhi Ren) and *Schisandrae Chinensis Fructus* (Wu Wei Zi) to astringe and supplement the kidney; for limp lower limbs, add *Taxilli Herba* (Sang Ji Sheng)

加减: 可加全蝎、乌梢蛇、川牛膝、桑枝、地鳖虫、川断等增强通经活络;若小便失禁,加桑螵蛸、山茱萸、肉桂、益智仁、五味子等补肾收涩;若下肢瘫软无力甚,加桑寄生、鹿筋补肾壮筋;若上肢偏废,加桂枝以通络;若患侧手足肿甚,加茯苓、泽泻、薏苡仁、防己等淡渗利湿;若兼见语言不利,加郁金、石菖

and *Musculus Cervi* (Lu Jin) to supplement the kidney and strengthen the sinews; for paralysis of upper limbs, add *Cinnamomi Ramulus* (Gui Zhi) to dredge collaterals; for heavy edema of affected parts, add *Poria* (Fu Ling), *Alismatis Rhizoma* (Ze Xie), *Coicis Semen* (Yi Yi Ren) and *Stephaniae Tetrandrae Radix* (Fang Ji) to eliminate dampness with its blander nature; for aphasia, add *Curcumae Radix* (Yu Jin), *Acori Tatarinowii Rhizoma* (Shi Chang Pu), *Polygalae Radix* (Yuan Zhi) to expel phlegm and disinhibit orifices; for accompanying facial distortion, add *Typhonii Rhizoma* (Bai Fu zi), *Scorpio* (Quan Xie) and *Bombyx Batryticatus* (Jiang Chan) to dispel wind and dredge collaterals; for numb limbs, add *Pinelliae Rhizoma* (Ban Xia), *Citri Reticulatae Pericarpium* (Chen Pi), *Poria* (Fu Ling), *Arisaema cum Bile* (Dan Nan Xing) to expel wind, dry dampness and dissolve phlegm; for constipation, add *Cannabis Fructus* (Huo Ma Ren), Semen Pruni (Yu Li Ren) and *Cistanchis Herba* (Rou Cong Rong) to moisten the intestines to promote defecation.

蒲、远志祛痰利窍；若兼口眼歪斜，加白附子、全蝎、僵蚕等祛风通络；若肢体麻木，加半夏、陈皮、茯苓、胆南星祛风燥湿化痰；若大便秘结，加火麻仁、郁李仁、肉苁蓉等润肠通便。

(2) Hyperactivity of Liver-yang, and Vessels and Collaterals Stasis

(2) 肝阳上亢，脉络瘀阻

Manifestations: Stiff and tense muscles in affected parts, headache and dizziness, dark red complexion and tinnitus; scartlet tongue with thin yellow tongue fur; powerful taut pulse.

证候: 患侧僵硬拘急，兼见头晕头痛，面赤耳鸣。舌红绛，苔薄黄，脉弦硬有力。

Treatment: To calm the liver and subdue yang; stop wind and dredge collaterals.

治法: 平肝潜阳，息风通络。

Formulas and Herbs: Modified *Gastrodia and Uncaria Decoction* (Tian Ma Gou Teng Yin), usually composed of *Gastrodiae Rhizoma* (Tian Ma), *Uncariae Ramulus cum Uncis* (Gou Teng) and

方药: 天麻钩藤饮加减。常用：天麻、钩藤、石决明平肝潜阳；黄芩、栀子清肝火；牛膝、杜仲、桑寄生补肝肾；

Haliotidis Concha (Shi Jue Ming) to calm the liver and subdue yang, *Scutellariae Radix* (Huang Qin) and *Gardeniae Fructus* (Zhi Zi) to clear away liver-fire; *Achyranthis Bidentatae Radix* (Niu Xi), *Eucommiae Cortex* (Du Zhong) and *Taxilli Herba* (Sang Ji Sheng) to supplement the liver and kidney; *Polygoni Multiflori Caulis* (Ye Jiao Teng) and Poria cum Ligno Hospite (Fu Shen) to nourish the heart and tranquilize the spirits.

夜交藤、茯神养心安神。

2.2.3.2 Aphasia

2.2.3.2 语言不利

(1) Wind-Phlegm Blocking Collaterals

(1) 风痰阻络

Manifestations: Stiff tongue and impeded speech, numb limbs; rolling taut pulse.

证候: 舌强语謇,肢体麻木。脉弦滑。

Treatment: To dispel wind and eliminate phlegm; release orifices and dredge collaterals.

治法: 祛风除痰,宣窍通络。

Formulas and Herbs: Modified *Speech-Returing Pills* (Jie Yu Dan), usually composed of *Gastrodiae Rhizoma* (Tian Ma), *Scorpio* (Quan Xie), *Arisaema cum Bile* (Dan Nan Xing) and *Typhonii Rhizoma* (Bai Fu zi) to calm the liver, stop wind and remove phlegm; *Polygalae Radix* (Yuan Zhi), *Acori Tatarinowii Rhizoma* (Shi Chang Pu) and *Aucklandiae Radix* (Mu Xiang) to release orifices, promote qi flow and dredge collaterals; *Notopterygii Rhizoma et Radix* (Qiang Huo) to dispel wind.

方药: 解语丹加减。常用:天麻、全蝎、胆南星、白附子等平肝息风祛痰;远志、石菖蒲、木香等宣窍行气通络;羌活祛风。

(2) Kidney Deficiency and Essence Exhaustion

(2) 肾虚精亏

Mainfestations: Loss of voice and disability to speak, palpitation, short breath and soreness in the wasit and knees.

证候: 音喑失语,心悸,短气及腰膝酸软。

Treatment: To nourish yin, invigorate the kidney and open orifices.

治法: 滋阴补肾利窍。

Formulas and Herbs: Modified *Rehmannia Decoction* (Di Huang Yin Zi), usually composed *Cinnamomi Cortex* (Rou Gui) and *Aconm Lateralis*

方药: 地黄饮子加减。常去肉桂、附子,加杏仁、桔梗、木蝴蝶开音利窍。

Radix Praeparata (Fu Zi) are deleted, and to which *Armeniacae Semen Amaru* (Ku Xing Ren), *Platycodi Radix* (Jie Geng) and *Oroxyli Semen* (Mu Hu Die) are added to restore voice and free orifices.

Modification: For hyperactivity of liver-yang and pathogenic phlegm blockig the orifices, use *Gastrodia and Uncaria Decoction* (Tian Ma Gou Teng Yin) or *Liver-Sedating and Wind-Eliminating Decoction* (Zhen Gan Xi Feng Tang), along with *Acori Tatarinowii Rhizoma* (Shi Chang Pu), *Polygalae Radix* (Yuan Zhi), *Arisaema cum Bile* (Dan Nan Xing), *Bambusae Concretio Siliceae* (Tian Zhu Huang) and *Scorpio* (Quan Xie) to calm the liver and subdue yang as well as remove phlegm and open orifices.

加减：若偏于肝阳上亢、痰邪阻窍，用天麻钩藤饮或镇肝熄风汤，加石菖蒲、远志、胆南星、天竺黄、全蝎平肝潜阳，化痰开窍

2.2.3.3 Deviated Eyes and Mouth

2.2.3.3 口眼歪斜

Manifestations: Deviated eyes and mouth.

证候：口眼歪斜

Treatment: To dispel wind, dissolve phlegm and dredge collaterals.

治法：祛风，除痰，通络。

Formulas and Herbs: Pull Aright Powder (Qian Zheng San), usually composed of *Sinapis Semen* (Jie Zi) to dispel wind, dissolve phlegm and dredge collaterals, *Bombyx Batryticatus* (Jiang Chan) and *Scorpio* (Quan Xie) to stop wind, dissolve phlegm and stop convulsion.

方药：牵正散。常用：白芥子祛风、化痰、通络；僵蚕、全蝎息风、化痰、镇痉。

Modification: For trembling eyes and mouth, add *Gastrodiae Rhizoma* (Tian Ma), *Uncariae Ramulus cum Uncis* (Gou Teng) and *Haliotidis Concha* (Shi Jue Ming) to calm the liver and stop wind.

加减：若口眼瞤动，加天麻、钩藤、石决明平肝息风。

Goiter

瘿　病

Goiter disease is a disease characterized by

瘿病是指颈前喉结两旁

lumps in the neck and both sides of the larynx.

结块肿大为主要临床特征的一类疾病。

1 Etilogy and Pathogenesis

1 病因病机

The major causes of goiter diseases are emotional and spiritual injuries, improper diet and failure to acclimatizing to a new environment. These factors lead to malfunctions of qi, blood and fluid. Then qi stagnation and phlegm accumulation obstructin the neck. That is the fundamental pathogenesis of the disease.

瘿病的病因主要是情志内伤、饮食和水土失宜。气血津液运行失常,气滞痰凝,壅结颈前为其基本病机。

1.1 Emotional and Spiriutal Injury, Depressive Qi and Phlegm Blockage

1.1 情志内伤,气郁痰阻

Prolonged worry, anger and depression make the liver fail to disperse, which impedes qi activities and turn accumulated fluid into phlegm. Qi stagnation and phlegm accumulation leads to goiter disease, which changes with emotions and spirits. When blood circulation is inhibited for long, the swollen goiter will turn hard or into nodes.

长期忧愁思虑或愤郁恼怒,肝失条达,气机不利,津聚成痰,气滞痰凝,瘿病乃成,其消长可随情志波动。日久血行亦受障碍,可致瘿肿较硬或有结节。

1.2 Improper Diet and Poor Acclimatization Injuring the Spleen and Stomach

1.2 饮食、水土失宜损伤脾胃

Improper diet or living in the mountainous areas for long, or failure to acclimatize to a new environment will not only make damge to the spleen and stomach but also influence the proper flow of qi and blood. Theformer will disenable the spleen to transport and to transform water-dampness, which generates phlegm; and the latter make phlegm accumulated in the neck, leading to goiter diseases.

饮食失调,或久居高山之地,水土失宜,一则影响脾胃功能,脾失健运,水湿不化,聚湿生痰,二则影响气血正常运行,痰气瘀结颈前,发为瘿病。

1.3 Constitutional Factors That Likely to Trigger the Diseases or Transform into Fire

1.3 体质因素影响发病或易于化火

Women's physiological features such as menstruation, pregnancy, childbirth and breastfeeding

妇女的经、孕、产、乳等生理特点与肝经气血密切相

are closely related to qi and blood of liver meridians. When affected by emotional and disturbance and improper diet, it will lead to qi depression and phlegm accumulation, qi stagnation and blood stasis, and depressed liver-qi transforming into fire. Therefore, women are more likely to have goiter diseases. Moreover, if one is innate yin deficient, then when depression and stasis of phlegm and qi transform into fire, it will make great damage to yin, complicate and prolong the disease.

关，遇情志、饮食等致病因素，常引起气郁痰结、气滞血瘀、肝郁化火等病理变化，故女性易患瘿病。另外，素有阴亏之人，痰气郁滞之后易于化火，阴伤更甚，常使病机复杂，病程缠绵。

1.4 Phlegm Accumulating with Stasis Due to Prolonged Illness

When qi stagnation and phlegm stasis remain long, it will hinder blood circulation and obstruct blood vessels, causing qi, phlegm and stasis to get entangled and accumulated in the neck in shape of hard lumps with nodes that do not disappear for long and sometimes with prominent red vessels or purple dark stasis spots on the tongue.

Goiste disease is mainly caused by entanglement of qi stagnation, phlegm accumulation and blood stasis in the neck. At the beginning, it is often due to depressed qi activity, accumulated phlegm and fluid, and phlegm and qi interwined in the neck. When it is prolonged, blood vessels are blocked. Qi, phlegm and stasis are the main causes. Goiter disease lies in the liver and spleen, but is also related to the heart. It pathological nature is more often than not, excess, which, when it lasts long, will turns into deficiency, including qi deficiency and yin deficiency and finally takes on the complication of excess and deficiency.

1.4 病久不化痰瘀互结

气滞痰凝日久，可使血行不畅，血脉瘀阻，致气、痰、瘀互相胶结，聚于颈前，可见颈前肿块，经久不消，且质硬或伴结节，甚至赤脉显露，还可兼见舌紫暗或有瘀点、瘀斑。

瘿病的基本病机是气滞、痰凝、血瘀壅结颈前，初期多为气机郁滞，津凝痰聚，痰气搏结颈前所致，日久引起血脉瘀阻，气、痰、瘀合而为患。主要病位在肝脾，与心也有关。病理性质以实证居多，久病由实致虚，气虚、阴虚等渐显而呈虚实夹杂之候。

2 Syndrome Differentiation and Treatment

2.1 Key Points of Syndrome Differentiation

To treat goiter disease, first doctors should identify the englargement of the goiters, including the size, location, symmetry, texture and slipperiness. Secondly, doctors should then identify excess from deficiency and distinguish the existence of heat and fire, and the complications of qi, phlegm and stasis. As goiter disease is likely to transform into fire, doctors should, along with signs of tongue and pulse, distinguish the existence of exuberant liver-fire and yin-deficiency and fire-excess of the heart and liver, which, if prolonged, will turn into deficiency and cuase pathological changes and symptoms of heart-and-liver yin-deficiency and spleen-qi deficiency, leading to the complication of both deficiency and excess. The treatment should be focused on regulating qi and dissolving phlegm, remove goiter and nodes. For hard goister or with nodes, treat with herbs that can promote blood flow and remove stasis. For heat transforming to toxin, treat with herbs that can purge fire and detoxify. Goiter diseases, when prolonged, will exhaust and damage healthy qi, for which treat with herbs that can strengthen healthy qi. For fire-depression consuming yin, nouish yin and subdue fire and focus on these two methods in light of the predominance of excessive fire or consumed yin. For deficiency of yin-blood and stirring up of liver-wind, it is better to nourish yin and subdue yang, calm the liver and stop wind. For innate weak stomach, or qi and blood exhaustion due to prolonged illness, and unpeaceful minds and spirits, it is advisable to

2 辨证论治

2.1 辨治要点

瘿病首辨瘿肿的情况。首先根据临床特点，如肿块的大小、单侧或双侧发病、对称与否及质地、光滑等情况辨证。其次辨证候虚实及火热有无，辨清气、痰、瘀之兼夹情况。由于瘿病易于化火，应综合舌脉症，辨别有无肝火亢盛与心肝阴虚火旺之象，日久转虚可见心肝阴虚或脾气虚的病理变化及症状，成为虚实夹杂之证。治以理气化痰，消瘿散结，瘿肿质地较硬或有结节者，应配合活血化瘀，热甚化毒者应参以泻火解毒。瘿病日久，多耗伤正气，应注意扶正；火郁伤阴者，当以滋阴降火为主，并根据火旺、阴伤之偏盛，侧重滋阴或降火。如阴血不足，肝风内动者，宜育阴潜阳，平肝息风。如脾胃素虚或病久气血耗伤，心神不宁者，应加强健脾益气，养血安神。

strengthen the spleen and boost qi, nourish blood and calm the spirits.

2.2 Therapeutic Methods for Different Patterns

2.2.1 Qi Depression and Phlegm Obstruction

Manifestations: Goister in the front of neck, suffusive, symmetrical, soft, slippery, no pain, distention in the neck, oppression in the chest, frequent sigh or dashing pain in the chest and hypochondria, changing with emotions and spirits; thin white tongue fur; taut pulse.

Treatment: To regulate qi and diperse depression; dissolve phlegm and eliminate goiter.

Formulas and Herbs: *Four Seas Depression-Soothing Pills* (Si Hai Shu Yu Wan), usually composed of Radix Dolomiaeae Berardioidis (Qing Mu Xiang) and *Citri Reticulatae Pericarpium* (Chen Pi) to disperse the liver and regulate qi; *Laminariae Thallus Eckloniae Thallus* (Kun Bu), *Herba Zosterae Marinae* (Hai Dai), *Sargassum* (Hai Zao), *Sepiae Endoconcha*(Hai Piao Xiao) and *Meretricis Concha Cyclinae Concha*(Hai Ha ke) to dissolve phlegm and soften the hardness, eliminate goiter and break up nodes.

Modification: For hypochondriac pain and oppression, add *Bupleuri Radix* (Chai Hu), *Cyperi Rhizoma* (Xiang Fu), *Aurantii Fructus*(Zhi Qiao) and *Curcumae Radix* (Yu Jin) to disperse the liver and regulate qi, *Acori Tatarinowii Rhizoma* (Shi Chang Pu), *Curcumae Radix* (Yu Jin) and *Trichosanthis Fructus* (Gua Lou) to break up depression and nodes; for discomfort in the throat and neck, and hoarse voice, add *Platycodi Radix*(Jie Geng), *Amomi Fructus* (Niu Bang Zi), *Oroxyli Semen* (Mu Hu Die) and *Belamecandae Rhizoma* (She Gan) to

2.2 分型论治

2.2.1 气郁痰阻

证候: 颈前正中肿大,弥漫对称,质软、光滑、不痛,颈部觉胀,胸闷、喜太息,或兼胸胁窜痛,病情随情志而波动。苔薄白,脉弦。

治法: 理气疏郁,化痰消瘿。

方药: 四海舒郁丸。常用:青木香、陈皮疏肝理气;昆布、海带、海藻、海螵蛸、海蛤壳化痰软坚、消瘿散结。

加减: 胁痛憋闷者,加柴胡、香附、枳壳、郁金疏肝理气,石菖蒲、郁金、瓜蒌开郁散结;咽颈不适及声音嘶哑者,加桔梗、牛蒡子、木蝴蝶、射干利咽消肿。

benefit the throat and eliminate swelling.

2.2.2 Phlegm Accumulation and Blood Stasis

Manifestations: Hard lump in the front of neck or sometimes with nodes which does not disappear for long, oppression in the chest, poor appetite; purple dark tongue with stasis spots; white thin tongue fur or white tongue fur; taut or uneven pulse.

Treatment: To regulate qi and activate blood circulation; dissolve phlegm and remove goiter.

Formulas and Herbs: *Sargassum Jade Flask Decoction* (Hai Zao Yu Hu Tang), usually composed of *Sargassum* (Hai Zao), *Laminariae Thallus Eckloniae Thallus* (Kun Bu) and *Herba Zosterae Marinae* (Hai Dai) to dissolve phlegm, soften hardness, eliminate goiter and break up nodes; *Citri Reticulatae Pericarpium Viride* (Qing Pi), *Citri Reticulatae Pericarpium* (Chen Pi), *Pinelliae Rhizoma* (Ban Xia), *Fritillariae Thunbergii Bulbus* (Zhe Bei Mu), *Forsythiae Fructus* (Lian Qiao), *Glycyrrhizae Radix et Rhizoma* (Gan Cao) to regulate qi, dissolve phlegm and break up nodes; *Angelicae Sinensis Radix* (Dang Gui) and *Chuanxiong Rhizoma* (Chuan Xiong) to nourish blood and active blood circulation.

Modification: For oppression and discomfort in the chest, add *Curcumae Radix* (Yu Jin), *Cyperi Rhizoma* (Xiang Fu) and *Aurantii Fructus* (Zhi Qiao) to regulate qi and break up depression; for prolonged depression transforming into heat with symptoms such as feverish sensations, red tongue, yellow tongue and rapid pulse, add *Prunellae Spica* (Xia Ku Cao), *Scrophulariae Radix* (Xuan Shen) and *Moutan Cortex* (Mu Dan Pi) to clear away heat

2.2.2 痰结血瘀

证候: 颈前出现肿块,按之较硬或有结节,肿块经久不消,胸闷,纳差,舌质紫暗或有瘀点、瘀斑。苔薄白或白腻,脉弦或涩。

治法: 理气活血,化痰消瘿。

方药: 海藻玉壶汤。常用:海藻、昆布、海带化痰软坚,消瘿散结;青皮、陈皮、半夏、贝母、连翘、甘草理气化痰散结;当归、川芎养血活血。

加减: 若胸闷不舒者,加郁金、香附、枳壳理气开郁;若郁久化热而见烦热、舌红、苔黄、脉数,加夏枯草、玄参、牡丹皮清热泻火;若纳差、便溏者,加白术、茯苓、薏苡仁、山药健脾益气;若结块较硬及有结节者,酌加三棱、莪术、丹参、穿山甲片等增强活

and purge fire; for poor appetite and loose stool, add *Atractylodis Macrocephalae Rhizoma* (Bai Zhu), *Poria* (Fu Ling), *Coicis Semen* (Yi Yi Ren) and *Dioscoreae Rhizoma* (Shan Yao) to strengthen the spleen and boost qi; for fairly hard nodes, add moderately *Sparganii Rhizoma* (San Leng), *Curcumae Rhizoma* (E Zhu), *Salviae Miltiorrhizae Radix et Rhizoma Radix* (Dan Shen) and *Manitis Squama* (Chuan Shan Jia) to strengthen the effects of activating blood circulation and softening hardness, removing goiter and breaking up nodes; for hard lump with little or no mobility, add moderately *Vespae Nidus* (Feng Fang), *Cremastrae Pseudobulbus Pleiones Pseudobulbus* (Shan Ci Gu), *Herba Duchesneae* (She Mei), *Semiaquilegiae Radix* (Tian Kui Zi) and *Scutellariae Barbatae Herba* (Ban Zhi Lian) or along with *Bovine Bezoar Pills* (Xi Huang Wan) to remove stasis, dredge collaterals, detoxify and eliminate swelling.

血软坚、消瘿散结的作用；若肿块坚硬、移动性小甚至不能移动者，可酌加露蜂房、山慈菇、蛇莓、天葵子、半枝莲等，或配合犀黄丸，以散瘀通络、解毒消肿。

2.2.3 Obstruction of Liver-fire

Manifestations: Light or moderate enlargement in the front of the neck, which is generally soft and slippery and moves with swallowing activity, feverish sensations, sweating, irritation, protruding eyes, trembling fingers, flushing face and bitter mouth; red tongue with yellow tongue fur; rapid taut pulse.

Treatment: To cleanse the liver and purge fire; calm the liver and stop wind.

Formulas and Herbs: *Gardenia Liver-Draining Decoction* (Zhi Zi Qing Gan Tang) and *Sargassum and Dioscoreae Bulbiferae Decoction* (Zao Yao Tang) to eliminate goister, break up nodes, cool blood and subdue fire. Pay attention that *Dioscoreae*

2.2.3 肝火旺盛

证候：颈前轻度或中度肿大，一般柔软光滑，可随吞咽动作活动，烦热，易汗出，性情急躁易怒，眼球突出，手指颤抖，面部烘热，口苦。舌红，苔黄，脉弦数。

治法：清肝泻火，平肝息风。

方药：栀子清肝汤合藻药散。常用：栀子、牡丹皮清泻肝火；柴胡、白芍药疏肝解郁；茯苓、甘草、当归、川芎益脾养血活血；牛蒡子散热利

Rhizoma Bulbiferae (Huang Yao Zi) cannot be taken for long and be prohibited from those who has damage in the liver.

咽消肿;海藻、黄药子消瘿散结,凉血降火。注意黄药子不能久服,需跟踪肝功能情况,肝损者忌服。

Modification: For exuberant wind-yang and trembling fingers, add *Haliotidis Concha* (Shi Jue Ming), *Uncariae Ramulus cum Uncis* (Gou Teng), *Tribuli Fructus* (Ji Li) and *Ostreae Concha* (Mu Li) to calm the liver to stop wind; for irritation and restlessness, add *Gentianae Radix et Rhizoma* (Long Dan), *Prunellae Spica* (Xia Ku Cao) *Scutellariae Radix* (Huang Qin) to cleanse the liver and purge fire; for excessive heat in the stomach with big appetite and likeliness to get hunger quickly, use along *White Tiger Decoction* (Bai Hu Tang) to purge heat in the stomach, invigorate the stomach and protect fluid.

加减: 若风阳内盛,手指颤抖者,加石决明、钩藤、白蒺藜、牡蛎平肝息风;若烦躁易怒者,加龙胆草、夏枯草、黄芩清肝泻火;兼见胃热内盛而见多食易饥者,合用白虎汤清泄胃热、益胃护津。

2.2.4 Yin Deficiency of the Heart and Liver

Manifestations: Big or small goiter, soft, slow onset, palpitation, irritation, sleeplessness, sweating, trembling fingers, dry eyes, vertigo, fatigue; red trembling tongue; fine rapid taut pulse.

Treatment: To nourish yin essence, cleanse the liver and calm the spirits.

Formulas and Herbs: *Water-Enriching Liver-Clear awaying Decoction* (Zi Shui Qing Gan Yin), usually composed of *Rehmanniae Radix Praeparata* (Shu Di Huang), *Angelicae Sinensis Radix Corpus* (Dang Gui Shen), *Paeoniae Radix Alba* (Bai Shao Yao) and *Corni Fructus* (Shan Zhu Yu) to nourish yin and soften the liver; *Bupleuri Radix* (Chai Hu), *Gardeniae Fructus* (Zhi Zi), *Moutan Cortex* (Mu Dan Pi) and *Alismatis Rhizoma* (Ze Xie) to cleanse

2.2.4 心肝阴虚

证候: 瘿肿或大或小,质软,病起较缓,心悸不宁,心烦少寐,易汗出,手指颤动,眼干目眩,倦怠乏力。舌质红,舌体颤动,脉弦细数。

治法: 滋养阴精,清肝宁心。

方药: 滋水清肝饮。常用:熟地黄、当归身、白芍药、山茱萸养阴柔肝,柴胡、山栀、牡丹皮、泽泻清肝泻火,茯苓、山药、枣仁益气安神。

the liver and purge fire; *Poria* (Fu Ling), *Dioscoreae Rhizoma* (Shan Yao) and *Ziziphi Spinosae Semen* (Zao Ren) to boost qi and calm the spirits.

Modification: For liver-yin deficiency and dull pain due to liver-collateral disharmony, use *An Ever Effective Decoction for Nourishing Liver and Kidney* (Yi Guan Jian) to nourish and disperse the liver; for remarkable palpitation and insomnia, use *Celestial Emperor Heart-Supplementing Elixir* (Tian Wang Bu Xin Dan) to nourish yin, cleanse the heart and calm the spirits; for stirring up of deficiency-wind, trembling fingers and tongue, add *Uncariae Ramulus cum Uncis* (Gou Teng) and *Tribuli Fructus* (Ji Li) to calm the liver and stop wind; for the spleen which fails to transport with symptoms such as loose and more frequent stool, add *Atractylodis Macrocephalae Rhizoma* (Bai Zhu), *Coicis Semen* (Yi Yi Ren) and *Hordei Fructus Germinatus* (Mai Ya) to strengthen the spleen and stomach; for kidney-yin deficiency, tinnitus and soreness in the waist and knees, add *Testudinis Carapax et Plastrum* (Gui Jia), *Taxilli Herba* (Sang Ji Sheng), *Achyranthis Bidentatae Radix* (Niu Xi) and *Cuscutae Semen* (Tu Si Zi) to nourish kidney-yin; for healthy qi exhausted due to prolonged illness, emaciation and fatigue due to deficiency of essence and blood, decreasing menstration or menopause and impotence, add moderately *Astragali Radix* (Huang Qi), *Lycii Fructus* (Gou Qi Zi) and *Polygoni Multiflori Radix* Praeparata (Zhi Shou Wu) to boost qi and nourish essence and blood.

加减: 若肝阴亏虚、肝络不和而见胁痛隐隐,用一贯煎养肝疏肝;若心悸失眠较显,可选天王补心丹养阴清心安神;虚风内动,手指及舌体颤抖者,加钩藤、白蒺藜平肝息风;若脾失健运,见大便稀溏、便次增加,加白术、薏苡仁、麦芽健运脾胃;若肾阴亏虚而见耳鸣、腰膝酸软者,加龟甲、桑寄生、牛膝,菟丝子滋补肾阴;若病久正气耗伤,精血不足而见消瘦乏力,女性月经量少或闭经,男子阳痿者,可酌加黄芪、枸杞子、制首乌等补益正气、滋养精血。

Chapter 5 Kidney System Diseases

第5章 肾系病证

Edema

Edema is a disease of dysfunction of the lung, spleen and kidney, characterized by swelling in the face, eyelid, limbs, back and even the whole body, as a result of unsmooth water channels and qi activities that causes water and fluid retention, penetrating into skin.

1 Etiology and Pathogenesis

Edema is usually caused by pathogenic wind attacking the exterior, sore-toxin attacking the interior, exogenous water-damp affection, improper diet, congenital defects, prolonged illness and fatigue. The pathogenesis is impairment of splenic movement and transformation, impairment of kidney's closing and opening, and disturbance of qi transformation in san jiao, which leads to water and fluid penetrating into the skin.

1.1 Pathogenic Wind Attacking and Impairment of Regulation of the Lung

Pathogenic wind attacks the exterior, blocking the lung-qi and impairing the regulation of the lung. When wind blocks water passage, edema is caused.

水　肿

水肿是由于肺、脾、肾功能失调，水道失畅，气化不利，导致体内水液潴留，泛滥肌肤，表现以头面、眼睑、四肢、腹背，甚至全身浮肿为特征的一类病证。

1 病因病机

水肿的病因主要有风邪袭表、疮毒内犯、外感水湿、饮食不节及禀赋不足、久病劳倦等，基本病机为肺失通调，脾失转输，肾失开阖，三焦气化不利，水液泛滥肌肤。

1.1 风邪外袭，肺失通调

风邪袭表，肺气闭塞，通调失职，风遏水阻，发为水肿。

1.2 Spreading of Sore-toxin Interiorly Attacking the Lung and Spleen

Scabies, boils and sore-toxin on the skin attacking the lung and spleen, impairing the qi activities of three jiaos, which leads to water retention inside and causes edema.

1.2 疮毒浸淫，内归肺脾

肌肤疖痈疮毒内归脾肺，导致三焦气化不利，水湿内停，发为水肿。

1.3 Water-damp Affection Encumbers the Spleen-earth

Being caught in the rain or living in damp places for long will lead to water-damp to attack inside and encumbers spleen-qi. When spleen-yang fails to move and transform, edema is caused.

1.3 水湿浸渍，困遏脾土

冒雨涉水，或久居潮湿之地，水湿内侵，脾气受困，脾阳不振，而成水肿。

1.4 Excessive Damp-heat Obstructing the Three jiaos

When damp-heat attacks inside or depressed dampness transforms into heat, three jiaos will be obstructed, which leads to obstruction of water passages, causing edema in the end.

1.4 湿热内盛，三焦壅滞

湿热内侵，或湿郁化热，三焦壅滞，水道不通，而成水肿。

1.5 Retention of Blood Stasis inside Causing Mutual Blocking of Stasis and Water

Edema due to proloned illness, water retention, dampness obstruction and blockade of the three Jiao causes qi stagnation and blood stasis. Stasis and water blocks each other, leading to intractable edema.

1.5 瘀血内停，瘀水交阻

久病水肿，水停湿阻，三焦壅塞，造成气滞血瘀，瘀水交阻，互为因果，而成难治性水肿。

1.6 Improper Diet and Overstrain Making Damages to the Spleen and Stomach

Irregular diet or overstrain will make damages to the spleen and stomach, resulting in hypoactivity of spleen-yang. When the spleen fails to transport and distribute water essence, water remains in the skin, causing edema.

1.6 饮食劳倦，损伤脾胃

饮食失常，或劳倦过度，损伤脾胃，脾阳不振，水精不能输布，水湿潴留肌肤发为水肿。

1.7 Excess of Sexual Intercourse Damaging Kidney-essence

Excess of sexual intercourse and childbirth will

1.7 房劳过度，内伤肾元

房劳过度，生育过多，损

damage kidney-essence, which causes kidney-qi deficiency and dysfunction of water transportation and distribution. Water remains in the skin, causing edema.

伤肾精，肾气不足，水湿输布失常，溢于肌肤，发为水肿。

Overall, edema is related to the lung, spleen and kidney, among which the kidney is critical. The pathological factors are pathogenic wind, water-damp, sore-toxin and blood stasis. In light of the difference of pathological factors and individual constitution, edema, by its pathological nature, can be grouped into yin edema and yang edema and they can be interchangeable and complicated. Yang edema is of excess type and is more likely to be caused by pathogenic wind, sore-toxin and water-damp, which lies in the lung and spleen. Meanwhile, yin edema pertains to deficiency type or complication type and is likely to be caused by improper diet, overstrain, innate deficiency and weakness due to prolonged illness, which lies in the spleen and kidney.

综上所述，其病位在肺、脾、肾，而关键在肾。病理因素为风邪、水湿、疮毒、瘀血。由于致病因素及体质的差异，水肿的病理性质有阴水、阳水之分，并可相互转换或夹杂：阳水属实，多由外感风邪、疮毒、水湿而成，病位在肺、脾；阴水属虚或虚实夹杂，多由饮食劳倦、禀赋不足、久病体虚所致，病位在脾、肾。

2 Syndrome Differentiation and Treatment

2 辨证论治

2.1 Key Points of Syndrome Differentiation

2.1 辨治要点

For edema, it should be first identifiedas yang edema or yin edema. Then, identify the pathological position.

水肿病证首先须辨阳水、阴水。其次应辨病变之脏腑。

First, identify yin edema from yang edema. Yang edema usually takes on shortly but lasts short, and is generally caused by pathogenic wind, damp-toxin, water and damp-heat. Swelling is more likely to start top-down from the head and face to the overall body. The affected skin is tense and shiny and bounces back quickly after being pressed. The symptoms are of exterior, excess and heat type. Pa-

先辨阴水、阳水：阳水，一般起病较快，病程较短，病因多为风邪、湿毒、水气、湿热。肿多从头面开始，由上而下，继及全身，肿处皮肤绷急光亮，按之凹陷即起，证见表、实、热证，患者一般情况较好，无正气大亏之象。阴

tients are generally well without signs of exhaustion of heathly-qi. On the other hand, yin edema takes on gradually and lasts long and is usually caused by imporper diet, overstrain and zang-fu organ injuries due to prenatal and postnatal factors. Swelling begins bottom-up, spreading to the overall body. The skin is loose and cannot bounce back quickly after being pressed, or even it feels like mud when pressed. The symptoms are of interior, deficiency and cold type. Patients are usually in poor conditions with remarkable injury in zang-fu organs. Yin edema and yang edema can interchange.

水，一般起病较慢，病程较长，病因多为饮食劳倦，先天或后天因素所致的脏腑亏损。肿多由下而上，继及全身，肿处皮肤松弛，按之凹陷不易恢复，甚则按之如泥，证见里、虚、寒证，患者一般情况较差，脏腑功能明显受损。阳水阴水亦可相互转化。其次辨病变之脏腑，在肺、脾、肾、心、肝之差异：肺水多并见咳逆；脾水多并见脘腹满闷而食少；肾水多并见腰膝酸软，或见肢冷，或见烦热；心水多并见心悸、怔忡；肝水多并见胸胁胀满。最后，对于虚实夹杂，多脏共病者，应仔细辨清本虚标实之主次。

Secondly, identify the pathological organs, the lung, spleen, kidney, heart or liver. Lung edema usually has cough while spleen edema witnesses fullness and oppression in the stomach and abdomen and little intake. Kidney edema has soreness in the waist and knees or cold limbs or feverish sensation. Heart edemausually has palpitation while liver edema sees distention and fullness in the chest and hypochondria. Finally, in case of complication of deficiency and excess and affection of more than one organ, it is important to distinguish carefully the primary and secondary conflict between deficiency and excess, the primary symptoms and the secondary symptoms. The treatment principle of edema should be to promote sweating, promote urination, and expel water by purgation. The specific treat-

水肿的治疗原则是发汗、利尿、泻下逐水，具体应用视阴阳虚实不同而异：阳水以祛邪为主，应予发汗、利水或攻逐，同时配合清热解毒、理气化湿等法；阴水当以扶正为主，健脾温肾，同时配以利水、养阴、活血、祛瘀等法；对于虚实夹杂者，则当兼顾，或先攻后补，或攻补兼施。

ments should be in accordance with difference between yin and yang, deficiency and excess. For yang edema, eliminate pathogenic factors by inducing perspiration, promoting urination, along with clearing away heat, detoxifying, regulating qi and dissipating dampness. For yin edema, it is most important to strengthen the healthy qi, invigorate the spleen and warm the kidney along with disinhibiting water, nourishing yin, activating blood and expelling stasis. For complication of deficiency and excess, both of them should be treated or treated by attacking method first and supplementing method next.

2.2 Therapeutic Methods for Different Patterns

2.2 分型论治

2.2.1 Yang Edema

2.2.1 阳水

2.2.1.1 Wind and Water Fights against Each Other

2.2.1.1 风水相搏

Manifestations: Swelling in the face and eyelid, spreading to limbs and torso in a short time with aversion to cold, fever, soreness in the joint, difficult urination; for relatively wind-heat type: swollen and sore throat, red tongue, and rapid floating rolling pulse; for wind-cold type: aversion to cold, cough and gasp, thin white tongue fur, floating rolling or floating taut pulse.

证候:眼睑浮肿,继则四肢及全身皆肿,来势迅速,多有恶寒,发热,肢节酸楚,小便不利等症。偏于风热者,伴咽喉红肿疼痛,舌质红,脉浮滑数。偏于风寒者,兼恶寒,咳喘。舌苔薄白,脉浮滑或浮紧。

Treatment: To disperse wind, clear away heat, disperse the lung and promote water movement.

治法:疏风清热,宣肺行水。

Formulas and Herbs: Spleen-Effusing Decoction Plus White Atractyodest (Yue Bi Jia Zhu Tang), usually composed of *Ephedrae Herba* (Ma Huang) and *Zingiberis Rhizoma Recens* (Sheng Jiang) to disperse the lung, relieve exterior symptoms and promote water movement; *Atractylodis Macrocephalae Rhizoma* (Bai Zhu) to strengthen the spleen to

方药:越婢加术汤。常用:麻黄、生姜宣肺解表行水;白术健脾制水;石膏解肌清热。

eliminate fluid retention; *Gypsum Fibrosum Fibrosum* (Shi Gao) to relieve muscles and clear away heat.

Modification: For predominance of wind-cold, delete *Gypsum Fibrosum Fibrosum* (Shi Gao) and add instead *Perillae Folium*(Zi Su Ye), *Cinnamomi Ramulus* (Gui Zhi) and *Saposhnikoviae Radix* (Fang Feng) to expel wind and cold; for predominance of wind-heat, add *Forsythiae Fructus* (Lian Qiao), *Platycodi Radix*(Jie Geng), *Isatidis Radix* (Ban Lan Gen) and fresh *Phragmitis Rhiamoma* (Lu Gen) to clear away heat and relieve the throat, detoxify and disperse binds; for sweating and aversion to wind and deficiency of defensive yang, use modified *Stephaniae Tetrandrae and Astragali Decoction* (Fang Ji Huang Qi Tang) to promote qi flow and water movement.

加减: 若风寒偏盛,去石膏,加苏叶、桂枝、防风祛风散寒;若风热偏盛,可加连翘、桔梗、板蓝根、鲜芦根,以清热利咽,解毒散结;如见汗出恶风,卫阳已虚,则用防己黄芪汤加减,以益气行水。

2.2.1.2　Spreading Damp-toxin

2.2.1.2　湿毒浸淫

Manifesatations: Swelling in the face and eyelid, spreading to the whole body, shiny skin, little urine in dark red, boils and sores over the body, even ulcerated, aversion to wind, fever; red tongue, thin yellow tongue fur; rapid floating pulse or rapid rolling pulse.

证候: 眼睑浮肿,延及全身,皮肤光亮,尿少色赤,身发疮痍,甚则溃烂,恶风发热。舌质红,苔薄黄,脉浮数或滑数。

Treatment: To disperse the lung and detoxify, remove dampness and eliminate edema.

治法: 宣肺解毒,利湿消肿。

Formulas and Herbs: *Ephedra, Forsythia, and Rice Bean Decoction* (Ma Huang Lian Qiao Chi Xiao Dou Tang) and *Five-Ingredient Toxin-Dispersing Beverage* (Wu Wei Xiao Du Yin). The former is usually composed of *Ephedrae Herba* (Ma Huang), *Mori Cortex* (Sang Bai Pi) and *Armeniacae Semen Amaru* (Ku Xing Ren) to disperse the lung and promote water movement; *Forsythiae Fructus* (Lian

方药: 麻黄连翘赤小豆汤合五味消毒饮。前方以麻黄、桑白皮、杏仁宣肺行水;连翘、赤小豆清热利水;后方用金银花、野菊花、蒲公英、紫花地丁、紫背天葵加强清热解毒之力。

Qiao) and *Vignae Semen*(Chi Xiao Dou) to clear away heat and promote urination while the latter is usually composed of *Lonicerae Japonicae Flos* (Jin Yin Hua), *Chrysanthemi Flos* Indici (Ye Ju Hua), *Taraxaci Herba* (Pu Gong Ying), *Violae Herba* (Zi Hua Di Ding) and *Herba Gynurae Bicoloris* (Zi Bei Tian Kui) to strengthen the effect of clear awaying away heat.

Modification: For excess of dampness and skin ulceration, add *Sophorae Flavescentis Radix* (Ku Shen) and *Smilacis Glabrae Rhizoma* (Tu Fu Ling); for red swollen due to blood-heat, add *Moutan Cortex* (Mu Dan Pi) and *Paeoniae Radix Rubra* (Chi Shao Yao); for skin itch due to excess of wind, add *Dictamni Cortex* (Bai Xian Pi) and *Kochiae Fructus* (Di Fu Zi).

加减: 湿盛皮肤糜烂者，加苦参、土茯苓；若血热而红肿，加牡丹皮、赤芍药；若风盛而皮肤瘙痒者，加白鲜皮、地肤子。

2.2.1.3 Spreading of Water-damp

Manifestations: Slow onset, long duration, edema all over the body, lower limb in particular, no mark after pressing, little and short urine, general heaviness, chest oppression, poor appetite, nausea; white greasy tongue fur; deep slow pulse.

Treatment: To invogirate the spleen to dry dampness, activate yang and drain water.

Formulas and Herbs: *Five Cortices Cool Decoction* (Wu Pi Yin) and *Poria Stomach Decoction* (Wei Ling Tang). The former is usually composed of *Mori Cortex* (Sang Bai Pi), *Arecae Pericarpium* (Da Fu Pi), *Cortex Poria* (Fu Ling Pi), *Citri Reticulatae Pericarpium* (Chen Pi) and *Cortex Zingiberis Recens* (Sheng Jiang Pi) to eliminate dampnes and drain water while the latter is usually composed of *Atractylodis Macrocephalae Rhizoma* (Bai Zhu) and *Poria* (Fu Ling) to invigorate the spleen and dis-

2.2.1.3 水湿浸渍

证候: 起病缓慢，病程较长，全身水肿，下肢明显，按之没指，小便短少，身体困重，胸闷，纳呆，泛恶，苔白腻，脉沉缓。

治法: 运脾化湿，通阳利水。

方药: 五皮饮合胃苓汤。前方以桑白皮、大腹皮、茯苓皮、陈皮、生姜皮化湿行水；后方用白术、茯苓健脾化湿，苍术、厚朴健脾燥湿，肉桂温阳化气，猪苓、泽泻利水消肿。

solve dampness, *Atractylodis Rhizoma* (Cang Zhu) and *Magnoliae Officinalis Cortex* (Hou Pu) to strengthen the spleen and eliminate dampness, *Cinnamomi Cortex* (Rou Gui) to warm yang and transform qi, *Polyporus* (Zhu Ling) and *Alismatis Rhizoma* (Ze Xie) to drain water and eliminate edema.

Modification: For swollen face and chest fullness so much as unable to lie down, add *Perillae Fructus* (Zi Su Zi) and *Descurainiae Semen Lepidii Semen* (Ting Li Zi) to lower qi and disperse water; for exogenous pathogenic wind affection, edema and even asthma, add *Ephedrae Herba* (Ma Huang) and *Armeniacae Semen Amaru* (Ku Xing Ren) to disperse the lung and stop asthma; for dampness encumbering zhong jiao and distention and fullness in the stomach and obdomen, add *Semen Zanthoxyli Pericarpium* (Chuan Jiao Mu), *Arecae Pericarpium* (Da Fu Pi) and *Zingiberis Rhizoma* (Gan Jiang).

加减: 若面肿,胸满,不得卧,加苏子、葶苈子降气行水;若外感风邪,肿甚而喘者,可加麻黄、杏仁宣肺平喘;若湿困中焦,脘腹胀满者,可加川椒目、大腹皮、干姜。

2.2.1.4　Excessive Damp-heat

2.2.1.4　湿热壅盛

Manifestations: Edema all the the body, tense, shiny skin, discomfort and oppression in the chest and stomach, feverish dysphoria, thirst, short and dark red urine or dry stool; red tongue with yellow greasy tongue fur; deep rapid or soft rapid pulse.

证候: 遍体浮肿,皮肤绷急光亮,胸脘痞闷,烦热口渴,小便短赤,或大便干结,舌红,苔黄腻,脉沉数或濡数。

Treatment: To clear away damp-heat.

治法: 分利湿热。

Formulas and Herbs: *Coursing and Piercing Decoction* (Shu Zao Yin Zi), usually composed of *Phytolaccae Radix* (Shang Lu) and *Arecae Semen* (Bing Lang) to attack and expel water retention to promote urination and defecation; *Notopterygii Rhizoma et Radix* (Qiang Huo) and *Gentianae Macrophyllae Radix* (Qin Jiao) to disperse wind, relieve exterior and drain water; *Alismatis Rhizoma* (Ze Xie), *Vignae Semen* (Chi Xiao Dou), *Akebiae*

方药: 疏凿饮子。常用:商陆、槟榔攻逐水饮,通利二便;羌活、秦艽疏风解表利水;泽泻、赤小豆、木通、椒目利尿消肿。全方共起解表、利尿、攻逐之效。

Caulis (Mu Tong) and *Semen Zanthoxyli* (Jiao Mu) to promote urination and eliminate edema. These two formulas together can relieve exterior symptoms, induce urination and expel damp-heat.

Modification: For continuous abdominal fullness and difficult defecation, add *Fangji, Zanthoxylum, Lepidium Descurainiae, and Rhubarb Pills* (Ji Jiao Li Huang Wan) to increase the strength of attacking and purging; for serious edema and gasping as much as unable to lie down, add *Descurainiae Semen Lepidii Semen* (Ting Li Zi) and *Mori Cortex* (Sang Bai Pi) to purge the lung and drain water; for overall severe edema, gasping, palpitation, ascites, difficult urination and deep strong pulse, use *Ten Jujubes Decoction* (Shi Zao Tang) which should be stop as soon as the symptoms are relieved.

加减：若腹满不减，大便不通者，可合己椒苈黄丸，以助攻泻之力；若肿势严重，兼见喘促不得平卧者，加葶苈子、桑白皮泻肺利水；若全身高度浮肿，气喘、心悸、腹水、小便不利、脉沉而有力者，可用十枣汤治疗，但应中病即止。

2.2.2 Yin Edema

2.2.2.1 Deficiency of Spleen-yang

Manifestations: Prolonged body edema, below the waist in particular, difficult to bounce back when pressed, distention and oppression in the stomach and abdomen, less intake, loose stool, lustreles face, lassitude and fatigue, tired limbs, little and short urine; pale tongue with white greasy or slippery tongue fur; deep slow or deep weak pulse.

Treatment: To strengthen the spleen, warm yang and drain water.

Formulas and Herbs: Modified *Spleen-Firming Decoction* (Shi Pi Yin), usually composed of *Aconiti Radix Lateralis Praeparata Secta* (Fu Pian), *Zingiberis Rhizoma* (Gan Jiang), *Atractylodis Macrocephalae Rhizoma* (Bai Zhu), *Magnoliae Officinalis Cortex* (Hou Po), *Tsaoko Fructus* (Cao Guo) and *Poria* (Fu Ling) to warm and invigorate spleen-

2.2.2 阴水

2.2.2.1 脾阳虚衰

证候：身肿日久，腰以下为甚，按之凹陷不易恢复，脘腹胀闷，纳减便溏，面色不华，神疲乏力，四肢倦怠，小便短少。舌质淡，苔白腻或白滑，脉沉缓或沉弱。

治法：健脾温阳利水。

方药：实脾饮加减。常用：附片、干姜、白术、厚朴、草果、茯苓温运脾阳；槟榔、木瓜、木香理气行水。

yang; *Arecae Semen* (Bing Lang), *Chaenomelis Fructus* (Mu Gua) and *Aucklandiae Radix* (Mu Xiang) to regulate qi and drain water.

Modification: For severe qi deficiency with symptoms such as short breath weak voice, add *Ginseng Radix et Rhizoma* (Ren Shen) and *Astragali Radix* (Huang Qi) to strengthen spleen and boost qi; for little and short urination, add *Cinnamomi Ramulus* (Gui Zhi) and *Alismatis Rhizoma* (Ze Xie) to help the bladder to transform qi to drain water; for damp-heat consuming yin due to prolonged illness, add *Rehmannia Radix* (Sheng Di Huang), *Ophiopogonis Radix* (Mai Men Dong) and *Anemarrhenae Rhizoma* (Zhi Mu) to nourish kidney-yin.

加减: 若气虚甚,症见气短声弱者,可加人参、黄芪以健脾益气;若小便短少,可加桂枝、泽泻,以助膀胱气化而行水;若病久湿热伤阴,加生地黄、麦门冬、知母滋养肾阴。

2.2.2.2 Declination of Kidney-yang

2.2.2.2 肾阳衰微

Manifestations: Coming and going edema in the face and body, in particular, the lower body, difficult to bounce back when pressed, less or more urine, cold-pain in the waist, cold limbs, fear for cold, lassitude, waxy pale complexion, even palpitation, gasping and unable to lie down, distention and fullness of the enlarged abdomen; pale enlarged tongue with white tongue fur; deep fine pulse or deep retarded powerless pulse.

证候: 水肿反复消长不已,面浮身肿,腰以下甚,按之凹陷不起,尿量减少或反多,腰酸冷痛,四肢厥冷,怯寒神疲,面色㿠白,甚者心悸胸闷,喘促难卧,腹大胀满,舌质淡胖,苔白,脉沉细或沉迟无力。

Treatment: To warm the kidney to boost yang, transform qi to disperse water.

治法: 温肾助阳,化气行水。

Formulas and Herbs: *Life Saver Kidney Qi Pills* (Ji Sheng Shen Qi Wan) and *True Warrior Decoction* (Zhen Wu Tang). The former is usually composed of *Dioscoreae Rhizoma* (Shan Yao), *Poria* (Fu Ling) and *Alismatis Rhizoma* (Ze Xie) to strengthen the spleen and eliminate dampness; *Rehmanniae Radix Praeparata* (Shu Di Huang) and

方药: 济生肾气丸合真武汤。前方用山药、茯苓、泽泻健脾利湿,熟地黄、山茱萸补肾滋阴,附子、肉桂温补肾阳;后方以附子、白术温补脾肾,茯苓、生姜利水发汗,白芍药和营养血。

Corni Fructus (Shan Zhu Yu) to supplement kidney and nourish yin, *Aconm Lateralis Radix Praeparata* (Fu Zi) and *Cinnamomi Cortex* (Rou Gui) to warm and supplement kidney-yang while the latter is usually composed of *Aconm Lateralis Radix Praeparata* (Fu Zi) and *Atractylodis Macrocephalae Rhizoma* (Bai Zhu) to warm and supplement the spleen and kidney; *Poria* (Fu Ling) and *Zingiberis Rhizoma Recens* (Sheng Jiang) to drain water and promote sweating; *Paeoniae Radix Alba* (Bai Shao Yao) to harmonize ying and nourish blood.

Modification: For clear, long urination in great amount, delete *Alismatis Rhizoma* (Ze Xie) and *Plantaginis Semen* (Che Qian Zi) and add *Cuscutae Semen* (Tu Si Zi) and *Psoraleae Fructus* (Bu Gu Zhi) to warm and consolidate the lower origin; for edema mainly in the face, indifferent facial expressions, slow movement, physical cold and cold limbs, use modified *Vital Gate Pills* (You Gui Wan) to warm and supplement spleen-yang; for continual edema, lassitude, soreness in the waist and spermatorhea, thirst and dry mouth, feverish dysphoria in the five certers, red tongue and weak fine pulse, use *Kidney Pills* (Zuo Gui Wan) plus *Alismatis Rhizoma* (Ze Xie), *Poria* (Fu Ling) and *Malvae Fructus* (Dong Kui Zi).

加减：若小便清长量多，去泽泻、车前子，加菟丝子、补骨脂以温固下元；若面部浮肿为主，表情淡漠、动作迟缓、形寒肢冷，治以温补肾阳为主，方用右归丸加减；若水肿反复发作，精神疲惫、腰酸遗精、口渴干燥、五心烦热、舌红、脉细弱者，治当滋补肾阴为主，方用左归丸加泽泻、茯苓、冬葵子。

2.2.2.3 Blood Stasis and Water Obstruction

Manifestations: Prolonged edema with different intensity in differe parts, edema in limbs or whole body, in particular lower body, stasis spots on the skin, sharp pain in the waist or with blood urine; dark purple tongue with white tongue fur; deep fine uneven pulse.

Treatment: To active blood movement to dispel

2.2.2.3 血瘀水阻

证候：水肿延久不退，肿势轻重不一，四肢或全身浮肿，以下肢为主，皮肤瘀斑，腰部刺痛，或伴血尿。舌紫暗，苔白，脉沉细涩。

治法：活血祛瘀，化气行

stasis, transform qi to disperse water.

水。

Formulas and Herbs: *Peach Pit, Safflower and Four Agents Decoction* (Tao Hong Si Wu Tang) and *Poria Five Powder* (Wu Ling San). The former is usually composed of *Persicae Semen* (Tao Ren), *Carthami Flos* (Hong Hua), *Angelicae Sinensis Radix* (Dang Gui) and *Chuanxiong Rhizoma* (Chuan Xiong) to activate blood movement to eliminate stasis while the latter is usually composed of *Cinnamomi Ramulus* (Gui Zhi) and *Atractylodis Macrocephalae Rhizoma* (Bai Zhu) to dredge yang and invigorate the spleen, *Poria* (Fu Ling), *Alismatis Rhizoma* (Ze Xie) and *Polyporus* (Zhu Ling) to promote urination and eliminate edema.

方药：桃红四物汤合五苓散。前方用桃仁、红花、当归、川芎等活血化瘀；后方以桂枝、白术通阳健脾，茯苓、泽泻、猪苓利尿消肿。

Modification: For serious edema all over the body, gasping, irritation, difficult urination, all of which pertains to symptoms of excess of blood stasis and water and upflow of lung-qi, add *Descurainiae Semen Lepidii Semen* (Ting Li Zi), *Semen Zanthoxyli Pericarpium* (Chuan Jiao Mu) and *Lycopi Herba* (Ze Lan) to expel stasis and purge the lung; for soreness in the waist and knees, lassitude and fatigue which pertains to symptoms of deficiency of spleen and kidney, use *Life Saver Kidney Qi Pills* (Ji Sheng Shen Qi Wan); for fatigue and cold limbs, less intake and loose stool, add *Astragali Radix* (Huang Qi) and *Aconm Lateralis Radix Praeparata* (Fu Zi).

加减：若全身肿甚，气喘烦闷、小便不利，此为血瘀水盛、肺气上逆，可加葶苈子、川椒目、泽兰以逐瘀泻肺；如见腰膝酸软、神疲乏力，乃为脾肾亏虚之象，可合用济生肾气丸；若有乏力肢冷、纳减便溏，可加黄芪、附子。

For edema due to prolonged illness, despite no remarkable stasis and obstruction, itis usual clinical practice to use *Leonuri Herba* (Yi Mu Cao), *Lycopi Herba* (Ze Lan), *Persicae Semen* (Tao Ren) and *Carthami Flos* (Hong Hua) to help to promote urination and eliminate edema.

对于久病水肿者，虽无明显瘀阻之象，临床上亦常合用益母草、泽兰、桃仁、红花等药，以加强利尿消肿的效果。

Stranguria Syndrome

淋 证

Stranguria syndrome patterns can be caused by many factors, characterized by damp-heat accumulated in xia jiao, impairment of qi transformation of the kidney and bladder. Clinically, the symptoms are frequent and urgent urination, dribble after urianation, roughness and pain in the urethra, tension in the lower abdomen or pain stretching to waist and abdomen.

淋证是由多种原因造成湿热蕴结下焦，肾与膀胱气化不利，临床表现为小便频急，淋沥不尽，尿道涩痛，小腹拘急或痛引腰腹为主症的一类病证。

1 Etiology and Pathogenesis

1 病因病机

By clinical manifestations, stranguria syndrome can be grouped into six types, and the major cause is damp-heat. The pathogenesis is damp-heat accumulated in xia jiao and impairment of qi transformation of the kidney and bladder.

淋证根据其临床表现分为六种，其病因主要是以湿热为主，基本病机是湿热蕴结下焦、肾与膀胱气化不利。

1.1 Damp-heat Pours Downward and Pathogenic Factors Stagnating in the Bladder

1.1 湿热下注，膀胱邪滞

Unclean vulva allows pathogenic damp-heat to make way into the bladder. Or over-intake of spicy, sweet and greasy food generate damp-heat inside which pours downward into the bladder which fails to transform qi, leading to stranguria syndrome.

外阴不洁，湿热之邪入侵膀胱；或过食辛辣肥甘，湿热内生，下注膀胱，膀胱气化不利而为淋证。

1.2 Emotional and Spirtual Dissatisfaction Causing Depressed Liver and Qi Stagnation

1.2 情志不遂，肝郁气滞

Depression, anger will disenable the liver to disperse or transform depressed qi into fire. When qi and fire depressed inxia jiao, the bladder fails to transform qi and leads to stranguria syndrome.

抑郁恼怒，肝失疏泄，或气郁化火，气火郁于下焦，膀胱气化不利而为淋证。

1.3 Weak Constitution and Strain for Long Making the Spleen and Kidney Deficient

1.3 体虚久劳，脾肾亏虚

Innate deficiency, aging, prolonged illness, o-

先天不足、年老久病、劳

ver strain or excess of sexual life will make the spleen and kidney go deficient. The kidney and bladder then cannot well transform qi, leading to stranguria syndrome.

累过度、房事不节等导致脾肾亏虚，肾与膀胱气化无权遂成淋证。

Overall, stranguria syndrome lie in the bladder and kidney but also are related to the liver and spleen. The pathogensis is damp-heat and its nature is pathogenic excess during the onset stage but can be turned into deficiency type or complicated type if prolonged.

综上所述，淋证其病位在膀胱与肾，发病亦与肝、脾有关。其病理因素主要为湿热之邪。病理性质在病初多为邪实之证，久病则由实转虚，或虚实夹杂。

2 Syndrome Differentiation and Treatment

2 辨证论治

2.1 Key Points of Syndrome Differentiation

2.1 辨治要点

Firstly, it is important to differentiate the six kinds ofstranguria syndrome. Generally speaking, heat stranguria takes on suddenly with fever sometimes, and has other symptoms like red hot urine and buring pain during urination. Stone stranguria refer to difficult urination dispite great urgency, sharp pain in the urethera, stretching to the lower abdomen which can only be relieved when sand stones are urinated. Qi stranguria has such symptoms as fullness, oppression, distention and pain in less abdomen, roughness and pain during urination or dropsy in the less abdomen and dribble after urination. Blood stranguria shows symptoms like scarlet or pale red blood urine or pain with blood clots. Chyloid stranguria refers to roughness and pain during urination and urine as turbid as milky or rice water. Overstrain stranguria syndrome has such symptoms as unremarkable roughness and pain during urination but dribble after urination and continuous soreness in the waist due to prolonged stranguria, which will be triggered and aggravated by overstrain

淋证首先应别六淋之类别：一般来说，热淋，起病多急，或伴发热，小便赤热，尿时灼痛；石淋，小便窘急不能卒出，尿道刺痛，痛引少腹，尿出砂石而痛止；气淋，少腹满闷胀痛，小便艰涩疼痛，或少腹坠胀，尿后余沥不尽；血淋，尿色鲜红或淡红或夹血块而痛；膏淋，小便涩痛，尿液浑浊如脂膏或米泔水；劳淋，久患淋证，遇劳倦、房事即加重或诱发，小便涩痛不显著，余沥不尽，腰痛缠绵。其次，须辨证候之虚实，辨别淋证虚实的主要依据：一是病程，新病初起或在急性发作阶段多实，久病者病程较长，病势缠绵多虚；二看疼痛程度，病急痛甚者多实，病缓痛轻者多虚；三看尿液，浑浊

and sexual intercourse. Secondly, it is necessary to differentiate deficiency from excess. There are two important aspects to do this. One is duration. Newly developed diseases or diseases during the onset stage are most likely to be execess type while proloned diseases are to be deficiency type. Second is intensity of pain. Acute pain is usually of excess type while light pain, deficiency type. Third is urine. Turbid yellow dark urine is due to excess of pathogenic damp-heat while pale, clear away and white urine is due to healthy qi deficiency or removal of pathogenic factors. For complication of deficiency and excess, it is important to distinguish the primary symptoms from the secondary symptoms, deficiency from excess along with the acuteness or chonicness of the disease.

黄赤多为湿热邪气盛,清白,色淡为正虚或邪退。虚实夹杂者,须分清标本虚实之主次,证情之缓急。

Treatment of stranguria syndrome should follow the principles of clearing away heat and promomting uriantion for excess type while supplementing for deficiency type. In details, for excess type, it is advisable to clear away heat and eliminate dampness for predominance of damp-heat in the bladder and to cool blood and stop bleeding for predominance of heat scorching blood collaterals. For sand stone accumulation as the primary cause, it is better to relieve stranguria syndrome and expel stone and to activate and disperse qi for qi stagnation. For deficiency type, if spleen deficiency is the primary cause, then strengthen the spleen and boost qi. If kidney deficiency is the cause, then supplement and invigorate the spleen. For complication of deficiency and excess, then dredge and supplement at the same time in term of the primary and secondary symptoms and the intensity of urgency.

淋证的基本治则为实则清利,虚则补益。具体而言,实证以膀胱湿热为主者,治宜清热利湿;以热灼血络为主者,治宜凉血止血;以砂石结聚为主者,治以通淋排石;以气滞不利为主者,治以利气疏导。虚证以脾虚为主者,治以健脾益气;以肾虚为主者,治宜补虚益肾。对虚实夹杂者,又当通补兼施,审其主次缓急,兼顾治疗。

2.2 Therapeutic Methods for Different Patterns

2.2.1 Heat Stranguria

Manifestations: Frequent short rough urination with sharp burning pain, urine in yellow and dark, tension and distention pain in the lower abdomen, or cold and fever, bitter mouth, nausea or soreness in the waist that refuses to be pressed upon, or dry stool; yellow greasy tongue fur; rolling rapid pulse.

Treatment: To clear away heat, eliminate dampness and relieve stranguria.

Formulas and Herbs: *Eight Corrections Powder* (Ba Zheng San), usually composed of *Dianthi Herba* (Qu Mai), *Polygoni Avicularis Herba* (Bian Xu), *Plantaginis Semen* (Che Qian Zi) and *Talcum* (Hua Shi) to clear away heat, eliminate dampness and relieve stranguria; *Rhei Radix et Rhizoma* (Da Huang) and *Gardeniae Fructus* (Zhi Zi) to purge damp-heat in the three jiaos.

Modification: For accompanying symptoms like cold and fever, bitter mouth and nausea, add *Scutellariae Radix* (Huang Qin) and *Bupleuri Radix* (Chai Hu) to harmonize and relieve shaoyang; for remarkable heat-toxin with such symptoms as high fever, pain in the waist and scarlet tongue, use *Coptis Detoxifying Decoction* (Huang Lian Jie Du Tang) and *Five-Ingredient Toxin-Dispersing Beverage* (Wu Wei Xiao Du Yin) to purge fire and detoxify; for damp-heat consuming yin with symptoms like dry mouth and throat, feverish dysphoria in the five centers and red tongue with little tongue fur, delete *Rhei Radix et Rhizoma* (Da Huang) and add *Rehmannia Radix* (Sheng Di Huang), *Anemarrhenae Rhizoma* (Zhi Mu) and *Imperatae Rhizoma* (Bai Mao Gen) to nourish yin and clear away heat.

2.2 分型论治

2.2.1 热淋

证候: 小便频数短涩,灼热刺痛,溺色黄赤,少腹拘急胀痛,或有寒热,口苦,呕恶,或有腰痛拒按,或有大便秘结。苔黄腻,脉滑数。

治法: 清热利湿通淋。

方药: 八正散。常用:瞿麦、萹蓄、车前子、滑石清热利湿通淋;大黄、栀子清泄三焦湿热。

加减: 若伴寒热、口苦、呕恶者,加黄芩、柴胡以和解少阳;若热毒显著,症见高热、腰痛、舌红绛,用黄连解毒汤合五味消毒饮以清热泻火解毒;若湿热伤阴者,见口干舌燥、五心烦热、舌红少苔,去大黄,加生地黄、知母、白茅根以养阴清热。

2.2.2 Stone Stranguria

Manifestations: Sand stones in urine, roughness and pain during urination or sudden stop during urination, tension and pain in the urethera, tension in the lower abdomen without expection, heavy twisting pain in the waist on one side, even stretching to vulva, blood in the urine; red tongue, thin yellow tongue fur; string pulse or rapid string pulse.

Treatment: To clear away heat and eliminate dampness, expel sand stones and relieve stranguria.

Formulas and Herbs: *Pyrrosia Powder* (Shi Wei San), usually composed of *Pyrrosiae Folium* (Shi Wei), *Dianthi Herba* (Qu Mai), *Talcum* (Hua Shi) and *Plantaginis Semen* (Che Qian Zi) to promote urination, relieve stranguria and expel sand stones; *Lysimachiae Herba* (Jin Qian Cao), *Lygodii Spora* (Hai Jin Sha) and *Galli Gigerii Endothelium Corneum* (Ji Nei Jin) to expel sand stones and soften the hard.

Modification: For twisting pain in the waist, add *Paeoniae Radix Alba* (Bai Shao Yao) and *Glycyrrhizae Radix et Rhizoma* (Gan Cao) to relieve the acuteness and stop pain; for blood in urine, add *Cirsii Herba* (Xiao Ji Cao), *Rehmannia Radix* (Sheng Di Huang) and *Nelumbinis Rhizomatis Nodus* (Ou Jie) to cool blood and stop bleeding; for distention and pain in the lower abdomen, add *Aucklandiae Radix* (Mu Xiang) and *Linderae Radix* (Wu Yao) to regulate qi and relieve stranguria.

If the stone is big enough to block the urethera and cause serious water accumulation in therenal pelvis, it is suggested patients have operation instead of herbal medicine.

2.2.2 石淋

证候:尿中夹砂石,排尿涩痛,或排尿时突然中断,尿道窘迫疼痛,少腹拘急,往往突发,一侧腰腹绞痛难忍,甚则牵及外阴,尿中带血。舌红,苔薄黄,脉弦或带数。

治法:清热利湿,排石通淋。

方药:石韦散。常用:石韦、瞿麦、滑石、车前子利尿、通淋排石;金钱草、海金沙、鸡内金排石软坚。

加减:若腰腹绞痛者,加白芍药、甘草以缓急止痛;若尿中带血,可加小蓟草、生地黄、藕节以凉血止血;若小腹胀痛加木香、乌药行气通淋。

若结石过大,阻塞尿路,肾盂严重积水者,不宜服用中药,宜手术治疗。

2.2.3 Blood Stranguria

Manifestations: For excess type, hot, rough urine in dark red color with sharp pain, or urine with blood clots and aggravated pain, fullness and tension, or dysphoria; red tongue tip with yellow tongue fur, rapid rolling pulse; for deficiency type, pale red urine with slight pain during urination or with soreness in the waist and knees, feverish dysphoria in the five centers, red tongue with little tongue fur, fine rapid pulse.

Treatment: To clear away heat and relieve stranguria, cool blood and stop bleeding.

Formulas and Herbs: *Cirsii Decoction* (Xiao Ji Yin Zi) for excess type, and *Anemarrhena, Phellodendron, and Rehmannia Pills* (Zhi Bai Di Huang Wan) for deficiency type. The former is usually composed of *Cirsii Herba* (Xiao Ji) and *Rehmannia Radix* (Sheng Di Huang) to cool blood and stop bleeding; *Nelumbinis Rhizomatis Nodus* (Ou Jie), *Typhae Pollen* (Pu Huang) and *Angelicae Sinensis Radix* (Dang Gui) to stop bleeding and dissolve stasis; *Glycyrrhizae Radix et Rhizoma Tenuis* (Sheng Cao Shao), *Gardeniae Fructus* (Zhi Zi), *Talcum* (Hua Shi) and *Lophatheri Herba* (Zhu Ye) to clear away heat and relieve stranguria. The latter is usually composed of *Rehmannia Pills with Six Ingredients* (Liu Wei Di Huang Wan) to nourish and supplement kidney-yin, *Anemarrhenae Rhizoma* (Zhi Mu) and *Phellodendri Chinensis Cortex* (Huang Bo) to clear away heat and cool blood.

Modification: For blood stasis and blood clots in the urine, dark tongue and uneven pulse, add *Notoginseng Radix et Rhizoma* (San Qi), *Achyranthis Bidentatae Radix* (Niu Xi) and *Persicae Semen* (Tao

2.2.3 血淋

证候：实证表现为小便热涩刺痛，尿色深红，或夹有血块，疼痛满急加剧，或见心烦，舌尖红，苔黄，脉滑数。虚证表现为尿色淡红，排尿疼痛轻微，可伴有腰膝酸软，五心烦热，舌红少苔，脉细数。

治法：清热通淋，凉血止血。

方药：实证用小蓟饮子；虚证用知柏地黄丸。前方用小蓟、生地黄凉血止血，藕节、蒲黄、当归止血化瘀，生草梢、山栀、滑石、竹叶清热通淋；后方以六味地黄丸滋补肾阴，知母、黄柏清热凉血。

加减：若有瘀血征象，见尿中有血块、舌暗脉涩，加三七、牛膝、桃仁以化瘀止血；若出血不止，可加仙鹤草、琥

Ren) to dissolve stasis and stop bleeding; for non-stop bleeding, add *Agrimoniae Herba* (Xian He Cao) and *Succinum* (Hu Po) Powder to astringe and stop bleeding; for spleen-deficieny and qi that is too weak to gather blood due to prolonged illness, with symptoms like lassitude and fatigue and lusterless face, use *Angelica Splenic Decoction* (Gui Pi Tang) plus *Agrimoniae Herba* (Xian He Cao), *Alismatis Rhizoma* (Ze Xie) and *Talcum* (Hua Shi) to boost qi, nourish blood and relieve stranguria.

珀粉以收敛止血;若久病脾虚气不摄血,症见神疲乏力、面色少华者,用归脾汤加仙鹤草、泽泻、滑石益气养血通淋。

2.2.4 Qi Stranguria

2.2.4 气淋

Manifestations: For excess type, roughness and stagnation during urination, disinhibited urination, distention and pain in the lower abdomen, pale red tongue with thin white tongue fur and string pulse, which usually takes place after emotional and spiritual dissatisfaction; for deficiency type, dropsy and distention in the lower abdomen, frequent urination, weak urination, lassitude and fatigue, pale tongue and weak fine powerless pulse.

证候: 实证表现为小便涩滞,排尿不畅,少腹胀满疼痛,舌淡红,苔薄白,脉弦,常发生在情志不畅之后;虚证表现为少腹坠胀,尿意频频,排尿无力,神疲乏力,舌质淡,脉虚细无力。

Treatment: To for excess type, disperse the live and regulate qi, and relieve stranguria and promote urination; for deficiency type, supplement zhong jiao and strengthen the spleen, and boost qi and raise the descending.

治法: 实证宜疏肝理气,通淋利尿;虚证宜补中健脾,益气升陷。

Formulas and Herbs: *Aquilaria Powder* (Chen Xiang San) for excess type and *Center-Supplementing qi-Boosting Decoction* (Bu Zhong Yi Qi Tang) for deficiency type. The former is usually composed of *Aquilariae Lignum Resinatum* (Chen Xiang), *Citri Reticulatae Pericarpium* (Chen Pi) and *Vaccariae Semen* (Wang Bu Liu Xing) to disperse the liver and regulate qi; *Angelicae Sinensis Radix* (Dang Gui) and *Paeoniae Radix Alba* (Bai Shao

方药: 实证用沉香散;虚证用补中益气汤。前方用沉香、陈皮、王不留行疏肝理气,当归、白芍药柔肝养血,石韦、滑石、冬葵子等清热利湿通淋;后方用补中益气汤益气健脾,升提中阳。

Yao) to soften the liver and nourish blood; *Pyrrosiae Folium* (Shi Wei), *Talcum* (Hua Shi) and *Malvae Fructus* (Dong Kui Zi) to clear away heat, eliminate dampness and relieve stranguria while the latter is to boost qi, strengthen the spleen and raise middle-yang.

Modification: For distention in the lower abdomen to hypochondria, add *Cyperi Rhizoma Praeparatum* (Zhi Xiang Fu), *Foeniculi Fructus* (Xiao Hui Xiang) and *Curcumae Radix* (Yu Jin) to disperse the liver and regulate qi; for blood stasis and remarkable sharp pain in the lower abdomen, add *Carthami Flos* (Hong Hua) and *Paeoniae Radix Rubra* (Chi Shao Yao).

加减: 若少腹胀满,上及于胁者,加制香附、小茴香、广郁金以疏肝理气;若见有血瘀,少腹刺痛显著者,加红花、赤芍药等。

2.2.5 Chyloid Stranguria

2.2.5 膏淋

Manifesations: For excess type, turbid urine like milk or rice water with oil coating, which when settled down, has floccules or blood in the urine, unremarkable heat and roughness in the urethera, difficult urination, dry mouth, red tongue with yellow greasy tongue fur, soft rapid pulse; for deficiency type, continual stranguria, creamy dribble, severe roughness and pain, emanciation, dizziness, fatigue, soreness in the wasit and knees, pale tongue with greasy tongue fur and fine powerless pulse.

证候: 实证表现为小便浑浊,色乳白或如米泔水,上有浮油,置之沉淀,或伴有絮状凝块物,或混有血液,尿道热涩疼痛,尿时阻塞不畅,口干,舌质红,苔黄腻,脉濡数;虚证表现为病久不已,反复发作,淋出如脂,涩痛不甚,形体日见消瘦,头昏无力,腰膝酸软,舌淡,苔腻,脉细无力。

Treatment: To for excess type, clear away heat, seperete the lucid from the turbid and purge the turbid ; for deficiency type, supplement the spleen, invigorate the kidney.

治法: 实证宜清热利湿,分清泄浊;虚证宜补脾益肾固涩。

Formulas and Herbs: Modified *Cheng's Fish Poison Yam Clear away-Turbid Separation Beverage* (Chen Shi Bi Xie Fen Qing Yin) for excess type and *Chyloid Stranguria Decoction* (Gao Lin Tang) for

方药: 实证用程氏萆薢分清饮加减;虚证用膏淋汤。前方用萆薢、石菖蒲分清泄浊,黄柏、车前子清热利湿,

deficiency type. The former consists of *Dioscoreae Hypoglaucae Rhizoma* (Bi Xie) and *Acori Tatarinowii Rhizoma* (Shi Chang Pu) to separate the lucid from the turbid and purge the turbid; *Phellodendri Chinensis Cortex* (Huang Bo) and *Plantaginis Semen* (Che Qian Zi) to clear away heat and eliminate dampness; *Atractylodis Macrocephalae Rhizoma* (Bai Zhu) and *Poria* (Fu Ling) to strengthen the spleen and dispel dampness. The latter consists of *Codonopsis Radix* (Dang Shen) and *Dioscoreae Rhizoma* (Shan Yao) to invigorate the spleen, *Rehmannia Radix* (Di Huang) and *Euryales Semen* (Qian Shi) to supplement the kidney; *Os Draconis* (Long Gu), *Ostreae Concha* (Mu Li) and *Paeoniae Radix Alba* (Bai Shao Yao) to absorb chyle.

白术、茯苓健脾除湿；后方用党参、山药健脾，地黄、芡实补肾，龙骨、牡蛎、白芍固摄脂液。

Modification: For blood in urine, add *Cirsii Herba* (Xiao Ji), *Nelumbinis Rhizomatis Nodus* (Ou Jie) and *Imperatae Rhizoma* (Bai Mao Gen) to cool blood and stop bleeding; for yellow dark urine with heat and pain, add *Glycyrrhizae Radix et Rhizoma Tenuis* (Gan Cao Shao), *Lophatheri Herba* (Zhu Ye) and *Tetrapanacis Medulla* (Tong Cao) to clear heart to subtract fire; for damp-heat consuming yin due to prolonged illness, with symptoms like dry mouth and throat, feverish dysphoria in the five centers, add *Rehmannia Radix* (Sheng Di Huang), *Ophiopogonis Radix* (Mai Men Dong) and *Anemarrhenae Rhizoma* (Zhi Mu) to nourish kidney-yin.

加减：伴有血尿，加小蓟、藕节、白茅根凉血止血；小便黄赤、热痛明显，加甘草梢、竹叶、通草清心导火；病久湿热伤阴，见口干舌燥、五心烦热、舌红少苔，加生地黄、麦门冬、知母滋养肾阴。

2.2.6 Overstrain Stranguria

Manifestations: Unremarkable darkness, roughness and pain during urination, but dribble after urination which comes and goes and is often triggered by strain, sorensss in the waist and knees, lassitude and fatigue, long duration; pale tongue; fine weak

2.2.6 劳淋

证候：小便不甚赤涩，溺痛不甚，但淋沥不已，时作时止，遇劳即发，腰膝酸软，神疲乏力，病程缠绵。舌质淡，脉细弱。

pulse.

Treatment: To supplement the spleen and invigorate the kidney.

Formulas and Herbs: *Matchless Dioscorea Pills* (Wu Bi Shan Yao Wan), usually composed of *Dioscoreae Rhizoma* (Shan Yao), *Poria* (Fu Ling) and *Alismatis Rhizoma* (Ze Xie) to strengthen the spleen and eliminate dampness; *Rehmanniae Radix Praeparata* (Shu Di Huang), *Corni Fructus* (Shan Zhu Yu), *Cuscutae Semen* (Tu Si Zi), *Eucommiae Cortex* (Du Zhong), *Morindae Officinalis Radix* (Ba Ji Tian), *Schisandrae Chinensis Fructus* (Wu Wei Zi) and *Halloysitum Rubrum* (Chi Shi Zhi) to supplement the kidney to strengthen absorption.

Modification: For kidney-yin deficiency, red tongue and little tongue fur, add *Rehmannia Radix* (Sheng Di Huang) and *Testudinis Carapax et Plastrum* (Gui Jia) to nourish kidney-yin; for yin deficiency and fire execss, red cheeks and feverish dysphoria, yellow dark urine with buring sensation, use *Anemarrhena, Phellodendron, and Rehmannia Pills* (Zhi Bai Di Huang Wan) to nourish yin and subtract fire; for kidney-yang deficiency, aversion to cold and cool limbs, add *Aconm Lateralis Radix Praeparata* (Fu Zi), *Cinnamomi Cortex* (Rou Gui) and *Cervi Cornu* (Lu Jiao) to warm and supplement kidney-yang.

治法：补脾益肾。

方药：无比山药丸。常用：山药、茯苓、泽泻健脾利湿；熟地黄、山茱萸、菟丝子、杜仲、巴戟天、五味子、赤石脂等补肾固摄。

加减：若肾阴虚，舌红苔少，加生地黄、龟版滋养肾阴；若阴虚火旺，面红烦热、尿黄赤伴有灼热不适者，可用知柏地黄丸滋阴降火；若肾阳虚，症见畏寒怕冷、四肢欠温者，加附子、肉桂、鹿角片等温补肾阳。

Bloody Urine

Bloody urine refers to blood or blood clots in the urine due to blood penetrating from vessels into water channels, which can be caused by many factors.

尿　血

尿血指各种原因所致血行脉外渗入水道，而见小便中混有血液甚或伴有血块的病证。

1 Etiology and Pathogenesis

Bloody urine is mainly caused by pathogenic heat injuring collaterals, prolonged illness andover-strain. Its pathogenesis is collaterals injured by pathogenic heat and unconsolidation of the spleen and kidney, which leads to blood deviation from regular meridians into water channels.

1.1 Injures of Blood Collaterals Due to Invasion of Exogenous Pathogenic Factors

Pathogenic heat or pathogenic dampness makes damages tocollaterals and vessels in the lower body, causing bloody urine.

1.2 Essence Consumption and Blood Heat Due to Overstrain and Prolonged Illness

Overstrain and prolonged illness makes damages to qi which fails tocontrol blood, or makes damages to yin, causing yin deficiency and fire excess, which forces blood to move frenetically, leading to bloody urine.

Overall, bloody urineslies in the kidney and bladder. Its pathological factors are mainly damp-heat, blood stasis, qi deficiency and yin deficiency. By nature, it comes into deficiency and excess types. Excess will turn into deficiency when bloody urine is prolonged.

2 Syndrome Differentiation and Treatment

2.1 Key Points of Syndrome Differentiation

It is necessary toidentify the pathological position and tell the difference of deficiency type and excess type in the bladder, kidney and spleen according to clinical manifestations. Meanwhile, identify deficiency type from excess type. Generally, newly developed bloody urine is of excess type

1 病因病机

尿血主要病因有热邪伤络,久病劳倦等,基本病机是热伤脉络及脾肾不固,血不循经,渗入水道。

1.1 感受外邪,损伤血络

热邪或湿邪损伤下部脉络,以致尿血。

1.2 劳倦久病,精亏血热

劳倦久病,损伤于气,统血失司;或损伤于阴,阴虚火旺,迫血妄行,以致尿血。

综上所述:其病位在肾及膀胱;病理因素主要有湿热、瘀血、气虚、阴虚;病理性质有虚实之分,实证久病亦可由实转虚。

2 辨证论治

2.1 辨治要点

尿血辨证应辨明病位,并分清虚实。尿血病位有膀胱、肾及脾的不同,应根据病史及临床表现注意辨明。同时应辨证候之虚实:一般初病多实,久病多虚;由火热迫

and the prolonged is of deficiency type. It is excess type if it is caused by fire-heat forcing blood to move frenetically while it is deficiency type if it is due to yin deficiency and fire excess which leads to qi deficiency and weakened yang-qi.

血所致者属实，由阴虚火旺，气虚不摄，甚至阳气虚衰所致者属虚。

The treatment of blood patterns has four principles: treat fire, treat qi, treat blood and treat deficiency. For excess fire, purge it. For deficiency fire, nourish yin to subdue fire. Forexcess type, purify and subdue qi while for deficiency type, supplement and boost qi. In addition, formulas that can cool blood to stop bleeding, astringe to stop bleeding, dispel stasis to stop bleeding can be used.

对血证的治疗可归纳为治火、治气、治血、治虚四个原则。实火当清热泻火，虚火当滋阴降火；实证当清气降气，虚证当补气益气。另适当地选用凉血止血、收敛止血或祛瘀止血的方药。

2.2 Therapeutic Methos for Different Patterns

2.2 分型论治

2.2.1 Damp-heat inxia jiao

2.2.1 下焦湿热

Manifestations: Yellow dark buring hot urine in scarlet color, irritation, dry mouth, red face, sores in the mouth, insomnia; red tongue; rapid pulse.

证候：小便黄赤灼热，尿血鲜红，心烦口渴，面赤口疮，夜寐不安。舌质红，脉数。

Treatment: To clear away heat and eliminate dampness, cool blood and stop bleeding.

治法：清热利湿，凉血止血。

Formulas and Herbs: Cirsii Decoction (Xiao Ji Yin Zi), usually composed of *Cirsii Herba* (Xiao Ji), *Rehmannia Radix* (Sheng Di Huang) and *Nelumbinis Rhizomatis Nodus* (Ou Jie)to cool blood and stop bleeding, *Gardeniae Fructus* (Zhi Zi), *Akebiae Caulis* (Mu Tong) and *Lophatheri Herba* (Dan Zhu Ye) to clear away heat and purge fire; *Talcum* (Hua Shi) and *Glycyrrhizae Radix et Rhizoma* (Gan Cao) to drain water and clear away heat as well as induce heat downward; *Angelicae Sinensis Radix* (Dang Gui) to nourish and activate blood.

方药：小蓟饮子。常用：小蓟、生地黄、藕节凉血止血；栀子、木通、淡竹叶清热泻火；滑石、甘草利水清热，导热下行；当归养血活血。

Modification: For excessive heat, irriration and thirst, add *Scutellariae Radix* (Huang Qin) and *Trichosanthis Radix* (Tian Hua Fen) to clear away heat

加减：热盛而心烦口渴者，加黄芩、天花粉清热生津；尿血较甚者，加槐花、白

and generate body fluid; for severe bloody urine, add *Sophorae Flos* (Huai Hua) and *Imperatae Rhizoma* (Bai Mao Gen) to cool blood and stop bleeding; for blood clots in the urine, add *Persicae Semen* (Tao Ren), *Carthami Flos* (Hong Hua) and *Achyranthis Bidentatae Radix* (Niu Xi) to activate blood and eliminate stasis.

茅根凉血止血;尿中夹有血块者,加桃仁、红花、牛膝活血化瘀。

2.2.2 Kidney Deficiency and Fire Excess

2.2.2 肾虚火旺

Manifestations: Short dark urine with blood, dizziness and tinnitus, lassitude, red cheeks, feverish sensations, sores in the waist and knees; red tongue; fine rapid pulse.

证候: 小便短赤带血,头晕耳鸣,神疲,颧红潮热,腰膝酸软。舌质红,脉细数。

Treatment: To nourish yin and subdue fire, cool blood and stop bleeding.

治法: 滋阴降火,凉血止血。

Formulas and Herbs: *Anemarrhena, Phellodendron, and Rehmannia Pills* (Zhi Bai Di Huang Wan), usually composed of *Anemarrhenae Rhizoma* (Zhi Mu) and *Phellodendri Chinensis Cortex* (Huang Bo) to nourish yin and subjugate fire; *Rehmannia Pills* (Di Huang Wan) to nourish and supplement kidney yin.

方药: 知柏地黄丸。常用:知母、黄柏滋阴降火,地黄丸滋补肾阴。

Modification: Add moderately *Ecliptae Herba* (Mo Han Lian), *Cirsii Japonici Herba* (Da Ji), *Cirsii Herba* (Xiao Ji), *Nelumbinis Rhizomatis Nodus* (Ou Jie) and *Typhae Pollen* (Pu Huang) to cool blood and stop bleeding; for red cheeks and feverish sensations, add *Lycii Cortex* (Di Gu Pi) and *Cynanchi Atrati Radix et Rhizoma* (Bai Wei) to clear away deficiency heat.

加减: 酌情加用墨旱莲、大蓟、小蓟、藕节、蒲黄等凉血止血;若颧红潮热者,加地骨皮、白薇清退虚热。

2.2.3 Dysfunction of the Spleen to Control Blood

2.2.3 脾不统血

Manifestations: Prolonged bloody urine, even with bleeding in teeth and bleeding in the flesh, little intake, fatigue, short breath, low voice, lusterless face; pale tongue; fine weak pulse.

证候: 久病尿血,甚或兼见齿衄、肌衄,食少,体倦乏力,气短声低,面色不华。舌质淡,脉细弱。

Treatment: To supplement zhong jiao and invigorate the spleen; boost qi to control blood.

治法: 补中健脾,益气摄血。

Formulas and Herbs: *Angelica Splenic Decoction* (Gui Pi Tang), usually composed of *Codonopsis Radix* (Dang Shen), *Astragali Radix* (Huang Qi), *Atractylodis Macrocephalae Rhizoma* (Bai Zhu) and *Poria* (Fu Ling) to strengthen the spleen and boost qi; *Ziziphi Spinosae Semen* (Suan Zao Ren), *Polygalae Radix* (Yuan Zhi) and *Longan Arillus* (Long Yan Rou) to calm the spirits and nourish the heart; *Angelicae Sinensis Radix* (Dang Gui) to supplement blood.

方药: 归脾汤。常用:党参、黄芪、白术、茯苓健脾益气,酸枣仁、远志、龙眼安神养心,当归补血。

Formulas and Herbs: For descending due to qi deficiency with dropsy in the lower abdomen, add *Cimicifugae Rhizoma*(Sheng Ma) and *Bupleuri Radix* (Chai Hu), along with *Codonopsis Radix* (Dang Shen), *Astragali Radix* (Huang Qi), *Atractylodis Macrocephalae Rhizoma* (Bai Zhu) in the formula to help to boost qi and raise yang.

加减: 气虚下陷症见少腹坠胀者,可加升麻、柴胡,配合原方中的党参、黄芪、白术,以起到益气升阳的作用。

2.2.4 Unconsolidation of Kidney-qi

2.2.4 肾气不固

Manifestations: Prolonged bloody urine in pale red color, dizziness and tinnitus, lassitude and fatigue, sore in the waist and spine; pale tongue; deep weak pule.

证候: 久病尿血,血色淡红,头晕耳鸣,精神困惫,腰脊酸痛。舌质淡,脉沉弱。

Treatment: To supplement and boost kidney qi; stop bleeding with astringent therapy.

治法: 补益肾气,固摄止血。

Formulas and Herbs: *Matchless Dioscorea Pills* (Wu Bi Shan Yao Wan), usually composed of *Rehmanniae Radix Praeparata* (Shu Di Huang), *Dioscoreae Rhizoma* (Shan Yao), *Corni Fructus* (Shan Zhu Yu) and *Achyranthis Bidentatae Radix* (Huai Niu Xi) to supplement the kidney and boost essence, *Cistanchis Herba* (Rou Cong Rong), *Cuscutae Semen*(Tu Si Zi) and *Morindae Officinalis Radix*

方药: 无比山药丸。常用:熟地黄、山药、山茱萸、怀牛膝补肾益精;肉苁蓉、菟丝子、巴戟天温肾助阳;茯苓、泽泻健脾利水;五味子、赤石脂益气固涩。

(Ba Ji Tian) to warm the kidney and strengthen yang; *Poria* (Fu Ling) and *Alismatis Rhizoma* (Ze Xie) to invigorate the spleen and drain water; *Schisandrae Chinensis Fructus* (Wu Wei Zi) and *Halloysitum Rubrum* (Chi Shi Zhi) to boost qi with their astringent nature.

Modification: For severe bloody urine, add *Ostreae Concha* (Mu Li), *Fructus Rosae Laevigatae* (Jin Yin Zi) and *Psoraleae Fructus* (Bu Gu Zhi) to stop bleeding with their astringent nature; for soreness in the waist and spine, and aversion to cold, add *Cervi Cornu* (Lu Jiao) and *Cibotii Rhizoma* (Gou Ji) to warm and supplement controling vessel.

加减: 尿血较重者,可再加牡蛎、金樱子、补骨脂等固涩止血;腰脊酸痛,畏寒肢冷者,加鹿角片、狗脊温补督脉。

Long Bi

Long bi is a disease of dribbling urine in very small amount, even blockage of urination due to the impairment of the kidney and bladder to transform qi. Difficult urination with little urine that develops gradually is called "Long" while block with no urine which develops acutely is called "Bi".

癃 闭

癃闭是由于肾和膀胱气化失司而导致小便量少,点滴而出,甚则小便闭塞不通为主症的一种病证。小便不利,点滴短少,病势较缓者称为"癃";小便闭塞,点滴全无,病势较急者称为"闭"。

1 Etiology and Pathogenesis

The major causes of the disease are accumulated damp-heat, lung heat and qi blockade, overstrain and improper diet, weak constitution due to aging or prolonged illness. Its pathogenesis is the dysfunction of the kidney and bladder to transform qi.

1 病因病机

癃闭的致病原因主要有湿热蕴结、肺热气壅、劳倦饮食不节、久病年老体虚等,基本病机肾及膀胱气化失常而产生本病。

1.1 Damp-heat Invading the Bladder and Impairing Qi Transformation

Over intake of spicy savoury food will disenable the spleen to transport, due to which damp-heat is generated or kidney-heat moves to the bladder.

1.1 湿热内侵膀胱,气化不利

或过食辛辣厚味,脾失健运,湿热内生,或肾热移于膀胱,湿热互结,下注膀胱,

Dampness and heat together pour downward to the bladder, causing the bladder unable to transform qi, which leads to the blockage of urination and finally *long bi*.

致膀胱气化不利，小便不通，而成癃闭。

1.2 Difficult Urination Due to Lung Heat and Qi Stagnation Causing by Invasion of Pathogenic Heat in the Upper Body

1.2 热邪上受，肺热气壅，水道不利

Heat injuries the lung and disenables the lung to disperse and descend, for which body fluid cannot be transported to the bladder. On the other hand, when heat moves downward to the bladder, the Upper Jiao andXia jiao both are blocked by heat, leading to *long bi*.

热伤肺气，肺气不能肃降，津液不能下输膀胱；又因热气下移膀胱，以致上、下焦均为热气闭阻，而成癃闭。

1.3 Failure of Yang to Rise Due to Overstrain and Improper Diet

1.3 劳倦饮食伤脾，清阳不升

Overstrain hurts the spleen. Improper diet causes spleen deficiency andclear qi unable to rise. Turbid yin cannot descend and body fluid cannot be transported regularly, leading to difficult in urine.

劳倦伤脾，或饮食不节，致脾虚而清气不升，浊阴难降，水津转输失调，致小便不利。

1.4 Powerlessness to Transform Qi Caused by Weak Constitution Due to Aging

1.4 年老体衰，气化无权

The bladder fails to transform qi and separate thelucid from the turbid due to aging, weak constitution, kidney-yang deficiency, heat accumulation in xia jiao damaging kidney-yin. Then *long bi* is resulted.

年老、久病体虚，肾阳不足，或下焦积热，耗伤肾阴，以致膀胱气化无权，分清泌浊失职，发为癃闭。

1.5 Depression of Liver-qi and Impairement of Dispersion of the Liver Due to Injury of the Seven Emotions Causes

1.5 七情内伤，肝气郁结，疏泄不及

Injury of the seven emotions disenables the liver to disperse qi, which affects the transformation and transportation of water and fluid of thethree jiaos, or blocks meridian-qi. All these will impair qi transformation of the bladder, leading to *long bi*.

七情内伤，肝失疏泄，影响三焦水液运化，或阻滞经气，影响膀胱气化，而致癃闭。

1.6 Difficulty in Urination Due to Blockage of the Urethra

Blood stasis, corruptive essence, or lumps and sand stones that blocks the urethra causes difficulty in urination, leading to *long bi*.

Overall, the disease lies in the bladder, but is closely related to thethree jiaos, lung, spleen and kidney. The pathological factors are damp-heat, heat-toxin, qi stagnation and phlegm stasis. According to the different pathogenesis, the pathological nature can be deficiency or excess, which can be interchangeable or complicated. For instance, excess type can be impairment of qi transformation of the bladder due to damp-heat in the bladder, lung-heat and qi blockade, depressed liver and qi stagnation or urethra blockage. Deficiency type can be impairment of qi transformation of the bladder due to unraised spleen-qi and weakened kidney-yang. The complication of deficiency and excess can be due to depressed liver and qi stagnation that tranforms into fire, consuming yin, or lingering damp-heat burning yin, which disenables water and fluid to pour down to the bladder.

1.6 尿道阻塞,水道不通

瘀血败精,或肿块结石,阻塞尿路,小便难以排出,而成癃闭。

综上所述,癃闭病位在膀胱,与三焦、肺、脾、肾关系密切。其病理因素有湿热、热毒、气滞及痰瘀。根据癃闭的病因不同,其病理性质有虚实之分,并常相互关联,或彼此兼夹。如:膀胱湿热、肺热气壅、肝郁气滞、尿路阻塞,以致膀胱气化不利者为实证;脾气不升、肾阳衰惫,导致膀胱气化无权者为虚证。又如肝郁气滞,化火伤阴;或湿热久恋,又易灼伤肾阴而使水液无以下注膀胱等,则表现为虚实夹杂之证。

2 Syndrome Differentiation and Treatment

2.1 Key Points of Syndrome Differentiation

For *long bi*, it is primary to identify deficiency from excess. Then identify the intensity of the urgency. First, identity deficiency from excess. Damp-heat accumulation, lung-heat and qi blockage, urethra blockage are usually of excess type while unraised spleen-qi, deficiency kidney-yang and weakened fire of the vital gate are usually of deficiency type. Sudden attack, short duration, good

2 辨证论治

2.1 辨治要点

癃闭的辨证首先要判别病之虚实。其次要了解病情之轻重缓急。先辨病之虚实:因湿热蕴结、肺热气壅、尿路阻塞所致者,多属实证;因脾气不升、肾阳不足、命门火衰多属虚证。起病急,病程短,体质较好,尿流窘迫,

constitution, precipitant urination, little reddish burring urine, distention and pain in the lower abdomen, yellow greasy or thin yellow tongue fur, and stringy uneven or rapid pulse are of excess type. Gradual onset, long duration, powerless urination, spiritual fatigue, lusterless face, short breath, low voice, pale tongue, deep fine weak pulse are of deficiency type. For excess type, it is necessary to differentiate the predominance of damp-heat, turbid-stasis, lung heat and depressed liver while for deficiency type, it is necessary to differentiate the weakness of the spleen and kidney, yin deficiency and yang deficiency. Next, know about the intensity of urgency and severity. Water accumulation in the bladder and urinary blockage are quite urgent but little dribbling urine with water accumulated in the bladder are not. It gets worse when "*long*" (dribbling) turns into "*bi*" (blockage) and it gets better when "*bi*"(blockage) turns into "*long*"(dribbling).

小便短赤灼热，小腹胀痛，苔黄腻或薄黄，脉弦涩或数，属于实证；起病慢，病程长，体质较差，尿流无力，精神疲乏，面色少华，气短声低，舌质淡，脉沉细弱，属于虚证。实证当辨湿热、浊瘀、肺热、肝郁之偏胜；虚证当辨脾、肾虚衰之不同，阴阳亏虚之差别。其次要了解病情之缓急，病势之轻重。水蓄膀胱，小便闭塞不通为急病；小便量少，但点滴能出，无水蓄膀胱者为缓证。由"癃"转"闭"为病势加重，由"闭"转"癃"为病势减轻。

The treatment should follow the principle of "dredging fu-organs" and change with the manifestations of deficiency and excess. For excess type, clear away pathogenic heat, activate qi activity and remove stasis and clots. For deficiency type, supplement the spleen and kidney to promote qi transformation. For water accumulation in the bladder (uroschesis), acupuncture, sneezing therapy, emetic therapy and urethral catheterization can be adopted to promote urination in emergent cases.

癃闭的治疗以"腑以通为用"为原则，并根据证候虚实之不同而异：实证宜清邪热，利气机，散瘀结；虚证宜补脾肾，助气化。对于水蓄膀胱之急症（尿潴留），应配合针灸、取嚏、探吐、导尿等法急通小便。

2.2 Therapeutic Methods for Different Patterns

2.2 分型论治

2.2.1 Damp-heat in the Bladder

2.2.1 膀胱湿热

Manifestations: Anuresis, or dribbling short dark burning urine in very small amount, distention

证候：小便点滴不通，或量极少而短赤灼热，小腹胀

and pain in the lower abdomen, bitter and sticky mouth, or thirst but without desire for drink, or difficult defecation; red tongue with yellow greasy tongue fur; rapid pulse.

满，口苦口黏，或口渴不欲饮，或大便不畅。舌质红，苔黄腻，脉数。

Treatment: To clear away and eliminate damp-heat; promote urination.

治法： 清利湿热，通利小便。

Formulas and Herbs: *Eight Corrections Powder* (Ba Zheng San), usually composed of *Polygoni Avicularis Herba* (Bian Xu), *Dianthi Herba* (Qu Mai), *Akebiae Caulis* (Mu Tong), *Plantaginis Semen* (Che Qian Zi) to drain and promte urine; *Gardeniae Fructus* (Zhi Zi) to purge damp-heat in the three jiaos; *Talcum* (Hua Shi) and *Glycyrrhizae Radix et Rhizoma* (Gan Cao) to clear away heat in xia jiao; *Rhei Radix et Rhizoma* (Da Huang) to promote defection and purge fire.

方药： 八正散。常用：萹蓄、瞿麦、木通、车前子通利小便；栀子清化三焦湿热；滑石、甘草清利下焦湿热，大黄通便泻火。

Modification: For dysphoria and sores and ulceration on the tongue and in the mouth, add *Heat-Abducting Powder* (Dao Chi San) to clear away heart-fire; for lingering damp-heat, burning kidney-yin which leads to dry mouth and throat, feverish sensations, night sweating, feverish sensation in sole hearts and palms and shiny red tongue, change for *Kidney Enriching Gate-Opening Pills* (Zi Shen Tong Guan Wan) plus *Rehmannia Radix* (Sheng Di Huang), *Plantaginis Semen* (Che Qian Zi) and *Achyranthis Bidentatae Radix* (Niu Xi) to nourish kidney and clear away damp-heat to promote qi transformation; for damp-heat accumulated in the three jiaos that causes impairment of qi transformation, little or no urine, dark dull complexion, chest oppression, xia jiao, nausea, vomiting, urinary smell in the mouth or even coma and dilirium, use *Coptis-Warming-Gallbladder Decoction* (Huang

加减： 若兼心烦、口舌生疮糜烂者，可合导赤散以清心火；若湿热久恋下焦，导致肾阴灼伤而出现口干咽燥、潮热盗汗、手足心热、舌光红，可改用滋肾通关丸加生地黄、车前子、牛膝等，以滋肾阴、清湿热，而助气化；若因湿热蕴结三焦，气化不利，小便量极少或无尿、面色晦滞、胸闷烦躁、恶心呕吐、口中有尿臭，甚则神昏谵语，宜用黄连温胆汤加车前子、通草、制大黄等，以降浊和胃、清热利湿。

Lian Wen Dan Tang) plus *Plantaginis Semen* (Che Qian Zi), *Tetrapanacis Medulla* (Tong Cao) and *Rhei Radix et Rhizoma* Praeparata (Zhi Da Huang) to subdue turbidity, harmonize the stomach, clear away heat and eliminate dampness.

2.2.2 Obstruction of Lung Heat

Manifestations: Difficulty in urination or dribbling even anuresis, dry throat, polydipsia with desire for drink, short breath or with cough; red tongue with thin yellow tongue fur; rapid pulse.

Treatment: To clear away and purge lung heat; dredge water channels.

Formulas and Herbs: *Lung Clear awaying Decoction* (Qing Fei Yin), usually composed of *Scutellariae Radix* (Huang Qin) and *Mori Cortex* (Sang Bai Pi) to clear away and purge lung heat; *Ophiopogonis Radix* (Mai Men Dong) to nourish lung-yin; *Plantaginis Semen* (Che Qian Zi), *Akebiae Caulis* (Mu Tong) and *Gardeniae Fructus* (Zhi Zi) to clear away heat and promote urination.

Modification: For stuffed nose, dizziness and floating pulse, add *Menthae Haplocalycis Herba* (Bo He) and *Platycodi Radix* (Jie Geng) to disperse the lung and relieve the exterior; for lung-yin deficiency with dry throat and mouth, red tongue with little tongue fur, add *Adenophorae Radix* (Nan Sha Shen), *Polygonati Rhizoma* (Huang Jing) and *Dendrobii Caulis* (Shi Hu); for accompanying dark burning urine and distention in the lower abdomen, use *Eight Corrections Powder* (Ba Zheng San) to treat together upward and downward.

2.2.3 Depressed Liver and Qi Stagnation

Manifestations: Anuresis or difficulty in urination, depressed minds and spirits or irritation and

2.2.2 肺热壅盛

证候：小便不畅或点滴不通，咽干，烦渴欲饮，呼吸急促，或有咳嗽。舌红，苔薄黄，脉数。

治法：清泄肺热，通利水道。

方药：清肺饮。常用：黄芩、桑白皮清泄肺热；麦门冬滋养肺阴；车前子、木通、栀子清利小便。

加减：有鼻塞、头痛、脉浮等表证者，加薄荷、桔梗宣肺解表；肺阴不足者，症见咽干口燥、舌红少苔，加沙参、黄精、石斛；兼尿赤灼热、小腹胀满者，合八正散上下并治。

2.2.3 肝郁气滞

证候：小便不通或通而不爽，情志抑郁，或多烦善

getting angry easily, distention and fullness in the abdomen and hypochondria; red tongue with thin yellow tongue fur; stringy pulse.

怒，胁腹胀满。舌红，苔薄黄，脉弦。

Treatment: To disperse and activate qi activity; promote urination.

治法: 疏利气机，通利小便。

Formulas and Herbs: *Aquilaria Powder* (Chen Xiang San), usually composed of *Aquilariae Lignum Resinatum* (Chen Xiang) and *Citri Reticulatae Pericarpium* (Ju Pi) to disperse the liver and regulate qi; *Angelicae Sinensis Radix* (Dang Gui) and *Vaccariae Semen* (Wang Bu Liu Xing) to promote qi and blood flow; *Pyrrosiae Folium* (Shi Wei), *Malvae Fructus* (Dong Kui Zi) and *Talcum* (Hua Shi) to dredge water channels.

方药: 沉香散。常用:沉香、橘皮疏肝理气;当归、王不留行行气活血;石韦、冬葵子、滑石通利水道。

Modification: For severe depressed liver and qi stagnation, add *Six Milled Ingredients Decoction* (Liu Mo Tang) to help disperse the liver and regulate qi; for depressed qi transforming to fire with red tongue and thin yellow tongue fur, add *Moutan Cortex* (Mu Dan Pi) and *Gardeniae Fructus* (Zhi Zi) to purge liver fire.

加减: 若肝郁气滞症状严重者，可合六磨汤以增强其疏肝理气的作用;若气郁化火，而见舌红、苔薄黄，可加牡丹皮、山栀以清肝泻火。

2.2.4 Turbid Stasis Blocking

2.2.4 浊瘀阻塞

Manifestations: Dribbling urine or urine flow as thin as thread or anuresis, distention, fullness and pain in the lower abdomen; purple dark tongue, or with stasis spots; uneven pulse.

证候: 小便点滴而下，或尿如细线，甚则阻塞不通，小腹胀满疼痛。舌紫暗，或有瘀点，脉涩。

Treatment: To dissolve stasis and break clots; dredge water channels.

治法: 化瘀散结，通利水道。

Formulas and Herbs: *Substitutive Dead-On Pills* (Dai Di Dang Wan), usually composed of of *Angelicae Sinensis Radix Extremitas* (Dang Gui Wei), *Manitis Squama* (Chuan Shan Jia), *Persicae Semen* (Tao Ren), *Rhei Radix et Rhizoma* (Da Huang) and *Natrii Sulfas* (Mang Xiao) to free stasis and re-

方药: 代抵当丸。常用:当归尾、穿山甲、桃仁、大黄、芒硝通瘀散结;生地黄凉血滋阴;肉桂助膀胱气化。

move clots; *Rehmannia Radix* (Sheng Di Huang) to cool blood and nourish yin; *Cinnamomi Cortex* (Rou Gui) to help the bladder to transform qi.

Modification: For severe blood stasis and remarkable sharp pain in the lower abdomen, add *Carthami Flos* (Hong Hua) and *Achyranthis Bidentatae Radix* (Niu Xi) to strengthen the effects of activating blood and eliminating stasis; for qi and blood deficiency due to proloned illness and lusterless face, it is advisable to add *Astragali Radix* (Huang Qi), *Salviae Miltiorrhizae Radix et Rhizoma Radix* (Dan Shen) and *Angelicae Sinensis Radix* (Dang Gui) to boost qi, nourish blood and dissolve stasis; for sand stones in the urethra, add *Lysimachiae Herba* (Jin Qian Cao), *Lygodii Spora* (Hai Jin Sha), *Malvae Fructus* (Dong Kui Zi), *Dianthi Herba* (Qu Mai) and *Pyrrosiae Folium* (Shi Wei) to expel stone and promote urination.

加减：若瘀血现象较重，小腹刺痛显著，可加红花、川牛膝以增强其活血化瘀作用；若病久气血两虚，面色不华，宜益气养血行瘀，可加黄芪、丹参、当归之类；若尿路有结石，可加金钱草、海金沙、冬葵子、瞿麦、石韦以通淋排石利尿。

2.2.5 Unraised Spleen-qi

Manifestations: Dropsy in the lower abdomen, desire for urination but inhibited or little in amount, lassitude and fatigue, poor appetite, short break and low voice; pale tongue, thin tongue fur; fine pulse.

Treatment: To raise the lucid and subdue the tubid; transform qi and drain water.

Formulas and Herbs: *Center-Supplementing qi-Boosting Decoction* (Bu Zhong Yi Qi Tang) and *Spring Pond Decoction* (Chun Ze Tang), usually composed of *Ginseng Radix et Rhizoma* (Ren Shen) and *Astragali Radix* (Huang Qi) to boost qi; *Atractylodis Macrocephalae Rhizoma* (Bai Zhu) to strengthen the spleen and transport dampness; *Cinnamomi Ramulus* (Gui Zhi) to activate yang;

2.2.5 脾气不升

证候：小腹坠胀，时欲小便而不得出，或量少而不畅，神疲乏力，食欲不振，气短而语声低微。舌淡，苔薄脉细。

治法：升清降浊，化气行水。

方药：补中益气汤合春泽汤。常用：人参、黄芪益气；白术健脾运湿；桂枝通阳，升麻、柴胡升清降浊；猪苓、泽泻、茯苓利水渗湿。

Cimicifugae Rhizoma (Sheng Ma) and *Bupleuri Radix* (Chai Hu) to raise the lucid and subdue the turbid; *Poria* (Fu Ling), *Polyporus* (Zhu Ling) and *Alismatis Rhizoma* (Ze Xie) to drain water and eliminate dampness.

Modification: For qi deficiency affecting yin, deficient spleen-yin, unraised clear qi, qi and yin deficiency with red tongue with little tongue fur, change for *Ginseng, Poria and Atractylodes Powder* (Shen Ling Bai Zhu San); for spleen deficiency affecting kidney, soreness in the waist and knees, physical cold and cold limbs, add *Life Saver Kidney Qi Pills* (Ji Sheng Shen Qi Wan) to warm and supplement the spleen and kidney, and transform qi and disinhibit water.

加减: 若气虚及阴,脾阴不足,清气不升,气阴两虚,症见舌红苔少,可改用参苓白术散;若脾虚及肾,兼有腰膝酸软、形寒肢冷,可合济生肾气丸以温补脾肾、化气利水。

2.2.6 Extreme Asthenia of Kidney-yang

Manifestations: Anuresis or dribbling powerless urination, waxy pale complexion, timid posture, aversion to cold, cold limbs, coldness, weakness and soreness in the waist and knees; pale enlarged tongue with thin white tongue fur; fine deep or weak pulse.

Treatment: To warm and supplement kidney-yang; transform qi and drain water.

Formulas and Herbs: *Life Saver Kidney Qi Pills* (Ji Sheng Shen Qi Wan), usually composed of *Aconm Lateralis Radix Praeparata* (Fu Zi) and *Cinnamomi Cortex* (Rou Gui) to warm and supplement kidney-yang; *Rehmanniae Radix Praeparata* (Shu Di Huang) and *Corni Fructus* (Shan Zhu Yu) to supplement the kidney and nourish yin; *Dioscoreae Rhizoma* (Shan Yao), *Poria* (Fu Ling) and *Alismatis Rhizoma* (Ze Xie) to strengthen the spleen and eliminate dampness.

2.2.6 肾阳衰惫

证候: 小便不通或点滴不爽,排出无力,面色㿠白,神气怯弱,畏寒肢冷,腰膝冷而酸软无力。舌淡胖,苔薄白,脉沉细或弱。

治法: 温补肾阳,化气利水。

方药: 济生肾气丸。常用:附子、肉桂温补肾阳;熟地黄、山茱萸补肾滋阴;山药、茯苓、泽泻健脾利湿。

Modification: For low-spiritedness, soreness in the waist and spine due to essence and blood deficiency and affected controling vessel, which can be often found on old people, use *Musk and Velvet Deerhorn Pills* (Xiang Rong Wan) to supplement and nourish essence and blood as well as promote yang and dredge orifices; for subtractd urine or even anuresis, vomiting, dysphoria, coma due to powerlessness to transform qi and turbid-yin accumulation caused by extreme asthenia of kidney-yang and decline of vital gate fire, use *Thousand-Gold Spleen-Warming Decoction* (Qian Jin Wen Pi Tang) and *Euodiae Decoction* (Wu Zhu Yu Tang) to warm and supplement the spleen and kidney, and harmonize the stomach to descend adverse flow of qi.

加减：若形神萎顿、腰脊酸痛，为精血俱亏，病及督脉，多见于老人，方用香茸丸补养精血、助阳通窍；若因肾阳衰惫，命火式微，致三焦气化无权，浊阴内蕴，小便量少，甚至无尿、呕吐、烦躁、神昏者，方用千金温脾汤合吴茱萸汤，以温补脾肾、和胃降逆。

2.3 External Treatment

The following methods can be adopted topromote urination in emergency case of water accumulated in the bladder in case water-toxin floods upward.

2.3 外治法

对于水蓄膀胱之急症，为图速效，以防水毒上泛之各种变证的出现，可用以下诸法速通小便，以解燃眉之急。

2.3.1 Sneezing and Emetic Therapy

Sneezing or vomiting can make way for lung qi, raise middle and dredge qi in xia jiao. It is an easy and efficient method to promote urination. The procedure is to put a sterilized cotton swab in the noise or throat to force sneezing or vomiting. Or blow 0.3 to 0.6 gram of Gleditsiae powder into the nose to force sneezing.

2.3.1 取嚏或探吐法

打喷嚏或呕吐，能开肺气，举中气，而通下焦之气，是一种简单而有效的通利小便的方法。其方法是用消毒棉签，向鼻中取嚏或喉中探吐；也可用皂角末0.3～0.6克，吹鼻取嚏。

2.3.2 External Application

(1) Take a bulb of garlic, 3 Gardeniae and some salt, crush them and spread them on the piece of paper. Apply the mixure onto the navel. It will take effect in a fairy long time.

2.3.2 外敷法

(1) 独头蒜头1个，栀子3枚，盐少许，捣烂，摊纸贴脐部，良久可通。

(2) Take 250 g of salt. Fry it and wrap it in cloth. Put it on the navel and abdomen. Fry it again when it gets cold.

（2）食盐 250 克，炒热，布包熨脐腹，冷后再炒热敷之。

2. 3. 3 Water-flow Association

The sound of water-flow will generate desire for urination in patients. This method can be applied to anuresis due to depression patterns.

2. 3. 3 流水诱导法

使患者听到水声，即可有尿意，而随之排出小便。此法适用于郁证患者所引起的尿闭。

2. 3. 4 Urethral Catheterization

If all the above methods fail andthe bladder is full of urination, which sounds dullness when knocked at the lower abdomen, give immediately to relieve the emergency.

2. 3. 4 导尿法

若经上述治疗无效，而小腹胀满特甚，叩触小腹膀胱区呈浊音，当用导尿法，以缓其急。

Impotence

阳　痿

Impotence is a disease characterized by sloppy penis incapable of erection, or slackness even when erected, or very short erection time that impairs normal sexual life, caused by ancestral sinew lacking in nourishing due to emptiness and deficiency of meridians and vessel, or obstruction and stagnation of meridians and collaterals. However, temporary erection inabilbity due to fever, overstrain and emotional abnormality cannot be regarded as impotence.

阳痿是指各种原因引起经脉空虚或经络阻滞，导致宗筋失养，临床表现为成年男子性交时，由于阴茎痿软不举，或举而不坚，或坚而不久，无法进行正常性生活的病证。但对发热、过度劳累、情绪反常等因素造成的一时性阴茎勃起障碍，不能视为病态。

1 Etilogy and Pathogenesis

The causes of impotence are mainly overstrain, injury, prolonged illness, improper diet, injury of the seven emotions and exogenous pathogenic affection. Its pathogenesis is injury of the liver, spleen, heart and spleen, emptiness and deficiency of meridians and vessels or obstruction and stagnation of

1 病因病机

本病的病因主要有劳伤久病，饮食不节，七情所伤，外邪侵袭。基本病机为肝、肾、心、脾受损，经脉空虚，或经络阻滞，导致宗筋失养而发为阳痿。

meridians and collaterals, which leads to poorly nourishd ancestral sinew, causinig impotence.

1.1 Damages to Essence and Qi Due to Indulgence in Sex or Masturbation

Indulgence in sex life or masturbation at young ages makes deficient essence and qi, decline of vital gate fire, which leads to erection inability of penis, and thin clear away cold sperm.

1.2 Injury of the Heart and Spleen Due to Anxiety

Worry and anxiety injuries the heart and spleen. Spleen and stomach deficiency causes qi and blood deficiency and poorly nourishd ancestral sinew, leading to impotence.

1.3 Impotence Due to Damages of Kidney by Fear

Fear can damage the kidney and fear can cause qi to move downward, which gradually will leads to erection inability, slack erection of penis and fianally impotence.

1.4 Unlifted Depression and Slack Ancestral Sinew

The liver controls the ancestral sinew. Penis is where ancestral sinew converges. Therefore, emotional and spiritual dissatisfaction, worry, depression and anger will impair the dispersion and purging of the liver, leading to the inability of the ancestral sinew.

1.5 Downward of Damp-heat Due to Alcohol and Sweet Savoury Food

Over intake of alcohol, spicy greasy savory food will accumulate dampness and generate heat, disenabling the spleen to transport. Then damp-heat pours downward and the ancestral sinew slackens,

1.1 纵欲手淫，精气虚损

房劳过度，或少年频犯手淫，以致精气虚损，命门火衰，引起阳事不举，精薄清冷。

1.2 思虑焦劳，损伤心脾

思虑焦劳，损伤心脾，脾胃虚以致气血两虚，宗筋失养，而成阳痿。

1.3 恐惧伤肾，阳痿不举

恐则伤肾，恐则气下，渐至阳痿不振，举而不刚，而致阳痿。

1.4 抑郁不舒，宗筋弛缓

肝主筋，阴器为宗筋之汇，若情志不遂，忧思郁怒，肝失疏泄条达，则宗筋无能。

1.5 酒热甘肥，湿热下注

过食酒热辛辣，肥甘厚腻，积湿生热，脾失健运，湿热下注，宗筋弛纵，而致阳痿。

causing impotence.

Overall, impotence lies in the ancestral sinew but pathogocial organs involve the liver, spleen, heart and spleen. Its pathological nature has the difference of deficiency and excess and often is complication of deficiency and excess, which can be interchangeable.

综上所述,阳痿之病位在宗筋,病变脏腑主要涉及肝、肾、心、脾。阳痿的病理性质,有虚实之分,且多虚实相兼,常可因实致虚,亦可因虚致实。

2 Syndrome Differentiation and Treatment

2 辨证论治

2.1 Key Points of Syndrome Differentiation

2.1 辨治要点

Since impotence comes into deficiency type, excess type and complication type, therefore, it is necessary to first identity its nature. For the secondary symptoms excess, distinguish qi stagnation from damp-heat; for the primary symptoms deficiency, distinguish qi, blood, yin and yang defiency as well as pathological changes of zang-organs. For complication type, first identify pathological zang-organ and then identify the pathogenic factors.

因本病有虚有实,亦有虚实夹杂者,故首先当辨虚实:标实者需区别气滞、湿热;本虚者应辨气血阴阳虚损之差别,病变脏器之不同;虚实夹杂者,先别虚损之脏器,后辨夹杂之病邪。

As for treatment, for excess type, it is advisable to disperse live depression, clear away and eliminate damp-heat. For deficiency type, warm and supplement for decline of vital gate fire together with nurturing essence; nourish and regulate qi and blood for blood deficiency of the heart and spleen together with warm and supplement to eliminate depression. For complication, treat both the primary and secondary symptoms.

阳痿的治疗原则为:实证者,肝郁宜疏通,湿热应清利;虚证者,命门火衰宜温补,结合养精,心脾血虚当调养气血,佐以温补开郁;虚实夹杂者需标本兼顾。

2.2 Therapeutic Methods for Different Patterns

2.2 分型论治

2.2.1 Decline of the Vital Gate Fire

2.2.1 命门火衰

Manifestations: Penis erection inability or slack erection, thin clear away cold sperm, lassitude and fatigue, aversion to cold, cold limbs, waxy pale complexion, dizziness, tinnitus, soreness in the

证候: 阳事不举,或举而不坚,精薄清冷,神疲倦怠,畏寒肢冷,面色㿠白,头晕耳鸣,腰膝酸软,夜尿清长。舌

waist and knees, clear away long urine at night; pale enlarged tongue, thin white tongue fur; fine deep pulse.

淡胖,苔薄白,脉沉细。

Treatment: To warm the spleen and invigorate yang.

治法: 温肾壮阳。

Formulas and Herbs: *Birth-Praising Pills* (Zan Yu Wan), usually composed of *Curculiginis Rhizoma* (Xian Mao), *Morindae Officinalis Radix* (Ba Ji Tian), *Epimedii Folium* (Yin Yang Huo), *Allii Tuberosi Semen* (Jiu Cai Zi), *Cnidii Fructus* (She Chuang Zi), *Eucommiae Cortex* (Du Zhong), *Cinnamomi Cortex* (Rou Gui), *Aconm Lateralis Radix Praeparata* (Fu Zi) to warm the kidney and invigorate yang, along with *Rehmanniae Radix Praeparata* (Shu Di Huang), *Angelicae Sinensis Radix* (Dang Gui), *Lycii Fructus* (Gou Qi Zi) and *Corni Fructus* (Shan Zhu Yu) to nourish blood and yin.

方药: 赞育丸。常用:仙茅、淫羊藿、巴戟天、韭菜籽、蛇床子、杜仲、肉桂、附子等温肾壮阳的药物,又伍以熟地黄、当归、枸杞、山茱萸等养血滋阴的药物以达到阴阳相济的目的。

Modification: For frequent spermatarrhea and thin cold sperm, add *Rubi Fructus* (Fu Pen Zi), *Fructus Rosae Laevigatae* (Jin Yin Zi) and *Alpiniae Oxyphyllae Fructus* (Yi Zhi Ren) to supplement the kidney and secure essence; for unremarkable decline of fire, weak essence and blood with symptoms like lusterless complexion, dizziness, dim sight, soreness in the waist and knees, use *Kidney Pills* (Zuo Gui Wan); for damp-heat consuming yin with such symptoms as dry throat and mouth, feverish dysphoria in five centers, red tongue with little tongue fur, add *Gardeniae Fructus* (Zhi Zi), *Phellodendri Chinensis Cortex* (Huang Bo) and *Talcum* (Hua Shi) to purge damp-heat and protect yin.

加减: 若滑精频繁,精薄精冷,可加覆盆子、金樱子、益智仁补肾固精;若火衰不甚,精血薄弱,症见面色少华、头晕眼花、腰膝酸软,可予左归丸治疗;若湿热伤阴,症见咽干口燥、五心烦热、舌红少苔,可加栀子、黄柏、滑石等清泄湿热而护阴。

2.2.2 Injury of the Heart and Spleen

2.2.2 心脾受损

Manifestations: Erection inability or slack erection, low spiritedness, palpitation, fearful throb-

证候: 阳事不举,或举而不坚,精神不振,心悸怔忡,

bing, insomnia, lusterless complexion, poor apetite; pale tongue with thin white tongue fur; stringy fine powerless pulse.

夜寐不安,面色不华,胃纳不佳。舌质淡,苔薄白,脉弦细无力。

Treatment: To supplement and invigorate the heart and spleen.

治法: 补益心脾。

Formulas and Herbs: *Angelica Splenic Decoction* (Gui Pi Tang), usually composed of *Codonopsis Radix* (Dang Shen), *Astragali Radix* (Huang Qi), *Atractylodis Macrocephalae Rhizoma* (Bai Zhu) and *Poria* (Fu Ling) to strengthen the spleen and boost qi; *Ziziphi Spinosae Semen* (Suan Zao Ren), *Polygalae Radix* (Yuan Zhi) and *Longan Arillus* (Long Yan Rou) to nourish the heart and calm the spirits; *Angelicae Sinensis Radix* (Dang Gui) to supplement blood.

方药: 归脾汤。常用:党参、黄芪、白术、茯苓健脾益气;酸枣仁、远志、龙眼养心安神;当归补血。

2.2.3 Injury of the Kidney Due to Fear

2.2.3 恐惧伤肾

Manifestations: Impotence, slack erection of penis or erection for short duration, palpitation, easily frightened, timidity, suspiciousness, insomnia, dribbling urine; thin tongue fur; string fine pulse.

证候: 阳痿不振,举而不坚,或坚而不久,心悸易惊,胆怯多疑,夜寐不安,小便淋漓。苔薄,脉弦细。

Treatment: To invigorate the spleen and calm the spirits.

治法: 益肾宁神

Formulas and Herbs: *Major Yuan (Primary) Qi-Reinforcing Decoction* (Da Bu Yuan Jian), usually composed of *Rehmanniae Radix Praeparata* (Shu Di Huang), *Corni Fructus* (Shan Zhu Yu), *Eucommiae Cortex* (Du Zhong) and *Lycii Fructus* (Gou Qi Zi) to invigorate the kidney; *Ginseng Radix et Rhizoma* (Ren Shen), *Angelicae Sinensis Radix* (Dang Gui) to supplement and boost qi and blood. *Ziziphi Spinosae Semen* (Suan Zao Ren), *Polygalae Radix* (Yuan Zhi) can be added to nourish the heart and calm the spirits.

方药: 大补元煎。常用:熟地黄、山茱萸、杜仲、枸杞益肾;人参、当归补益气血。本方还可加用酸枣仁、远志养心安神。

Modification: For qi descendance due to fright, add *Cimicifugae Rhizoma*(Sheng Ma) and *Bupleuri Radix* (Chai Hu) to raise yang.

加减: 因受惊恐而致气下者,可佐以升麻、柴胡以升阳。

2.2.4 Depression of the Liver

2.2.4 肝郁不舒

Manifestations: Erection inability, poor libido, depression or low moods, irritation, easily angered, oppression and discomfort in the chest, distention and oppression in the hypochondria, frequent sigh, little intake, loost stool; pale tongue with thin tongue fur; stringy pulse.

证候: 阳痿不举,性欲淡漠,情绪抑郁或低落,烦躁易怒,胸闷不舒,胁肋胀闷,常喜叹息,食少便溏。舌淡,苔薄,脉弦。

Treatment: To disperse the liver and resolve depression.

治法: 疏肝解郁。

Formulas and Herbs: *Free Wanderer Powder* (Xiao Yao San), usually composed of *Bupleuri Radix* (Chai Hu), *Paeoniae Radix Alba* (Bai Shao Yao) and *Angelicae Sinensis Radix* (Dang Gui) to disperse the liver and resolve depression as well nourish and harmonize blood; *Atractylodis Macrocephalae Rhizoma* (Bai Zhu), *Poria* (Fu Ling) and *Glycyrrhizae Radix et Rhizoma* (Gan Cao) to strengthen the spleen to help transport; which means excess earth controls wood.

方药: 逍遥散。常用:柴胡、白芍药、当归疏肝解郁,养血和血;白术、茯苓、甘草健脾助运,实土御木。

Modification: For irritation and easily angered, dry and bitter mouth, insomnia, short dark urine, add *Gentianae Radix et Rhizom* (Long Dan Cao), *Moutan Cortex* (Mu Dan Pi) and *Gardeniae Fructus* (Zhi Zi) to purge liver-fire; for dark purple tongue, uneven pulse, stasis spots on the body, add *Salviae Miltiorrhizae Radix et Rhizoma Radix* (Dan Shen), *Chuanxiong Rhizoma* (Chuan Xiong), *Persicae Semen* (Tao Ren) and *Carthami Flos* (Hong Hua) to activate blood and resolve stasis.

加减: 若见急躁易怒、口干口苦、夜寐不宁、小便短赤,可加用龙胆草、牡丹皮、山栀以清泻肝火;若见舌暗紫、脉涩、身有瘀点,可加丹参、川芎、桃仁、红花活血化瘀。

2.2.5 Dowward Flow of Damp-heat

2.2.5 湿热下注

Mainfestations: Slack and sloppy penis, or erec-

证候: 阴茎萎软,或勃而

ted but slack, damp stinky scrotum, soreness and fatigue of the lower limbs, yellow dark urine, or with slippery turbid spermatarrhea; yellow greasy tongue fur; soft or rapid pulse.

不坚，阴囊潮湿、骚臭，下肢酸困，小便黄赤，或伴遗精滑浊。苔黄腻，脉濡或数。

Treatment: To clear away heat and eliminate dampness.

治法：清热利湿。

Formulas and Herbs: *Gentian Liver-Draining Decoction* (Long Dan Xie Gan Tang), usually composed of *Gentianae Radix et Rhizom* (Long Dan Cao), *Scutellariae Radix* (Huang Qin), *Gardeniae Fructus* (Zhi Zi) and *Bupleuri Radix* (Chai Hu) to clear away heat and purge fire, *Akebiae Caulis* (Mu Tong), *Plantaginis Semen* (Che Qian Zi) and *Alismatis Rhizoma* (Ze Xie) to clear away and eliminate damp-heat, *Angelicae Sinensis Radix* (Dang Gui) and *Rehmannia Radix* (Sheng Di Huang) to nourish yin, activate and cool blood.

方药：龙胆泻肝汤。常用：龙胆草、黄芩、栀子、柴胡清热泻火；木通、车前子、泽泻清利湿热；当归、生地黄养阴活血凉血。

Modification: For erection in the dream, spermatarrhea when erected, night sweating, feverish sensation in five centers, soreness in the waist and knees, red tongue with little fluid, string fine rapid pulse, use *Anemarrhena, Phellodendron, and Rehmannia Pills* (Zhi Bai Di Huang Wan) and *Great Yin Supplementation Pills* (Da Bu Yin Wan).

加减：若见梦中阳举、举则遗精，寐则盗汗，五心烦热，腰膝酸软，舌红少津，脉弦细数，可用知柏地黄丸合大补阴丸。

Chapter 6 Diseases of Qi, Blood, and Body Fluid

第6章 气血津液病证

Obstruction of Dampness

湿 阻

Obstruction of dampness is a disease characterized by fullness and oppression in the stomach and abdomen, heavy body, tastelessness, poor appetite and greasy tongue fur due to dampness obstructing and stagnating zhong jiao and poor function of transformation and transportation of the spleen and stomach.

湿阻主要因湿邪阻滞中焦,脾胃运化功能减弱而导致的以脘腹满闷、肢体困重、口淡纳呆、苔腻等为主要症状的病证。

1 Etiology and Pathogenesis

1 病因病机

Dampness obstruction iszhong jiao obstructed by dampness, irregular ascendance and descendance, dysfunction of transformation and transportation, mainly caused by pathogenic dampness and improper diet.

湿阻的发生主要是由于感受湿邪,饮食不当,导致湿阻中焦,升降失常,脾胃运化障碍。

1.1 Blockage of Qi Activity Due to Invasion of Exogenous Dampness

1.1 感受外湿,阻遏气机

Exogenous pathogenic dampness penetrates into the body via skin due to continuous rain, humid air, humid habitation, working in water, wet clothes after sweating. Dampness belongs to pathogenic yin. Heavy turbid sticky exogenous dampness can easily

阴雨连绵,空气潮湿,或久居潮湿之地,或涉水作业,或汗出沾衣,外湿之邪,从体表肌肤而入。湿为阴邪,湿性重浊黏腻,感受外湿之邪,

attack yang-qi and obstruct qi acitivity, which leads to block and discomfort.

易伤人体阳气，阻遏气机运行，而成痞塞不通之证。

1.2 Impairment of Transportation of the Spleen Due to Improper Diet

1.2 饮食不当，脾失健运

Uncontrolled intake of cold and raw food, alcohol, greasy and sweat food, irregular mealtime will make damge to the spleen and stomach, which fail to transform and transport body fluid, generating dampness. On the other hand, injuried spleen and stomach are prone to exogenous dampness invasion. Therefore, exogenous and endogenous pathogenic factors will surely make the situation worse.

恣食生冷，酒醴肥甘，或饥饱失常，以致脾胃受损，运化功能失职，津液不得正常运化转输，酿成内湿而致病。脾胃受损又易招致外湿的侵袭，内外合邪，必然加重病情。

Dampness lies usually in zhong jiao, spleen and stomach. As matters with same nature tend to go together, the exogenous dampness or endogenous dampness will accumulate in the spleen since the spleen is damp earth in TCM. Dampness is controled the spleen and can injure the spleen. Exogenous dampness invades into the body via skin and flesh while endogenous dampness is caused by injuried spleen and stomach failing to transform and transport. The pathogenesis is dampness obstructing zhong jiao, irregular ascendance and descendance, dysfunction of transformation and transportation. The pathological nature is mainly complication of deficiency and excess. Though pathogenic dampness is the cause, it usually originates from spleen deficiency and therefore, the secondary symptoms are of excess and the primary symptoms are of deficiency. Dampness during the onset stage is excess but will turn into complication when prolonged.

湿阻病位以中焦脾胃居多。因脾为湿土，不论外湿、内湿伤人，必同气相求，故湿必归脾而害脾。外湿从体表、肌肤侵入人体；内生之湿，因脾胃受损，运化失常所致。湿阻的病机主要是湿阻中焦，升降失常，运化失司。病理性质以实证及虚实夹杂为主。虽湿邪为致病之因，但多缘于脾虚，故其标为实，其本为虚，病初多实，久病则多虚实夹杂。

Dampness obstruction generally comes into two pathological changes: cold type and heat type. Innately weak cold spleen and stomach, and over in-

湿阻一般分寒化和热化两种病理变化：凡素体脾胃虚寒，或过食生冷则易为寒

take of cold and raw food is likely to be damp-cold. Meanwhile, innately accumulated heat in the stomach and intestines, or yin deficiency, or over intake of sweat and greasy food tends to be damp-heat. Moveover, during treatment, doctors should pay attention not to over use herbs with cold and cooling nature to turn dampness into damp-cold and in the same way, do not over use warming and drying herbs to turn dampness into damp-heat.

湿之证;凡素体肠胃积热或阴虚火旺或过食肥甘之品，则易为湿热之证。此外,在治疗过程中,过用寒凉之品可使湿从寒化,过用温燥之药可使湿从热化。

2 Syndrome Differentiation and Treatment

2 辨证论治

2.1 Key Points of Syndrome Differentiation

2.1 辨治要点

To treat dampness obstruction, first distinguish cold and heat, that is, cold-dampness and damp-heat. The common manifestations are oppression in the stomach, general heaviness, poor appetite, greasy tongue fur, soft pulse and others. The difference is as follows. Cold-dampness has the manifestations of general heaviness, aversion to cold, discomfort and oppression in the stomach and abdomen which favors pressing, tastelessness or sweet taste, loose stool, white greasy tongue fur, soft slow pulse while damp-heat has the manifestations of general heaviness, fever, discomfort in the stomach like pain which refuses pressing, dry sticky mouth, dark urine, yellow greasy tongue fur and soft rapid pulse. Next, according to tongue manifestations and accompanying symptoms, differentiate the major and minor conflicts between pathogenic dampness and spleen deficiency. Generally speaking, during the onset stage of dampness obstruction, it is most likely to be caused by exogenous damp affection and of excess type. Thick greasy tongue fur of damp-cold or damp-heat is mainly due to pathogenic excess of re-

湿阻辨治要点首先在于分清寒热。即寒湿证与湿热证,湿阻的共同表现为脘闷、身重、纳呆、苔腻、脉濡等。不同的是:寒湿证表现为身重而恶寒,脘腹痞闷,喜按,口淡无味,或有甜味,便溏,舌苔白腻,脉濡缓;湿热证表现为身重而有热,脘痞似痛,不喜按,口苦黏腻,尿赤,舌苔黄腻,脉濡数。其次根据舌象及伴随症状分清湿邪与脾虚的主次关系。一般来说,湿阻初起,多为感受外湿,以实证为多见。若见舌苔厚腻,无论内湿外湿致病,均以湿浊停留,困阻中焦的邪实为主;若除四肢困重、脘闷纳呆外,伴有面色萎黄,且舌苔薄或薄腻而舌质淡胖者,则多以脾虚气弱为主。治疗上以除湿健脾为原则,

tention of damp-turbid which blocks and stagnates zhong jiao. General heaviness of limbs, oppression in the chest, poor appetite, sallow yellow complexion, thin or thin greasy tongue fur and pale enlarged tongue are manifestations of spleen deficiency and qi weakness. In terms of treatment, in addition to the principle of eliminating dampness and strengthening spleen, identify and weigh over the major and minor conflicts of spleen deficiency and pathogenic dampness and give treatments correspondingly. For excess type, first eliminate dampness. For deficiency type, it is important to strengthen the spleen. The herbs should be lucid and have compatibility with warming and clear awaying effects.

根据脾虚与湿邪孰为主孰为次,权衡轻重,灵活施治。实证以除湿为先,虚证以健脾为要,用药贵在清灵,注意温清配伍。

2.2 Therapeutic Methods for Different Patterns

2.2 分型论治

2.2.1 Dampness Encumbering the Spleen and Stomach

2.2.1 湿困脾胃

Manifestations: Heaviness of fatigue of the limbs, or heavy head as if swathed, oppression in the chest and distention in the abdomen, tastelessness, sticky in the mouth or with sweet taste, loose stool; white greasy tongue fur; soft rolling pulse.

证候: 肢体困重乏力,或头重如裹,胸闷腹胀,纳食不香,口中黏淡无味,或有甜味,便溏。舌苔白腻,脉濡滑。

Treatment: To resolve dampness by aromatization.

治法: 芳香化湿。

Formulas and Herbs: *Agastachis-Restoring Healthy Energy Powder* (Huo Xiang Zheng Qi San), usually composed of *Pogostemonis Herba* (Huo Xiang), *Perillae Fructus* (Zi Su Zi), *Citri Reticulatae Pericarpium* (Chen Pi) and *Angelicae Dahuricae Radix* (Bai Zhi) to resolve dampness by aromatization, *Magnoliae Officinalis Cortex* (Hou Pu), *Pinelliae Rhizoma* (Ban Xia) and *Atractylodis Macrocephalae Rhizoma* (Bai Zhu) to dry dampness with their bitter and warm nature; *Arecae Pericarpium* (Da Fu

方药: 藿香正气散。常用:藿香、紫苏、陈皮、白芷芳香化湿;厚朴、半夏、白术苦温燥湿;大腹皮、茯苓淡渗利湿。该方诸药集芳香、苦温、淡渗三法于一方,并配合桔梗宣通肺气、甘草甘缓和中。

Pi) and *Poria* (Fu Ling) to eliminate dampness with their bland nature. This formular combines aromatization, bitterness and warmth, blandness along with *Platycodi Radix* (Jie Geng) to disperse the lung qi and *Glycyrrhizae Radix et Rhizoma* (Gan Cao) to harmomize zhong jiao with sweetness gradually.

Modification: For accompanying food stagnation, add *Crataegi Fructus* (Shan Zha), *Massa Fermentata Medicinalis* (Shen Qu) and *Galli Gigerii Endothelium Corneum* (Ji Nei Jin) to promote digestion to eliminate stagnation; for accompanying exterior symptoms, add *Schizonepetae Herba* (Jing Jie) and *Saposhnikoviae Radix* (Fang Feng) to disperse the pathogenic exterior with acridity; for distention and fullness in the chest and abdomen, loose stool, white greasy tongue fur, use *Poria Stomach Decoction* (Wei Ling Tang) to strengthen the effects of drying dampness, strengthening the spleen, disinhibiting dampness with blander percolation.

加减: 兼见食滞,可加山楂、神曲、鸡内金消食化滞;兼有表证加荆芥、防风辛散表邪;若见胸腹胀满、大便溏薄、舌苔白而厚腻,可用胃苓汤以增强燥湿健脾、淡渗分利的作用。

2.2.2 Damp-heat Blocking the Middle

Manifestations: Heaviness and fatigue of the limbs, bitter sticky greasy mouth, poor appetite, oppression in the chest and distention in the abdomen, thirst but no desire for drink, dark urine, loose sticky stool, or with low fever; yellow greasy tongue fur; soft rapid pulse.

Treatment: To clear away heat and dry dampness.

Formulas and Herbs: *Coptis and Officinal Magnolia Bark Beverage* (Lian Pu Yin), usually composed of *Coptidis Rhizoma* (Huang Lian) and *Gardeniae Fructus* (Zhi Zi) to dry dampness with their bitter nature; *Pinelliae Rhizoma* (Ban Xia),

2.2.2 湿热中阻

证候: 四肢困重,口苦黏腻,纳呆,胸闷腹胀,口渴不欲饮,尿赤,大便溏烂不爽,或有低热。苔黄腻,脉濡数。

治法: 清热化湿。

方药: 连朴饮。常用:黄连、山栀以苦化湿热;半夏、厚朴、豆豉化湿除满;石菖蒲、芦根和中清热。亦可合用甘露消毒丹,以清热化湿、

Magnoliae Officinalis Cortex (Hou Pu) and *Sojae Semen Praeparatum* (Dan Dou Chi) to dry dampness and eliminate fullness, *Acori Tatarinowii Rhizoma* (Shi Chang Pu) and *Phragmitis Rhiamoma* (Lu Gen) to harmonize zhong jiao and clear away heat. *Sweet Dew Toxin-Dispersing Elixir* (Gan Lu Xiao Du Dan) can be also added to clear away heat and resolve dampness, resolve turbidity with their aroma.

芳香化浊。

Modification: For unremarkable heat pattern, unremarkable fever and greasy tongue fur, modified *Three Kernels Decoction* (San Ren Tang) can also be used; for in summer, thirst and frequent drink, frequent long urine, no sweating or little, continuous fever, oppression in the chest, poor appetite, lassitude and fatigue, greasy tongue fur and rapid pulse, use fresh *Pogostemonis Herba* (Huo Xiang), fresh *Nelumbinis Folium* (He Ye), *Bombycis Bombyx* (Can Jian), *Isatidis Radix* (Ban Lan Gen) and *Six-To-One power* (Liu Yi San) to clear away and eliminate summer heat and constrain urine.

加减：若热象不盛，身热不扬，苔不甚腻，亦可选用三仁汤加减；若盛夏季节，出现口渴多饮、尿频而长、无汗或出汗甚少、发热不退、胸闷纳呆、神疲乏力、苔腻、脉数，可用鲜藿香、鲜荷叶、蚕茧、板蓝根、六一散等清化暑湿兼摄小便。

2.2.3 Stagnation of Dampness Due to Spleen Deficiency

2.2.3 脾虚湿滞

Manifestations: Sallow yellow complexion, lassitude and fatigue, heaviness and fatigue of the limbs, discomfort in the stomach and abdomen, tastelessness, aversion to grease, loose stool or diarrhea; thin greasy tongue fur or pale enlarged tongue; soft slow pulse.

证候：面色萎黄，神疲乏力，四肢困重，脘腹不舒，纳食不香，厌食油腻，大便溏薄或泄泻。苔薄腻或舌质淡胖，脉濡缓。

Treatment: To strengthen the spleen and dry dampness.

治法：健脾化湿。

Formulas and Herbs: *Aucklandia, Amomum and Six Nobles Decoction* (Xiang Sha Liu Jun Zi Tang), usually composed of *Codonopsis Radix* (Dang Shen), *Atractylodis Macrocephalae Rhizoma*

方药：香砂六君子汤。常用：党参、白术、茯苓、甘草以健脾益气；半夏、陈皮以理气化湿；木香、砂仁和胃醒

(Bai Zhu), *Poria* (Fu Ling) and *Glycyrrhizae Radix et Rhizoma* (Gan Cao) to strengthen the spleen and boost qi; *Pinelliae Rhizoma* (Ban Xia) and *Citri Reticulatae Pericarpium* (Chen Pi) to regulate qi and eliminate dampness; *Aucklandiae Radix* (Mu Xiang) and *Amomi Fructus* (Sha Ren) to harmonize the stomach and invigorate the spleen.

脾。

Modification: For diarrhea with rumbling noise in the intestines due to spleen deficiency and unraised clear away qi, add *Puerariae Lobatae Radix* (Ge Gen), *Cimicifugae Rhizoma* (Sheng Ma) and *Pogostemonis Herba* (Huo Xiang) to raise clear away qi and dry dampness to stop diarrhea; for facial and limb edema due to deficiency of the spleen which fails to dam water and leads to retention of water-damp, add *Astragali Radix* (Huang Qi), *Lablab Semen Album* (Bai Bian Dou) and *Coicis Semen* (Yi Yi Ren) to boost qi and resolve dampness to eliminate edema; for dull pain in the abdomen, aversion to cold and cold limbs, add *Zingiberis Rhizoma* (Gan Jiang) and *Cinnamomi Ramulus* (Gui Zhi) to warm the middle, disperse cold and stop pain.

加减: 泄泻肠鸣者为脾虚清气不升所致,可加葛根、升麻、藿香升清化湿以止泻;如面浮肢肿者,为脾虚不能制水,水湿停聚所致,可加黄芪、扁豆、薏苡仁益气化湿以消肿;腹中隐痛,畏寒肢冷者,可加干姜、桂枝温中散寒止痛。

Depressive Disorder

郁 证

Depressive disorder is a disease caused by stagnation of qi activity due to depressed emotions and spirits, which features depressing mood, unpeacefulness, fullness and oppression in the chest, distention and pain in the abdomen or irritation and easy cry, for felling like things choked in the throat.

郁证是由于情志不舒引起气机郁滞,临床以心情抑郁、情绪不宁、胸部满闷、胁肋胀痛,或易怒喜哭,或咽中如有异物梗塞等症为主要临床表现的一类病证。

1 Etiology and Pathogenesis

1 病因病机

The main causes of depression are injury of the

郁证的主要病因是七情

seven emotions, worry, overstrain and innate zang-qi deficiency. Its pathogenesis is dysfunction of the liver to disperse and lung to transport, poorly nourishd heart and unregulated yin, yang, qi and blood of zang-fu organs.

所伤、思虑劳倦、脏气素虚。基本病机是肝失疏泄、脾失健运、心失所养、脏腑阴阳气血失调。

1.1 Depression of Liver-qi Due to Depressed Emotions

1.1 情志不畅,肝气郁结

When the seven emotions go extreme, liver-qi will be depressed into qi depression, which, if prolonged, will affect blood and lead to inhibited blood flow and blood depression. If qi depression turns into fire and liver-fire inflames upward, leading to fire depression. Qi stagnation and inhibited fluid will turn into accumulated phlegm, which, along with qi, turns into phlegm depression.

七情过极,肝气郁结,而成气郁;气郁日久,影响及血,血行不畅成为血郁;气郁化火,肝火上炎,则成火郁;气滞津行不畅,聚而成痰,痰气互结,而成痰郁。

1.2 Failure of Transportation of the Spleen Due to Worry and Overstrain

1.2 思虑劳倦,脾失健运

Worry and overstrain will hurt the spleen and disenable the spleen to transport. Food retention will then turn into food depression. Dampness will be accumulated into phlegm, leading to phlegm depression.

思虑、劳倦伤脾,脾失健运,食积不化成为食郁;湿聚成痰,而成痰郁。

1.3 Consumption of the Heart and Spirits Due to Innate Zang-qi Deficiency

1.3 脏气素虚,心神耗伤

Innate deficiency of the heart and gallbladder, burdened by worry and sorrow is likely to hurt heart-qi and heart yin, impairing the nourishment of the heart and spirits.

心胆素虚,复遇忧思悲愁,易损心气心阴,以致心神失养。

Overall, depressive disorder is most related to the liver and also related to the heart and spleen. Its pathological nature is deficiency and excess. Excess depression refers to qi stagnation mainly at the beginning, along with blood stasis, fire transformation, phlegm clots and food retention, which,

综上所述,郁证的发病与肝的关系最为密切,其次涉及心、脾。病理性质有虚实两端:初起以气滞为主,兼血瘀、化火、痰结、食滞等,属实证。后期或因火郁伤阴而

might turn into yin deficiency and fire excess later and yin deficiency of the heart and kidney if fire depression injuries yin. Or inadequate qi and blood transformation, and poorly nourishd heart and spirits due to spleen injury lead to deficiency of both the heart and spleen, which means excess now turns into deficiency of yin and blood. Among the six depressive disorders, qi depression always comes first, followed by other patterns of dampness, phlegm, heat, blood and food. These six patterns are interdetermined and complicated.

导致阴虚火旺、心肾阴虚之证;或因脾伤气血生化不足,心神失养,而导致心脾两虚之证。由实转虚,转为阴亏血虚。六郁中总以气郁为先,而后才有湿、痰、热、血、食诸郁,且六郁相因,互为兼夹。

2　Syndrome Differentiation and Treatment

2　辨证论治

2.1　Key Points of Syndrome Differentiation

2.1　辨治要点

It is of primary importance to identify the relationship between affected zang-fu organs and the six depressive disorders. Generally speaking, qi depression, blood depression and fire depression are related to the liver. Food depression, stagnation of dampness and phlegm depression are related to the spleen. Meanwhile, deficiency pattern is most related to the heart, then the liver, spleen and kidney. Next, identify excess from deficiency. Excess depressions usually last short and have manifestations of depressed spirits, distention and pain in the chest and hypochondria, choke in the throat, sigh, stringy or rolling pulse while deficiency depressions last long with manifestations such as low spiritedness, unpeacefulness, panic, deficiency irritation, insomnia, sorrow, easy cry, fine for fine rapid pulse.

首先辨明受病脏腑与六郁的关系。一般说来:气郁、血郁、火郁主要关系于肝;食郁、湿郁、痰郁主要关系于脾;而虚证则与心的关系最为密切,其次是肝、脾、肾的亏虚。其次辨别证候虚实:实证病程较短,表现精神抑郁,胸胁胀痛,咽中梗塞,时欲太息,脉弦或滑;虚证则病已久延,症见精神不振、心神不宁、心慌、虚烦不寐、悲忧善哭、脉细或细数等。

The treatment should follow the principle of regulating qi and resolving depression, disinhibiting qi activity, distracting attention and changing tem-

郁证的治疗原则是理气开郁、调畅气机、怡情易性是治疗郁病的基本原则。对于

perament. It is first to regulate qi and break depression for excess depressions while for deficiency depressions, supplement according to injuried zang-fu organs and the deficiency intensity of qi, blood, yin and essence. For complication of deficiency and excess, treat together in light of predominance of deficiency and excess.

实证,首当理气开郁;虚证则应根据损及的脏腑及气血阴精亏虚的不同情况而补之;对于虚实夹杂者,则又当视虚实的偏重而虚实兼顾。

2.2 Therapeutic Methods for Different Types of Depressions

2.2 分型论治

2.2.1 Depression of Liver-qi

2.2.1 肝气郁结

Manifestations: Spiritual depression, unpeaceful mind, fullness and oppression in the chest, distention and pain in the hypochondria with no fixed spots, oppression in the stomach and burping, no desire for food and drink, irregualar stool; thin greasy tongue fur; stringy pulse.

证候: 精神抑郁,情绪不宁,胸部满闷,胁肋胀痛,痛无定处,脘闷嗳气,不思饮食,大便不调。苔薄腻,脉弦。

Treatment: To disperse the liver and resolve depression; regulate qi and disperse zhong jiao.

治法: 疏肝解郁,理气畅中。

Formulas and Herbs: *Bupleurum-Dispersing-Liver Powder* (Chai Hu Shu Gan San), usually composed of *Bupleuri Radix* (Chai Hu), *Cyperi Rhizoma* (Xiang Fu) and *Aurantii Fructus*(Zhi Qiao) to disperse the liver and regulate qi; *Chuanxiong Rhizoma* (Chuan Xiong), *Paeoniae Radix Alba* (Bai Shao Yao) and *Glycyrrhizae Radix et Rhizoma* (Gan Cao) to activate blood and relieve urgency.

方药: 柴胡疏肝散。常用:柴胡、香附、枳壳疏肝理气;川芎、白芍药、甘草活血、缓急止痛。

Modification: For frequent burping and discomfort in the stomach, add *Inulae Flos* (Xuan Fu Hua), *Haematitum* (Zhe Shi), *Pinellinae Rhizoma Praeparatum* (Fa Ban Xia) to harmonize the stomach and descend adverse flow of qi; for liver-qi exploiting the spleen with symptoms like distention and pain in the abdomen and diarrhea, add *Atractylodis Rhizoma* (Cang Zhu), *Magnoliae Officinalis*

加减: 若见嗳气频作、脘闷不舒,可加旋覆花、代赭石、法半夏和胃降逆;若肝气乘脾而见腹胀、腹痛、腹泻,可加苍术、厚朴、茯苓、乌药健脾化湿,理气止痛;若兼有血瘀而见胸胁刺痛、舌质有瘀点瘀斑,可加当归、丹参、

Cortex (Hou Po), *Poria* (Fu Ling) and *Linderae Radix* (Wu Yao) to strengthen the spleen and dry dampness as well as regulate qi and stop pain; for accompanying sharp pain in the chest and sides due to blood stasis, stasis spots and macules on the tongue, add *Angelicae Sinensis Radix* (Dang Gui), *Salviae Miltiorrhizae Radix et Rhizoma Radix* (Dan Shen), *Curcumae Radix* (Yu Jin) and *Carthami Flos* (Hong Hua) to activate blood and eliminate blood stasis.

郁金、红花活血化瘀。

2.2.2　Qi Depression Transforms into Fire

Manifestations: Unpeaceful mind, irritation, easy anger, distention and fullness in the chest and hypochondria, bitter dry mouth, or headache, reddish eyes, tinnitus, or gastric upset and acid regurgitation, dry stool; red tongue with yellow tongue fur; stringy rapid pulse.

Treatment: To disperse the liver and resolve depression; cleanse the liver and purge fire.

Formulas and Herbs: *Moutan Cortex and Gardeniae- Free Wanderer Powder* (Dan Zhi Xiao Yao San), usually composed of *Moutan Cortex* (Mu Dan Pi) and *Gardeniae Fructus* (Zhi Zi) to cleanse the liver and purge fire; *Bupleuri Radix* (Chai Hu) and *Menthae Haplocalycis Herba* (Bo He) to disperse the liver and resolve depression; *Angelicae Sinensis Radix* (Dang Gui) and *Paeoniae Radix Alba* (Bai Shao Yao) to soften the liver and nourish blood; *Atractylodis Macrocephalae Rhizoma* (Bai Zhu) and *Poria* (Fu Ling) to strengthen the spleen and help to transport.

Modification: For severe heat patterns, bitter mouth and constipation, add *Gentianae Radix et Rhizom* (Long Dan) and *Rhei Radix et Rhizoma*

2.2.2　气郁化火

证候：情绪不宁，急躁易怒，胸胁胀满，口苦而干，或头痛，目赤，耳鸣，或嘈杂吞酸，大便秘结。舌质红，苔黄，脉弦数。

治法：疏肝解郁，清肝泻火。

方药：丹栀逍遥散。常用：牡丹皮、栀子清肝泻火；柴胡、薄荷疏肝解郁；当归、白芍药柔肝养血，白术、茯苓健脾助运。

加减：热势较甚，口苦、大便秘结者，可加龙胆草、大黄泻热通腑；肝火犯胃而见

(Da Huang) to purge fire and dredge fu-organs; for sharp pain in the hypochondria due to liver-fire attacking the stomach, bitter mouth, gastric upset, acid regurgitation, burping, vomiting, add *Coptidis Rhizoma* (Huang Lian) and *Euodiae Fructus* (Wu Zhu Yu) [*Coptis and evodia Pills* (Zuo Jin Wan)] to cleanse the liver and purge fire as well as descend adverse flow of qi to stop vomiting; for excess heat consuming yin with such symptoms as red tongue with little tongue fur and fine rapid pulse, delete warming and drying herbs like *Angelicae Sinensis Radix* (Dang Gui), *Atractylodis Macrocephalae Rhizoma* (Bai Zhu) and *Coptis and evodia Pills* (Zuo Jin Wan), and add moderately *Rehmannia Radix* (Sheng Di Huang), *Ophiopogonis Radix* (Mai Men Dong) and *Dioscoreae Rhizoma* (Shan Yao) to nourish yin and strengthen the spleen, or change for *Water-Enriching Liver-Clear awaying Beverage* (Zi Shui Qing Gan Yin).

胁肋疼痛、口苦、嘈杂吞酸、嗳气、呕吐者,可加黄连、吴茱萸(即左金丸)清肝泻火、降逆止呕;若热盛伤阴,而见舌红少苔、脉细数者,可去原方中当归、白术、生姜之温燥,酌加生地黄、麦门冬、山药滋阴健脾,或改用滋水清肝饮养阴清火。

2.2.3 Depression of Phlegm-qi

Manifestations: Spiritual depression, oppression and obstruction in the chest, distention and fullness in the hypochondrai, feeling choked in the throat that cannot be swallowed or coughed out; white greasy tongue fur; stringy rolling pulse. It is called "plum-pit qi" according to "Therapeutic Methods for Treating Qi" from *The Golden Mirror of Medicine* (Yi Zong Jin Jian).

Treatment: To promote qi flow and break up depression; resolve phlegm and dissipate stagnation.

Formulas and Herbs: *Pinellia and Officinal Magnolia Bark Decoction* (Ban Xia Hou Pu Tang), usually composed of *Pinelliae Rhizoma* (Ban Xia), *Magnoliae Officinalis Cortex* (Hou Pu) and *Poria*

2.2.3 痰气郁结

证候: 精神抑郁,胸部闷塞,胁肋胀满,咽中如有物梗塞,吞之不下,咯之不出。苔白腻,脉弦滑。《医宗金鉴》将本证称为"梅核气"。

治法: 行气开郁,化痰散结。

方药: 半夏厚朴汤。常用:半夏、厚朴、茯苓降逆化痰;紫苏、生姜理气散结。

(Fu Ling) to descend adverse flow of qi and resolve phlegm; *Perillae Fructus* (Zi Su Zi) and *Zingiberis Rhizoma Recens* (Sheng Jiang) to regulate qi and dissipate stagnation.

Modification: For stagnation of dampness and qi stagnation along with discomfort and oppression in the chest and stomach, burping and greasy tongue fur, add *Cyperi Rhizoma* (Xiang Fu), *Citri Saroodactylis Fructus* Sectus (Fo Shou Pian) and *Atractylodis Rhizoma* (Cang Zhu) to regulate qi and eliminate dampness; for phlegm-depression transforming into heat with irriation, red tongue and yellow tongue fur, add *Bambusae Caulis in Taenias* (Zhu Ru), *Trichosanthis Fructus* (Gua Lou), *Scutellariae Radix* (Huang Qin) and *Coptidis Rhizoma* (Huang Lian) to clear away and resolve phlegm-heat; for prolonged illness affecting collaterals and blood stasis symptoms, sharp pain in the chest and hypochondria, purple dark tongue with spots or macules, and uneven pulse, add *Curcumae Radix* (Yu Jin), *Salviae Miltiorrhizae Radix et Rhizoma Radix* (Dan Shen) and *Dalbergiae Odoriferae Lignum* (Jiang Xiang), *Curcumae Longae Rhizoma* (Jiang Huang) to activate blood and eliminate blood stasis.

加减: 湿郁气滞而兼胸脘痞闷、嗳气、苔腻者,加香附、佛手片、苍术理气除湿;痰郁化热而见烦躁、舌红苔黄者,加竹茹、瓜蒌、黄芩、黄连清化痰热;病久入络而有瘀血征象,胸胁刺痛、舌质紫暗或有瘀点瘀斑、脉涩者,加郁金、丹参、降香、姜黄活血化瘀。

2.2.4　Poor Nourishment of the Heart and Spirits

Manifestations: Trance, unpeaceful mind, suspiciousness, easily frightened, sorrow, worry, easy cry, or frequent pandiculation, or dancing around or swear and shout; pale tongue; stringy pulse. It is often found in women and likely to be triggered by mental stress. Its clinical maninfestations vary, but each patient has several similar symptoms every time he/she relapses. It is refered as "visceral agitation" in "Treatment for Women's Miscellaneous

2.2.4　心神失养

证候: 精神恍惚,心神不宁,多疑易惊,悲忧善哭,喜怒无常,或时时欠伸,或手舞足蹈,骂詈喊叫等,舌质淡,脉弦。此种证候多见于女性,常因精神刺激而诱发。临床表现多种多样,但同一患者每次发作多为同样几种症状的重复。《金匮要略》将

Diseases and Pulse Patterns" from *Essential Prescriptions of the Golden Coffer* (Jin Kui Yao Lue).

此种证候称为"脏躁"。

Treatment: To relieve urgency with sweet and moist herbs; nourish the heart and calm the spirits.

治法: 甘润缓急,养心安神。

Formulas and Herbs: *Liquorice, Wheat and Jujube Decoction* (Gan Mai Da Zao Tang), usually composed of *Glycyrrhizae Radix et Rhizoma* (Gan Cao) to relieve urgency, *Semen Tritici* (Huai Xiao Mai) to supplement and boost heart-qi, *Jujubae Fructus* (Da Zao) to strengthen the spleen and nourish the heart. *Albiziae Flos* (He Huan Hua) and *Ziziphi Spinosae Semen* (Suan Zao Ren) to break up depression and calm the spirits.

方药: 甘麦大枣汤。常用:甘草缓急;淮小麦补益心气;大枣健脾养心。还可加合欢花、酸枣仁开郁安神。

Modification: For wriggling or convulsion of hands and feet due to hemopenia engendering wind, add *Angelicae Sinensis Radix* (Dang Gui), *Rehmannia Radix* (Sheng Di Huang), *Margaritifera Concha* (Zhen Zhu Mu) and *Uncariae Ramulus cum Uncis* (Gou Teng) to nourish blood and stop wind; for agitation leading to insomnia, add *Ziziphi Spinosae Semen* (Suan Zao Ren), *Platycladi Semen* (Bai Zi Ren), *Poria cum Ligno Hospite* (Fu Shen) and *Polygoni Multiflori Radix Praeparat*a (Zhi Shou Wu) to nourish the heart and calm the spirits; for dyspnea and adverse qi flow, add *Five Milled Ingredients Decoction* (Wu Mo Yin Zi) to eliminate depression and dissipate stagnation, regulate qi and descend adverse flow of qi.

加减: 血虚生风而见手足蠕动或抽搐者,加当归、生地黄、珍珠母、钩藤养血息风;躁扰失眠者,加酸枣仁、柏子仁、茯神、制首乌等养心安神;喘促气逆者,可合五磨饮子开郁散结、理气降逆。

2.2.5 Deficiency of the Heart and Spleen

2.2.5 心脾两虚

Mainfestations: Unpeaceful mind, inquiring mind, suspiciousness, dizziness, lassitude, palpitation, forgetfulness, poor appetite, lusterless face; pale tongue with white thin tongue fur; fine pulse.

证候: 情绪不宁,多思善疑,头晕神疲,心悸胆怯,失眠健忘,纳差,面色不华。舌质淡,苔薄白,脉细。

Treatment: To strengthen the spleen and nour-

治法: 健脾养心,补益气

ish the heart; supplement qi and blood.

Formulas and Herbs: *Angelica Splenic Decoction* (Gui Pi Tang), usually composed of *Codonopsis Radix* (Dang Shen), *Astragali Radix* (Huang Qi), *Atractylodis Macrocephalae Rhizoma* (Bai Zhu) and *Poria* (Fu Ling) to boost qi and strengthen the spleen; *Angelicae Sinensis Radix* (Dang Gui) and *Longan Arillus* (Long Yan Rou) to nourish the heart and supplement blood; *Ziziphi Spinosae Semen* (Suan Zao Ren), *Polygalae Radix* (Yuan Zhi) and *Poria cum Ligno Hospite* (Fu Shen) to nourish the heart and calm the spirits.

Modification: For fullness and oppression in the heart and chest, depressed emotions and minds, add *Curcumae Radix* (Yu Jin) and *Citri Saroodactylis Fructus Sectus* (Fo Shou Pian) to regulate qi and break up depression; for headache, add *Chuanxiong Rhizoma* (Chuan Xiong) and *Tribuli Fructus* (Ji Li) to activate blood and dispel wind to stop pain.

2.2.6 Deficiency-Yin of the Heart and Kidney

Manifestations: Unpeaceful mind, palpitation, forgetfulness, dreaminess, insomnia, feverish sensation in five centers, night sweating, dry mouth and throat; red tongue with little fluid.

Treatment: To nourish the heart and kidney.

Formulas and Herbs: *Celestial Emperor Heart-Supplementing Elixir* (Tian Wang Bu Xin Dan) and *Rehmannia Pills with Six Ingredients* (Liu Wei Di Huang Wan), in which *Ginseng Radix et Rhizoma* (Ren Shen), *Dioscoreae Rhizoma* (Shan Yao) and *Poria* (Fu Ling) are used to supplement and boost heart-qi; *Rehmannia Radix* (Di Huang), *Corni Fructus* (Shan Zhu Yu), *Ophiopogonis Radix* (Mai Men Dong), *Asparagi Radix* (Tian Dong),

血。

方药: 归脾汤。常用:党参、黄芪、白术、茯苓益气健脾;当归、龙眼肉养心补血;酸枣仁、远志、茯神养心安神。

加减: 心胸满闷、情志不舒者,加郁金、佛手片理气开郁;头痛者,加川芎、白蒺藜活血祛风而止痛。

2.2.6 心肾阴虚

证候: 情绪不宁,心悸,健忘,失眠,多梦,五心烦热,盗汗,口咽干燥。舌红少津,脉细数。

治法: 滋养心肾。

方药: 天王补心丹合六味地黄丸。常用:人参、山药、茯苓补益心气;地黄、山茱萸、麦门冬、天门冬、玄参、阿胶补肾养阴;五味子、远志、酸枣仁、柏子仁养心安神。

Scrophulariae Radix (Xuan Shen) and *Asini Corii Colla* (E Jiao) are used to supplement the kidney and nourish yin; *Schisandrae Chinensis Fructus* (Wu Wei Zi), *Polygalae Radix* (Yuan Zhi), *Ziziphi Spinosae Semen* (Suan Zao Ren) and *Platycladi Semen* (Bai Zi Ren) to nourish the heart and calm the spirits.

Modification: For irritation and insomnia, dreaminess and spermatarrhea, due to heart and kidney failing to interact, add *Coordination Restoring Pills* (Jiao Tai Wan), which is composed of *Coptidis Rhizoma* (Huang Lian) and *Cinnamomi Cortex* (Rou Gui) to help the heart and kidney to interact; for frequent spermatarrhea, add *Euryales Semen* (Qian Shi), *Nelumbinis Stamen* (Lian Xu) and *Fructus Rosae Laevigatae* (Jin Yin Zi) to supplement the kidney to secure and astrict.

加减: 心肾不交而见心烦失眠、多梦遗精者,可合交泰丸(黄连、肉桂)交通心肾;遗精较频者,可加芡实、莲须、金樱子补肾固涩。

Consumptive Thirst

消　渴

Consumptive thirst refers to patterns characterized by more drink, more food, and more urine but less weight or sweat in urine.

消渴是指多饮、多食、小便多,久则身体消瘦,或尿有甜味等位主要症状的一类病证。

1 Etiology and Pathogenesis

Consumptive thirst is caused by exhaustion and deficiency of yin and body fluid, and predominance of dryness and heat due to congenital defects, improper diet, disharmony of emotions and minds, over strain and too much sexual life.

1 病因病机

消渴的病因有禀赋不足,饮食不节,情志失调,五志过极,劳欲过度等导致阴津亏损,燥热偏胜而成。

1.1 Accumulation of Heat Burning and Consuming the Lung and Stomach Due to Improper Diet and Emotional and Spiritual Disharmony

Improper diet generates heat accumulation in

1.1 饮食不节,情志失调,积热消灼肺胃

饮食不节,积热于胃,胃

the stomach. And stomach-heat fumes the lung. Or mental stress for a long time causes depressed liver-qi which turns into fire and consumes, and scorches the yin and body fluid of the lung and stomach, leading to consumptive thirst.

热熏热于肺；或长期过度精神刺激，肝气郁结，郁久化火，消灼肺胃阴津而成消渴。

1.2 Failure of the Spleen and Stomach to Separate the Lucid from the Turbid Due to Improper Diet and Overstrain

1.2 饮食劳倦，脾胃虚弱，清浊不分

Improper diet and overstrain makes damage to the spleen and stomach. Weakened spleen and stomach are unable to transform and transport. Water, grain and essence then flow directly downward and out with urine without nurturing the overall body, leading to turbid urine and emaciation of the patient.

饮食劳倦，伤及脾胃，致脾胃虚弱，运化失司，水谷精微不养周身而直趋于下，随小便而出，故见消瘦而尿浊。

1.3 Decline of Kidney Essence Due to Innate Deficiency, Overstrain and Too much Sexual Life

1.3 禀赋不足，劳欲过度，肾元虚衰

Innate deficiency or over-consumption will comsume kidney essence, causing deficiency fire which will broil the heart and lung, scorch the spleen and stomach, and impair the opening and closing of the kidney. Then the kidney fails to secure and astrict, leading to more drink, food and urine.

先天禀赋不足，或耗损过度，肾阴亏损，虚火内生，上燔心肺，中灼脾胃，且肾之开阖失司，固摄失权，故多饮、多食、多尿乃成。

1.4 Of Several Zang-organs Involved, Kidney Being the Root

1.4 涉及多脏，以肾为本

Consumptive thirst shows differently in the lung, spleen and stomach, and kidney, but they are mutually affected and will inevitably turn into lung dryness and stomach heat, spleen deficiency and kidney exhaustion. Of the three zang-organs, the kidney is the most important for prolonged weakness of other organs will eventually make damages to yin and yang of the kidney.

消渴虽有肺、脾胃、肾之分，但常相互影响，终成肺燥胃热，脾虚肾亏。三脏中以肾最为重要，他脏虚弱日久，最终无不损及肾之阴阳。

1.5 Transmutated Patterns Due to Prolonged Illness without Proper Treatment and Care

1.5.1 Welling-and Flat-abscesses

Entangled dry-heat kidnaps ying and yin, resulting in stagnation and obstruction of collaterals and vessels, bringing about accumulation of toxin which turns into pus and forms sores which are not easy to heel.

1.5.2 Cateract, Night Blindness and Deaf

Prolonged consumptive thirst will result in deficiency of both the liver and kidney, damage essence, consme blood, leading to poorly nourishd orifices of the liver and kidney.

1.5.3 Pulmonary Consumption

Excess dry-heat fumes and scorches the lung, consumes and injuries qi and yin and weakens the healthy qi, which makes the lung prone to be infected with turbucolosis germs, leading to pulmonary consumption.

1.5.4 Edema

During the late stage of consumptive thirst, the weak spleen and kidney fails to steam and distribute water, leading to water retention inside which penetrates into skin and cause edema with creamy turbid sweat urine.

1.5.5 Blood Stasis

Prolonged consumptive thirst affecting the collaterals causes stagnation of blood stasis. Or dry-heat due to yin deficiency consumes and burns fluid, causing unsmooth flow of blood. Or dry-heat for long consumes and injuries qi-yin, which leads to slack movement of qi and blood. Or weakened yin affects yang which results in deficiency and cold coagulation, leading to blood stasis. By the position of blood stasis, there can be seen chest obstruction, palpitation, vertigo, stroke and limb paralysis.

1.5 久病失治，不知调摄，变证百出

1.5.1 痈疽

燥热内结，营阴被劫，络脉瘀阻，蕴毒成脓，且溃后不易收口。

1.5.2 白内障、雀目、耳聋

消渴日久，肝肾两亏，伤精耗血，不能上承，肝肾二窍失养。

1.5.3 肺痨

本病燥热素盛，熏灼于肺，耗伤气阴，正气衰弱，易感痨虫，而成肺痨。

1.5.4 水肿

消渴后期，脾肾虚衰，水失输布蒸化，水饮内停，泛溢肌肤，而成水肿，并可见小便浑浊如脂膏，尿甘。

1.5.5 瘀血证

消渴久病入络，瘀血阻滞，或阴虚燥热，耗津灼液，血运不畅，或燥热日久，耗伤气阴，气虚血行无力，或阴损及阳，阳虚寒凝，均可导致瘀血产生，根据停留部位各异，可见胸痹、心悸、眩晕、中风、肢体麻木等。

1.5.6 Shock

When yin and fluid are exhausted, deficient yang floats and escapes. Patients will faint due to consumption of yin and escape of yang with shock symptoms of cold limbs and fine weak disappearing pulse.

The pathological factors are deficiency fire and stasis-turbidity. Its nature isprimary deficiency and secondary excess. Yin deficiency is the primary and dry-heat is the secondary. These two are interdetermined. The more deficient yin is, the more excessive dry-heat will be, and vice versa. The pathological positions are the lung, stomach and kidney, among which, the kidney is the major one.

1.5.6 厥脱

若阴津极度耗损，虚阳浮越，最终阴竭阳脱而见昏迷，四肢厥冷，脉微细欲绝等厥脱危相。

本病病理因素主要为虚火、瘀浊。病理性质为本虚标实，阴虚为本，燥热为标，两者互为因果，阴越虚，燥热越盛；反之亦然。病位为肺、胃、肾，以肾为主。

2 Syndrome Differentiation and Treatment

2.1 Key Points of Syndrome Differentiation

It is first to identify the position of consumptive thirst. Tough the three "more" usually coexist, in terms of their severity, consumptive thirst is grouped into upper, middle, lower consumptive thirst. Upper consumptive thirst is featured by lung dryness and more drink. Middle consumptive thirst is characterized by stomach-heat and more food. Lower consumptive thirst is featured by kidney deficiency and more urine. Then, distinguish deficiency from excess. Yin deficiency is the primary symptoms and dry-heat, the secondary symptoms. These two are interdetermined and predominate by duration and severity. The onset stage is mainly dry-heat and as the disease lasts, it turns into complication of deficiency and excess. When prolonged, yin deficiency predominates and injuries yin and yang, leading to yin and yang deficiency. Next, distinguish the consumptive thirst from complicating dis-

2 辨证论治

2.1 辨治要点

消渴首辨病位。因消渴的“三多”症，往往同时存在，但根据程度轻重不同，又有上中下消之分：上消以肺燥为主，多饮症状突出；中消以胃热为主，多食症状突出；下消以肾虚为主，多尿症状突出。其次辨标本。消渴以阴虚为本，燥热为标，两者互为因果，根据病程长短及病情轻重，各有侧重，初病燥热为主，病程较长两者互见，日久则阴虚为主，进而阴损及阳，导致阴阳两虚。再者需辨本症与并发症。本症为“三多一少”，而消渴又易现诸多并发症，一般以主症为主为先，并发症随病情进展而出现，

eases. Consumptive thirst is characterized by "three more and one less" and usually has many complicating diseases. Generally speaking, the major disease dominates and other complicating diseases follow as the disease develops. But a few patients and old patients do not have very remarkable manifestations of consumptive thirst. Instead, welling-and flat-abscesses, eye diseases, heart, head and kidney diseases are clues to diagnose consumptive thirst. Therefore, to treat consumptive thirst, it is wise to clear away heat, moist dryness, nourish yin and generate fluid. Doctors should pay attention to boost qi, nourish yin, strengthen the healthy qi and secure the basis. Take cautions to use attacking bitter and cold herbs which can easily resolve dryness and injury yin or injure the spleen and stomach. At the same time, distinguish the clear away from the turbid by starting from the spleen treatment. To treat the three kinds of consumptive thirst, never let go the kidney. Blood acitivation and stasis resolving should be applied all the way through. Do pay attention to treating the same complicating diseases.

其为次。但少数患者和老年患者,可有本症不显,而因痈疽、眼疾、心脑肾病证等为线索,最后确定而本病。故消渴以清热润燥、养阴生津为治疗大法,注重益气养阴,扶正固本,慎用易化燥伤阴或损伤脾胃的攻伐苦寒之品;同时当从脾论治而分清泌浊,治分三消而立足于肾,活血化瘀当贯穿始终。并注意针对并发症的治疗。

2.2 Therapeutic Methods for Different Patterns

2.2 分型论治

2.2.1 Dry-heat of the Lung and Stomach

2.2.1 肺胃燥热

Manifestations: Irritation, thirst for drink, quick digestion of grain and quick hunger, frequent urine in greater amount, yellow turbid urine, emaciation; red tongue with thin yellow tongue fur; rapid rolling pulse.

证候: 烦渴引饮,消谷善饥,小便频数量多,尿黄浊,形体消瘦。舌红苔薄黄,脉滑数。

Treatment: To clear away heat, generate fluid and stop thirst.

治法: 清热生津止渴。

Formulas and Herbs: *Consumptive thirst Formula* (Xiao Ke Fang), usually composed of *Trichosanthis Radix* (Tian Hua Fen) to clear away heat,

方药: 消渴方。常用:天花粉清热生津止渴;黄连清热降火;生地黄、藕汁、牛乳

generate fluid and stop thirst, *Coptidis Rhizoma* (Huang Lian) to clear away heat and subjugate fire; *Rehmannia Radix* (Sheng Di Huang), *Nelumbinis Rhizomatis Recentis Succus* (Ou Zhi) and milk to nourish yin, increase fluid and moisten dryness.

养阴增液润燥。

Modification: For irriation and thirst, dry throat and nose, or feverish sensations and night sweating, a little cough with little phlegm, red cheeks, short breath, obstructed breath, discomfort in the chest and sides, reddish tongue with little fluid and dry tongue fur, fine rapid girdling pulse, use *Asparagus and Ophiopogonis Radix Decoction* (Er Dong Tang) or *Fine Jade Paste* (Qiong Yu Gao) to clear away heat and nourish the lung; for yin injury affecting qi with symptoms such as short breath, lassitude and fatigue, spontaneous sweating and aversion to cold, tender pale tongue, vacuous pulse, use *Pulse-Engendering Powder* (Sheng Mai San) or *Fluid-Generating Sweat Beverage* (Sheng Jin Gan Lu Yin) to boost qi and nourish yin; for kidney-water consumption, along with soreness in the waist and knees, spermatarrhea, feverish sensations, night sweating, short breath when strained, dry throat at midnight, little tongue fur with dried fluid, fine rapid pulse, use *Modified Two Yin Meridians Decoction* (Jia Jian Er Yin Jian), *Astragal Decoction* (Huang Qi Tang) or *Lily Metal-Consolidating Decoction* (Bai He Gu Jin Tang) to supplement the lung and kidney as well as cleanse the stomach; for dry intestines and drained fluid, but more food and easy hunger, thirst for drink, dry stool, red tongue with little fluid, dry yellow tongue fur, excess powerful pulse, use *Humor-Increasing Purgative Decoction* (Zeng Ye Cheng Qi Tang) to nourish yin and

加减：若心烦口渴，咽燥鼻干，或潮热盗汗，微咳少痰，颧红，气短，呼吸不畅，胸胁不舒，舌质略红少津，苔燥，脉细带数，用二冬汤或琼玉膏清热养肺；若阴伤及气，兼见气短、神倦乏力、自汗畏寒、舌淡嫩、脉虚，用生脉散或生津甘露饮益气养阴；若耗及肾水，兼见腰膝酸软、梦遗滑精、潮热盗汗、劳则气短、夜半咽干、苔少津干、脉细数，用加减二阴煎、黄芪汤或百合固金汤双补肺肾，兼清其胃；若肠燥津枯，而见多食易饥、口渴引饮、大便燥结、舌红少津、苔黄燥、脉实有力，用增液承气汤滋阴养液、润肠通腑。

nourish fluid, moisten the intestines and dredge fu-organs.

2. 2. 2 Qi Deficiency of the Spleen and Stomach

Maninfestations: Thirst for drink, good appetite and loose stool, or less intake, lassitude, limb fatigue; pale tongue with white dry tongue fur; fine weak powerful pulse.

Treatment: To strengthen the spleen and boost qi, generate fluid and stop thirst.

Formulas and Herbs: *Seven Ingredients Plus Atractylodes Powder* (Qi Wei Bai Zhu San), usually composed of *Ginseng Radix et Rhizoma* (Ren Shen), *Poria* (Fu Ling), *Atractylodis Macrocephalae Rhizoma* (Bai Zhu) and *Glycyrrhizae Radix et Rhizoma* (Gan Cao) to strengthen the spleen and boost qi; *Puerariae Lobatae Radix* (Ge Gen) to increase fluid and stop thirst; *Aucklandiae Radix* (Mu Xiang) and *Pogostemonis Herba* (Huo Xiang) to promote qi flow to remove and resolve turbidity.

Modification: For qi deficiency of the spleen and stomach for long, which is very likely to generate dampness that encumbers the spleen, with symtoms like discomfort and oppression in the stomach and abdomen, poor appetite, loose stool, enlarged tongue with teeth marks, white greasy tongue fur, use *Aucklandia, Amomum and Six Nobles Decoction* (Xiang Sha Liu Jun Zi Tang).

2. 2. 3 Consumption and Deficiency of Kidney-yin

Manifestations: Frequent urine in greater amount as turbid as cream or sweat urine, soreness in the waist and knees, fatigue, dizziness, tinnitis, dreaminess, spermatarrhea, dry skin, itching all over; red tongue with little tongue fur; fine rapid pulse.

2. 2. 2 脾胃气虚

证候: 口渴引饮,能食与便溏并现,或饮食减少,精神不振,四肢乏力。舌淡,苔白而干,脉细弱无力。

治法: 健脾益气,生津止渴。

方药: 七味白术散。常用:人参、茯苓、白术、甘草补脾益气;葛根升津止渴;木香、藿香行气去陈化浊。

加减: 脾胃气虚日久,极易生湿困脾,而见脘腹痞闷、纳呆、便溏、苔白腻而胖且舌有齿印,用香砂六君子。

2. 2. 3 肾阴亏虚

证候: 尿频量多,混浊如膏脂,或尿甜,腰膝酸软,乏力,头晕耳鸣,多梦遗精,皮肤干燥,全身瘙痒。舌红少苔,脉细数。

Treatment: To nourish kidney-yin, invigorate essence and supplement blood, moisten dryness and stop thirst.

Formuals and Herbs: *Rehmannia Pills with Six Ingredients* (Liu Wei Di Huang Wan) or *Kidney Yin-Reinforcing Drink* (Zuo Gui Yin), usually composed of *Dioscoreae Rhizoma* (Shan Yao) in great amount to nourish spleen-yin and asctrict essence, *Corni Fructus* (Shan Zhu Yu) to supplement the kidney and consolidate essence; *Rehmanniae Radix Praeparata* (Shu Di Huang) and *Lycii Fructus* (Gou Qi Zi) to supplement the kidney and supplement fluid; *Poria* (Fu Ling) and *Glycyrrhizae Radix et Rhizoma* (Gan Cao) to nourish yin and purge heat with their sweat and bland nature; *Alismatis Rhizoma* (Ze Xie) and *Moutan Cortex* (Mu Dan Pi) to dredge, induce and purge heat.

Modification: For ministerial fire of xia jiao floating over the lung with short breath, feverish sensations, dry throat, dry cough, steamed bones and feverish sensations, red cheeks or coughing blood, add *Pulse-Engendering Powder* (Sheng Mai San) or *Wheat Flavor Rehamnnia Pills* (Mai Wei Di Huang Wan) and *Rehmannia Decoction* (Di Huang Yin Zi) to nourish water and clear metal; for kidney-yin deficiency, yangming meridians, exuberant heat, irritation, thirst, quick digestion of grain, easy hunger, headache, toothache, rolling rapid powerful pulse, use *Jade Lady Decoction* (Yu Nü Jian) to nourish the kidney and cleanse the stomach.

2.2.4 Deficiency of Both Yin and Yang

Mainfestations: Frequent urine as turbid as paste even one drink and one urine, feverish palms

治法: 滋养肾阴,益精补血,润燥止渴。

方药: 六味地黄丸或左归饮。常用药:重用山药养脾阴,摄精微;山茱萸补肾固精;熟地黄、枸杞子补肾滋液;茯苓、甘草甘淡育阴泄热;泽泻、牡丹皮通利泄热。

加减: 若下焦相火浮游于肺,兼见气短、潮热、咽燥、干咳、骨蒸潮热、颧红或咳嗽咯血,合用生脉散或用麦味地黄丸、地黄饮子滋水清金;若肾阴亏虚,阳明热炽,兼见烦渴干渴、消谷善饥、头痛牙疼、脉滑数有力,可选玉女煎滋肾清胃。

2.2.4 阴阳两亏

证候: 小便频数,混浊如膏,甚至饮一溲一,手足心

and soles, dry throat and mouth, sallow face, withered helix, dark complexion, soreness in the waist and knees, averion to cold, cold limbs, even impotence; pale white dry tongue fur; deep fine powerless pulse.

热，咽干口燥，面容憔悴，耳轮干枯，面色黧黑，腰膝酸软，四肢欠温，畏寒肢冷，甚至阳痿，舌苔淡白而干，脉沉细无力。

Treatment: To warm yang, nourish yin and supplement the kidney.

治法： 温阳滋阴补肾。

Formulas and Herbs: *Golden Chamber Kidney Qi Pills* (Jin Kui Shen Qi Wan) or *Vital Gate Pills* (You Gui Wan), usually composed of *Rehmannia Pills with Six Ingredients* (Liu Wei Di Huang Wan) to nourish yin and supplement the kidney, *Aconm Lateralis Radix Praeparata* (Fu Zi) and *Cinnamomi Ramulus* (Gui Zhi) to warm yang and kidney, or delete *Moutan Cortex* (Mu Dan Pi), *Poria* (Fu Ling) and *Alismatis Rhizoma* (Ze Xie), add *Lycii Fructus* (Gou Qi Zi), *Achyranthis Bidentatae Radix* (Niu Xi), *Cuscutae Semen* (Tu Si Zi), *Eucommiae Cortex* (Du Zhong), *Glycyrrhizae Radix et Rhizoma Praeparata* (Zhi Gan Cao), *Cervi Cornus Colla* (Lu Jiao Jiao) and *Angelicae Sinensis Radix* (Dang Gui) to warm the kidney and supplement deficiency.

方药： 金匮肾气丸或右归丸。常用：六味地黄丸滋阴补肾；附子、桂枝温阳暖肾；或去牡丹皮、茯苓、泽泻，加枸杞子、牛膝、菟丝子、杜仲、炙甘草、鹿角胶、当归温肾补虚。

Modification: For urine in great amount and turbid, add *Alpiniae Oxyphyllae Fructus* (Yi Zhi Ren), *Mantidis Ootheca* (Sang Piao Xiao), *Rubi Fructus* (Fu Pen Zi) and *Fructus Rosae Laevigatae* (Jin Yin Zi) to invigorate the kidney with their astringent nature; for general fatigue and tiredness, short breath, add *Codonopsis Radix* (Dang Shen), *Astragali Radix* (Huang Qi) and *Polygonati Rhizoma* (Huang Jing) to supplement and boost healthy qi; for impotence, add *Morindae Officinalis Radix* (Ba Ji Tian), *Epimedii Folium* (Yin Yang Huo) and *Cistanchis Herba* (Rou Cong Rong) to warm

加减： 若尿量多而混浊，加益智仁、桑螵蛸、覆盆子、金樱子益肾收摄；若身体困倦、气短乏力，加党参、黄芪、黄精补益正气；若阳痿，加巴戟天、淫羊藿、肉苁蓉温阳起痿；若兼有面色㿠白、头晕乏力，阴阳气血俱虚，用鹿茸丸温肾填精、益气养血；若见舌质紫暗或有瘀斑、瘀点、脉涩或结或代等瘀血证候，加丹参、川芎、郁金、红花、泽兰、

yang and improve erection; for waxy pale complexion, dizziness, fatigue, deficiency of yin, yang, qi and blood, use Velvet Deerhorn Pills to warm the kidney and fulfill essence, boost qi and nourish blood; for blood stasis patterns like purple dark tongue with spots and macules, uneven pulse or knot intermitten pulse, add *Salviae Miltiorrhizae Radix et Rhizoma Radix* (Dan Shen), *Chuanxiong Rhizoma* (Chuan Xiong), *Curcumae Radix* (Yu Jin), *Carthami Flos* (Hong Hua), *Lycopi Herba* (Ze Lan), *Euonymi Ramulus* (Gui Jian Yu) and *Crataegi Fructus* (Shan Zha) to activate blood and resolve stasis.

鬼箭羽、山楂活血化瘀。

2.2.5　Transmutated Patterns

For cateract, night blindness and deaf, use *Lycium, Chrysanthemun and Rehmannia Pills* (Qi Ju Di Huang Wan) to nourish and supplement the liver and kidney, invigorate essence and nourish blood; for usually complicating sores, welling and flat-abscess, use *Five-Ingredient Toxin-Dispersing Beverage* (Wu Wei Xiao Du Yin) to clear away heat and detoxify, dissolve welling and abscess; for pulmonary consumption, edema and stroke, refer to respective chapters; for shock, adopt first-aid measure of both western medicine and Tranditional Chinese Medicines by establish vein passage and give transfusion, nosal feeding and oral intake of herbal medicine, use *Pulse-Engendering Powder* (Sheng Mai San) plus *Os Draconis* (Long Gu) and *Ostreae Concha* (Mu Li), or *Triple-Armored Pulse-Restorative Decoction* (San Jia Fu Mai Tang) to boost qi, nourish yin and stem desertion.

2.2.5　变证

若见白内障、雀目、耳聋，用杞菊地黄丸滋补肝肾，益精养血；若并发疮毒痈疽，用五味消毒饮清热解毒，消散痈肿；并发肺痨、水肿、中风，则参考本书相应章节辨证论治；如发生厥脱重症，宜采取中西综合抢救措施，建立静脉通路及时充分补液，中药可鼻饲灌服，选方生脉散加龙骨、牡蛎，或三甲复脉汤等益气养阴固脱。

Abnormal Perspiration (Sweating)

Abnormal perspiration refer to irregular loss of sweat and fluid. Regardless of environmental factors, day or night, patients sweat, which will easily turns into spontaneous sweating in movement. Sweating over night which stops after patienets wake up is known as night sweating, also called bed sweating.

Normal sweating is a physiology sign but spontaneous sweating and night sweating are pathological.

1 Etiology and Pathogenesis

The cause of abnormal perspiration is impairment of controlance of the exterior and Wei (Defense) due to lung-qi deficiency and disharmony between the exterior and Wei (Defense). Or due to deficiency of heart blood, or deficient yin and fire excess, pathogenic heat forces fluid to leak outside. These three all can lead to irregular loss of sweat.

1.1 Deficiency of Ying (Nutrient) and Wei (Defense) Due to Weak Constitution and Prolonged Illness

Innately weak constitution, or overstrain or prlonged illness will consume and injure qi, blood, yin and yang, leading to deficiency of Ying (Nutrient) qi and Wei (Defensive) qi. The weakness and strength of yin and yang, or a little invasion of pathogenic wind in a body of exterior deficiency, will cause disharmony between Ying (Nutrient) qi and Wei (Defense) qi. Wei (Defensive) fails to

汗　证

汗证是指汗液外泄失常的病证。不因外界环境因素的影响，白昼时时汗出，动辄益甚者，成为自汗；寐中汗出，醒来自止者，称为盗汗，亦称为寝汗。

正常的出汗，是人体的生理现象。这里的自汗、盗汗均为病理现象。

1 病因病机

汗证的病因为肺气不足、营卫失和导致表卫失司；或心血不足导致心液不藏；或阴虚火旺、邪热郁蒸从而逼津外泄，三者均可导致汗液外泄失常。

1.1 体虚久病，营卫不足

素体不强，或劳欲太过或久病耗伤气血阴阳，均可使营卫不足。由于体内阴阳的偏盛、偏衰，或表虚之人微受风邪，以致营卫不和，卫外失司，而致汗出。

control outside, leading to loss of sweat.

1.2 Injury of the Spleen and Stomach Due to Improper Diet

1.2 饮食不节,损伤脾胃

Spicy sweet savoury food will hurt the spleen and stomach and generate dampness which turns into heat. When damp-heat is accumulated inside, it will force fluid to leak outside.

嗜食辛辣厚味,损伤脾胃,酿湿成热,湿热内蕴,迫津外泄。

1.3 Injury of the Heart and Spleen Due to Emotional and Spirtual Disharmony

1.3 情志失调,心脾受损

Emotional and spiritual dissatisfaction and too much worry injure the heart and spleen. Or blood deficiency andpoorly nourishd blood due to blood patterns will lead to defiency of heart blood. As sweat is the fluid of the heart, when blood doesn't nourish the heart and heart fluid is not held and leaks out, spontaneous sweating and night sweating are caused.

由于情致不舒,思虑太过,损伤心脾,或血证之后,血虚失养,均可导致心血不足。汗为心之液,血不养心,心液不藏而外泄,引起自汗或盗汗。

Overall, the general pathogenesis is irregular loss of sweat and fluid due to disharmony between yin and yang, and unsecured barrier of the skin. It is related to the liver, spleen, stomach, lung and kidney. Sweat is the fluid of the heart that cannot be over consumed, otherwise will exhaust qi and injure fluid and such symptoms like spiritual lassitude, palpitation and short breath will turn up.

总之,本病总的病机是由于阴阳失调,腠理不固,而致汗液外泄失常,与肝、脾、胃、肺、肾有关。而汗为心之液,不可过泄,久之耗气伤津,则出现神情倦怠、心慌气短等心气耗伤之证。

2 Syndrome Differentiation and Treatment

2 辨证论治

2.1 Key Points of Syndrome Differentiation

2.1 辨治要点

For abnormal perspiration, first yin and yin, deficiency and excess. In most case, it is deficiency type. Spontaneous sweating is likely to be unconsolidation due to qi deficiency while night sweating is more likely to be inner heat due to yin deficiency. However, sweating due to retention and fumigation

汗证首辨阴阳虚实,以属虚者为多。自汗多属气虚不固,盗汗多属阴虚内热。但因肝火、湿热等邪热郁蒸所致者,则属实证。病程久者,或病变重者,则会出现阴

of pathogenic heat such as liver-fire and damp-heat belongs to excess type. Long duration or aggravation of the disease will become complication of deficiency and excess. Prolonged spontaneous sweating injuries yin while prolonged night sweating injuries yang. Deficiency of qi and yin or deficiency of yin and yang, retention and fumigation of pathogenic heat, prolonged illness consuming yin and consuming qi are patterns of complication of deficiency and excess. In term of treatment, for deficiency type, boost qi, supplement blood, nourish yin and harmonize yin and Wei (Defensive) qi. For excess type, cleanse the liver and purge heat, dry dampness and harmoninze Ying (Nutrient) Phase. For complication, treat both aspects according to the conflicting relationship.

阳虚实错杂的情况。自汗久则伤阴,盗汗久则伤阳,出现气阴两虚,或阴阳两虚之证,邪热郁蒸,久病伤阴耗气,则见虚实兼夹之证。治当分虚实;虚证以益气、补血、养阴,调和营卫;实证当清肝泄热、化湿和营;虚实夹杂者,则根据虚实的主次而适当兼顾。

2.2 Therapeutic Methods for Different Patterns

2.2 分型论治

2.2.1 Unconsolidation of Lung and Wei (Defense) Phase

2.2.1 肺卫不固

Manifestations: Sweating, aversion to wind, easily catching cold, more sweating after strain, lusterless complexion; fine weak pulse.

证候: 汗出恶风,易于感冒,稍劳汗出尤甚,面色少华,脉细弱。

Treatment: To boost qi and consolidate the exterior.

治法: 益气固表。

Formulas and Herbs: Modified *Jade screen Powder* (Yu Ping Feng San), usually composed of *Astragali Radix* (Huang Qi) to boost qi and consolicate the exterior, *Atractylodis Macrocephalae Rhizoma* (Bai Zhu) to strengthen the spleen; *Saposhnikoviae Radix*(Fang Feng) to expel wind.

方药: 玉屏风散加味。常用黄芪益气固表,白术健脾,防风祛风。

Modification: For heavy sweating, add *Fructus Tritici Levis* (Fu Xiao Mai), *Radix Oryzae Glutinosae* (Nuo Dao Gen) and *Ostreae Concha* (Duan Mu Li) to consolidate the exterior and arrest sweating;

加减: 汗出多者,加浮小麦、糯稻根、煅牡蛎固表敛汗;气虚甚者,加党参、黄精益气固摄;兼见阴虚,舌红、

for serious qi deficiency, add *Codonopsis Radix* (Dang Shen) and *Polygonati Rhizoma* (Huang Jing) to boost and arrest qi; for accompanying yin deficiency, red tongue and fine rapid pulse, add *Ophiopogonis Radix* (Mai Men Dong) and *Schisandrae Chinensis Fructus* (Wu Wei Zi) to nourish yin and arrest sweat.

脉细数者,加麦门冬、五味子养阴敛汗。

2. 2. 2 Disharmony between Ying (Nutrient) Qi and Wei (Defensive) Qi

2. 2. 2 营卫不和

Manifestations: Aversion to wind, ache all over, heat and cold from time to time, sweating in half a body or some parts; white thin tongue fur; slow pulse.

证候: 汗出恶风,周身酸楚,时寒时热,半身或某些局部出汗。舌苔薄白,脉缓。

Treatment: To harmonize ying and wei.

治法: 调和营卫。

Formulas and Herbs: Modified *Cinnamon-Twig Decoction* (Gui Zhi Tang), usually composed of *Cinnamomi Ramulus* (Gui Zhi) and *Paeoniae Radix Alba* (Bai Shao Yao) to harmonize Ying (Nutrient) Qi and Wei (Defensive) Qi; *Glycyrrhizae Radix et Rhizoma Praeparata* (Zhi Gan Cao) and *Jujubae Fructus* (Da Zao) to harmonize zhong jiao and boost qi.

方药: 桂枝汤加减。常用:桂枝、白芍药调和营卫;炙甘草、大枣和中益气。

Modification: For heavy sweating, add *Os Draconis Calcinata* (Duan Long Gu) and *Ostreae Concha* (Duan Mu Li) to arrest sweat; for no desire to talk due to asthenia of qi and fatigue, add *Astragali Radix* (Huang Qi), *Ginseng Radix et Rhizoma* (Ren Shen), *Pseudostellariae Radix* (Tai Zi Shen) and *Atractylodis Macrocephalae Rhizoma* (Bai Zhu) to strengthen the spleen, boost qi and consolidate the exterior; for accompanying yang deficiency, add *Aconm Lateralis Radix Praeparata* (Fu Zi) to warm yang and arrest sweat.

加减: 汗出多者,可加煅龙骨、煅牡蛎固涩敛汗;少气懒言、乏力等气虚者,加黄芪、人参、太子参、白术健脾益气固表;兼阳虚者,加附子温阳敛汗。

2.2.3 Deficiency of Heart-blood

Manifestations: For spontaneous sweating or night sweating, palpitation, insomnia, lassitude, short breath, lusterless face; pale tongue; fine pulse.

Treatment: To supplement blood and nourish the heart.

Formulas and Herbs: Modified *Angelica Splenic Decoction* (Gui Pi Tang), usually composed of *Ginseng Radix et Rhizoma* (Ren Shen), *Scutellariae Radix* (Huang Qin) and *Angelicae Sinensis Radix* (Dang Gui) to boost qi and nourish blood; *Atractylodis Macrocephalae Rhizoma* (Bai Zhu), *Poria* (Fu Ling) to strengthen the spleen; *Polygalae Radix* (Yuan Zhi) and *Longan Arillus* (Long Yan Rou) to nourish the heart, calm the spirits and stop palpitation.

Modification: For heavy sweating, add *Schisandrae Chinensis Fructus* (Wu Wei Zi) and *Fructus Tritici Levis* (Fu Xiao Mai) to arrest sweating; for blood deficiency, add *Polygoni Multiflori Radix Praeparata* (Zhi Shou Wu), *Lycii Fructus* (Gou Qi Zi) and *Rehmanniae Radix Praeparata* (Shu Di Huang) to supplement and invigorate essence and blood.

2.2.4 Exuberant Fire Due to Yin Deficiency

Manifestations: Night sweating or spontaneous sweating, feverish sensation in five centers, red cheeks, thirst; red tongue with little tongue fur; fine rapid pulse.

Treatment: To nourish yin and subjugate fire.

Formulas and Herbs: Modified *Yellow Sextet plus Angelica Decoction* (Dang Gui Liu Huang Tang), usually composed of fresh *Rehmannia Radix*

2.2.3 心血不足

证候: 自汗或盗汗,心悸少寐,神疲气短,面色不华,舌质淡,脉细。

治法: 补血养心。

方药: 归脾汤加减。常用:人参、黄芪、当归益气养血;白术、茯苓健脾;远志、龙眼肉养心安神定悸。

加减: 汗多者,加五味子、浮小麦收涩敛汗;血虚者,加制何首乌、枸杞子、熟地黄补益精血。

2.2.4 阴虚火旺

证候: 夜寐盗汗,或有自汗,五心烦热,潮热颧红,口渴。舌红少苔,脉细数。

治法: 滋阴降火。

方药: 当归六黄汤加减。以生地黄、熟地黄、当归滋阴养血;黄连、黄柏、黄芩清热

(Di Huang), *Rehmanniae Radix Praeparata* (Shu Di Huang) and *Angelicae Sinensis Radix* (Dang Gui) and to nourish yin and blood; *Coptidis Rhizoma* (Huang Lian), *Phellodendri Chinensis Cortex* (Huang Bo), *Scutellariae Radix* (Huang Qin) to clear away heat; *Astragali Radix*(Huang Qi) to tonify qi and streng then exterior.

泻火。

Modification: For heavy sweating, add *Ostreae Concha* (Duan Mu Li), *Fructus Tritici Levis* (Fu Xiao Mai) and *Radix Oryzae Glutinosae* (Nuo Dao Gen) to astrict and astringe sweating; for feverish sensation, add *Gentianae Macrophyllae Radix* (Qin Jiao), *Stellariae Radix* (Yin Chai Hu) and *Cynanchi Atrati Radix et Rhizoma* (Bai Wei) to clear away and retreat deficiency heat.

加减: 汗出多者,加煅牡蛎、浮小麦、糯稻根固涩敛汗;潮热甚者,加秦艽、银柴胡、白薇清退虚热。

2. 2. 5 Retention and Fumigation of Pathogenic Heat

2. 2. 5 邪热郁蒸

Manifestations: Steaming sweating, hot face, irritation, bitter mouth; thin yellow tongue fur; rapid stringy pulse.

证候: 蒸蒸汗出,面赤烘热,烦躁,口苦。苔薄黄,脉弦数。

Treatment: To cleanse the liver and purge heat; resolve dampness and harmonize Ying (Nutrient) Phase.

治法: 清肝泄热,化湿和营。

Formulas and Herbs: Modified *Gentian Liver-Draining Decoction* (Long Dan Xie Gan Tang), usually composed of *Gentianae Radix et Rhizom* (Long Dan Cao), *Gardeniae Fructus* (Zhi Zi) and *Scutellariae Radix* (Huang Qin) to clear away liver-heat; *Alismatis Rhizoma* (Ze Xie), *Plantaginis Semen* (Che Qian Zi) and *Clematidis Armandii Caulis* (Chuan Mu Tong) to dredge and eliminate damp-heat; *Bupleuri Radix* (Chai Hu) to disperse the liver; *Rehmannia Radix* (Sheng Di Huang) and *Angelicae Sinensis Radix* (Dang Gui) to nourish yin-blood.

方药: 龙胆泻肝汤加减。常用:龙胆草、山栀子、黄芩清肝热;泽泻、车前子、川木通利湿热;柴胡疏肝;生地黄、当归养阴血。

Modification: For short dark urine (serious interior heat), add *Lophatheri Herba* (Zhu Ye) and *Phellodendri Chinensis Cortex* (Huang Bo).

加减：小便短赤，加竹叶、黄柏加强清心泄热。

Fever Due to Internal Injury

内伤发热

Interal-injury fever refers to heat due to internal injuries which usually takes on gradually and lasts long, characterized by low or high fever. Some patients feel feverish or feverish sensations in five centers without increase of body temperatute, which also belongs to this category.

内伤发热指以内伤为病因，所导致的发热。一般起病较缓，病程较长，临床上表现为低热及高热。某些患者仅自觉发热或五心烦热，而体温并无升高，亦属于内伤发热的范畴。

1 Etiology and Pathogenesis

1 病因病机

Internal-injury fever can be caused by emotional and spiritual discomfort, improper diet, overstrain, prolonged illness hurting heatlthy qi. Its pathogenesis is deficiency of qi, blood, yin and yang, and disharmony bwetween zang-fu organs. The affected organs vary with different patterns.

内伤发热的病因，主要有情志不舒、饮食失调、劳倦过度、久病伤正等方面，基本病机为气血阴阳亏虚、脏腑功能失调，病及的脏腑则随各种证型而有所不同。

1.1 Heat of Liver Meridians Due to Emotional and Spiritual Injury

1.1 情志所伤，肝经郁热

Depressed emotions and spiritscauses the liver-qi to fail to be dispersed. When qi depression turns into fire and lead to fever, or extreme anger causes excessive liver-fire, leading to fever.

情志抑郁，肝气不能条达，气郁化火而发热，或恼怒过度，肝火内盛以致发热。

1.2 External Injury, Bleeding and Stagnation of Blood Stasis

1.2 外伤、出血，瘀血阻滞

External injuries, bleeding or emotional and spiritual problems ans strain will cause blood deviated from channels which remains in the body, leading to blood stasis stagnating and obstructing the collaterals and meridians, resulting in fever.

由于外伤、出血或情志、劳倦等原因而产生离经之血，停滞体内或血行不畅，瘀血阻滞经络，壅阻不通，因而引起发热。

1.3 Decline of the Spleen and Stomach Due to Improper Diet

Improper diet or lack in regulation due to prolonged illness will causedecline of the spleen and stomach, middle-qi deficiency, primordial qi descendance, which leads to yin-fire and then fever.

1.4 Deficiency of Both Yin and Yang Due to Strain and Weak Constitution

Innate yin deficiency or consumed yin due to strain or prolonged heat diseases, or over bleeding, or over use and wrong use of warming and drying herbs will all lead to consumption and exhaustion of yin essence. When yin goes weak, yang will exuberates as water cannot control fire any longer, fever is caused.

Overall, the most important pathogenesis of interal-injury fever is emotional and spiritual injuries, improper diet, strain and weak constitution. Thse factors can lead to deficiency of qi, blood, yin and yang or qi depression, blood stasis and stagnation of dampnes. Among them, fever due to deficiency of qi, blood, yin and yang belongs to deficiency type while fever due to qi depression, blood stasis and stagnation of dampness belongs to excess type.

2 Syndrome Differentiation and Treatment

2.1 Key Points of Syndrome Differentiation

For interal-injury fever, it is first to identify excess from deficiency. After the disease is diagnosed, identify exess from deficiency in terms of clinical history, manifestations and pulse. Interal-injury fever due to qi depression, blood stasis and dampness retention is of excess type while that due to qi deficiency, blood deficiency, yin deficiency

1.3 饮食失调，脾胃虚弱

饮食失调，或久病失于调理，以致脾胃虚弱，中气不足，元气下陷以致阴火内生而引起发热。

1.4 劳倦体弱，阴阳亏虚

若素体阴虚，或劳倦伤阴，或热病日久伤阴，或失血过多，或过度、误用温燥药物等，导致阴精亏耗，阴衰则阳盛，水不制火而引起发热。

总之，内伤发热最重要的病因病机为情志所伤、饮食失调、劳倦体弱等因素，导致气血阴阳亏虚，或气郁、血瘀、湿郁。其中气血阴阳亏虚所致者属虚，气郁、血瘀、湿郁者都属实。

2 辨证论治

2.1 辨治要点

内伤发热首先辨虚实，在确诊为内伤发热的前提下，应先依据病史、症状、脉象等辨明其属虚属实：由气郁、血瘀、湿停所致者属实；由气虚、血虚、阴虚、阳虚所致者属虚。但也有虚实夹杂

and yang deficiency is of deficiency type. Of course, there is cases of complication. Next, identify the intensity. Long duration, frequent relapses, deficiency of stomach-qi and healthy qi or complication are manifestation of severity. In terms of treatment, for excess fire, purge it. For deficiency fire, supplement it. Adopt proper therapeutic methods for different manifestations and pathogenesis. Do mind not to use exterior relieving herbs with bitter cold nature to purge fire in case of every fever, because for interal-injury fever, dispersing herbs will be very likely to exhaust qi and hurt body fluid while bitter cold herbs will easily injure the spleen and stomach, or hurt yin while resolving dryness. These herbs will prolonger or aggravate the disease.

者。其次辨轻重，病程长久，反复发作，经治不愈，胃气衰败，正气虚甚，以及兼夹其他病证者，为病情较重的表现，否则反之。治当以实火宜泻，虚火宜补，并根据证候病机的不同而分别采用针对性的治法，切不可一见发热便用发散解表及苦寒泻火之剂。对内伤发热来说，发散易于耗气伤津，苦寒则易伤败脾胃以及化燥伤阴，使病情缠绵或加重。

2.2 Therapeutic Methods for Different Types

2.2 分型论治

2.2.1 Interal-injury fever due to Liver Depression

2.2.1 肝郁发热

Manifestations: For low fever or feverish sensation in the afternoon, fever changing with emotions, spiritual depression, fullness and distention in the chest and hypochondria or with irregular menstruation, breast distention, restlessness, irritation, bitter and dry mouth; yellow tongue fur; stringy rapid pulse.

证候：低热或午后潮热，热势常随情绪波动而起伏，精神抑郁，胸胁胀满，或兼月经不调，乳房发胀，烦躁易怒，口苦而干。苔黄，脉弦数。

Treatment: To disperse the liver to relieve depression; cleanse the liver to purge heat.

治法：疏肝解郁，清肝泻热。

Formulas and Herbs: Modified *Moutan Cortex and Gardeniae- Free Wanderer Powder* (Dan Zhi Xiao Yao San), usually composed of *Moutan Cortex* (Mu Dan Pi) and *Gardeniae Fructus* (Zhi Zi) to cleanse the liver; *Bupleuri Radix* (Chai Hu) to disperse the liver, *Angelicae Sinensis Radix* (Dang Gui) and *Paeoniae Radix Alba* (Bai Shao Yao) to nourish blood and soften the liver; *Poria* (Fu Ling)

方药：丹栀逍遥散加减。常用：牡丹皮、栀子清肝；柴胡疏肝；当归、白芍药养血柔肝；茯苓、白术健脾。

and *Atractylodis Macrocephalae Rhizoma* (Bai Zhu) to strengthen the spleen.

Modification: For severe fever, red tongue, dry mouth and constipation, subtract *Atractylodis Macrocephalae Rhizoma* (Bai Zhu) and add *Scutellariae Radix* (Huang Qin) and *Gentianae Radix et Rhizom* (Long Dan) to cleanse the liver and purge fire; for qi stagnation of the liver meridians with serious pain in the chest and hypochondria, add *Toosendan Fructus* (Chuan Lian Zi) and *Curcumae Radix* (Yu Jin) to regulate qi and stop pain.

加减： 热象较甚，舌红口干便秘者，可去白术，加黄芩、龙胆草清肝泻火；肝经气滞而见胸胁疼痛重着者，加川楝子、郁金理气止痛。

2. 2. 2　Internal-injury Fever Due to Blood Stasis

2. 2. 2　瘀血发热

Manifestations: Fever in the afternoon or at night, or feeling feverish in some body parts, dry throat but no great desire for drink, pain in fixed spots or lumps in the torso or limbs, coarse skin, yellowish or dark complexion; purple dark tongue with spots and macules; uneven pulse.

证候： 午后或夜晚发热，或自觉身体某些局部发热，口干咽燥但不多饮，躯干或四肢有固定痛处或肿块，肌肤甲错，面色微黄或黯黑。舌质紫黯或有瘀点、瘀斑，脉涩。

Treatment: To activate blood and resolve blood stasis.

治法： 活血化瘀。

Formulas and Herbs: Modified *Sanguine Mansion Stasis-Expelling Decoction* (Xue Fu Zhu Yu Tang), usually composed of *Persicae Semen* (Tao Ren), *Carthami Flos* (Hong Hua), *Paeoniae Radix Rubra* (Chi Shao) and *Chuanxiong Rhizoma* (Chuan Xiong) to activate blood; *Rehmannia Radix* (Sheng Di Huang) and *Moutan Cortex* (Mu Dan Pi) to cool blood; *Aurantii Fructus* (Zhi Qiao) regulate qi and *Achyranthis Bidentatae Radix* (Niu Xi) to induce blood downward.

方药： 血府逐瘀汤加减。常用：桃仁、红花、赤芍药、川芎活血；生地黄、牡丹皮凉血；枳壳理气；牛膝引血下行。

Modification: For high fever, add *Cynanchi Atrati Radix et Rhizoma* (Bai Wei) and *Moutan Cortex* (Mu Dan Pi) to cool blood and clear away heat, for

加减： 发热较甚者，可加白薇、牡丹皮清热凉血；肢体肿痛者，可加丹参、郁金、延

swelling pain in the torso and limbs, add *Salviae Miltiorrhizae Radix et Rhizoma Radix* (Dan Shen), *Curcumae Radix* (Yu Jin) and *Corydalis Rhizoma* (Yan Hu Suo) to cool blood, activate blood, relieve swelling and stop pain.

胡索凉血活血、散肿定痛。

2.2.3 Internal-injury Fever Due to Stagnation of Dampness

2.2.3 湿郁发热

Manifestations: Low fever which goes high in the afternoon, oppression in the chest, general heaviness, but desire for food, thirst but no desire for drink, even nausea; white or yellow greasy tongue fur; soft rapid pulse.

证候: 低热或午后热甚，胸闷身重，不思饮食，渴不欲饮，甚或呕恶。舌苔白腻或黄腻，脉濡数。

Treatment: To clear away heat and eliminate dampness.

治法: 清热利湿。

Formulas and Herbs: Modified *Three Kernels Decoction* (San Ren Tang), usually composed of *Armeniacae Semen Amaru* (Ku Xing Ren), *Amomi Fructus Rotundus* (Dou Kou) and *Coicis Semen* (Yi Yi Ren) to eliminate damp-heat and disperse qi activity of the three jiaos; *Pinelliae Rhizoma* (Ban Xia) and *Magnoliae Officinalis Cortex* (Hou Pu) to promote qi flow and eliminate dampness with acrid and bitter nature; *Talcum* (Hua Shi), *Lophatheri Herba* (Zhu Ye) and *Tetrapanacis Medulla* (Tong Cao) to eliminate dampness and clear away heat with their sweet, cold and bland nature.

方药: 三仁汤加减。常用:杏仁、白蔻仁、薏苡仁宣上、畅中、渗下而清利湿热，宣畅三焦气机;半夏、厚朴辛开苦降而行气化湿;滑石、竹叶、通草甘寒淡渗而利湿清热。

Modification: For nausea, add *Bambusae Caulis in Taenias* (Zhu Ru), *Pogostemonis Herba* (Huo Xiang) and *Citri Reticulatae Pericarpium* (Chen Pi) to harmonize the stomach and lower reversal flow; for chest oppression, tongue fur depression, add *Curcumae Radix* (Yu Jin) and *Eupatorii Herba* (Pei Lan) to resolve pathogenic dampness with aromatization; for severe heat, red tongue, rapid pulse and

加减: 呕恶者加竹茹、藿香、陈皮和胃降逆;胸闷、苔腻者加郁金、佩兰芳香化湿邪;热势较甚、舌红、脉数、口渴者，加茵陈、黄芩清利湿热。

thirst, add *Artemisiae Scopariae Herba* (Yin Chen) and *Scutellariae Radix* (Huang Qin) to clear away heat and eliminate dampness.

2. 2. 4 Internal-injury Fever Due to Qi Deficiency

Mainfestations: Fever going low and high which often attacks or worsens after overstrain, dizziness, fatigue, no desire to talk due to asthenia of qi, spontaneous sweating, prone to cold, little intake, loose stool; pale tongue with thin white tongue fur; weak pulse.

Treatment: To boost qi and strengthen the spleen, eliminate heat by sweet and warm herbs.

Formulas and Herbs: Modified *Center-Supplementing qi-Boosting Decoction* (Bu Zhong Yi Qi Tang), usually composed of *Astragali Radix* (Huang Qi) and *Codonopsis Radix* (Dang Shen) to boost qi; *Atractylodis Macrocephalae Rhizoma* (Bai Zhu) and *Citri Reticulatae Pericarpium* (Chen Pi) to strengthen the spleen; *Angelicae Sinensis Radix* (Dang Gui) to nourish blood, *Bupleuri Radix* (Chai Hu) and *Cimicifugae Rhizoma* (Sheng Ma) to raise yang; *Glycyrrhizae Radix et Rhizoma* Praeparâta (Zhi Gan Cao), *Zingiberis Rhizoma Recens* (Sheng Jiang) and *Jujubae Fructus* (Da Zao) to boost qi and harmonize zhong jiao.

Modification: For serious spontaneous sweating, add *Ostreae Concha* (Duan Mu Li), *Fructus Tritici Levis* (Fu Xiao Mai) and *Radix Oryzae Glutinosae* (Nuo Dao Gen) to arrest sweating; for intermitten cold and fever, sweating and aversion to wind, add *Cinnamomi Ramulus* (Gui Zhi) and *Paeoniae Radix Alba* (Bai Shao Yao) to regulate and harmonize Ying (Nutrient) qi and Wei (Defensive) qi; for chest oppression, stomach discomfort and

2. 2. 4　气虚发热

证候: 热势或低或高,发热常在劳累后发生或加剧,头晕乏力,短气懒言,自汗,易于感冒,食少便溏。舌质淡,苔薄白,脉弱。

治法: 益气健脾,甘温除热。

方药: 补中益气汤加减。常用:黄芪、党参益气;白术、陈皮健脾;当归养血;柴胡、升麻升阳;炙甘草、生姜、大枣益气和中。

加减: 自汗多者,加煅牡蛎、浮小麦、糯稻根固表敛汗;时冷时热、汗出恶风者,加桂枝、白芍药调和营卫;胸闷、脘痞、苔腻者,加苍术、厚朴、藿香健脾燥湿。

greasy tongue fur, add *Atractylodis Rhizoma* (Cang Zhu), *Magnoliae Officinalis Cortex* (Hou Pu) and *Pogostemonis Herba* (Huo Xiang) to strengthen the spleen and dry dampness.

2.2.5 Interal-injury Fever Due to Blood Deficiency

Manifestations: Fever, often low fever, dizziness and dazzling eyes, fatigue, palpitation, pale lips; pale tongue; fine pulse.

Treatment: To boost qi and nourish blood.

Formulas and Herbs: Modified *Angelica Splenic Decoction* (Gui Pi Tang), usually composed of *Ginseng Radix et Rhizoma* (Ren Shen), *Scutellariae Radix* (Huang Qin) and *Angelicae Sinensis Radix* (Dang Gui) to boost qi and nourish blood; *Atractylodis Macrocephalae Rhizoma* (Bai Zhu), *Poria* (Fu Ling) to strengthen the spleen; *Polygalae Radix* (Yuan Zhi) and *Longan Arillus* (Long Yan Rou) to nourish the heart, calm the spirits and stop palpitation.

Modification: For serious blood deficiency, add moderately *Rehmanniae Radix Praeparata* (Shu Di Huang), *Lycii Fructus* (Gou Qi Zi), *Polygoni Multiflori Radix Praeparata* (Zhi Shou Wu) and *Spatholobi Caulis* (Ji Xue Teng) to help nourish and engender blood; for blood deficiency due to chonic bleeding with a little bleeding at the moment, add moderately *Notoginseng Radix et Rhizoma* (San Qi) powder, *Agrimoniae Herba* (Xian He Cao), *Rubiae Radix et Rhizoma* (Qian Cao) and *Trachycarpi Petiolus* (Zong Lü Pi) to stop bleeding.

2.2.6 Interal-injury Fever due to Yin Deficiency

Manifestations: Fever in the afternoon or at night, hot palms and soles, osteopyrexia and fever,

2.2.5 血虚发热

证候: 发热,多表现为低热,头晕眼花,体倦乏力,心悸不宁,口唇色淡。舌质淡,脉弱。

治法: 益气养血。

方药: 归脾汤加减。常用:人参、黄芪、当归益气养血,白术、茯苓健脾;远志、龙眼肉养心定悸。

加减: 血虚甚者,酌加熟地黄、枸杞子、制首乌、鸡血藤以增强滋养生血的作用;由慢性失血所导致的血虚,若仍有少出血者,可酌加三七粉、仙鹤草、茜草、棕榈皮等止血。

2.2.6 阴虚发热

证候: 午后或夜间发热,手足心热,骨蒸潮热,心烦失

irritation, insomnia, dreaminess, night sweating, dry mouth and throat, dry stool and little urine; red dry tongue with little or no tongue fur; fine rapid pulse.

眠，多梦盗汗，口干咽燥，便干尿少。舌红而干，少苔甚至无苔，脉细数。

Treatment: To nourish yin and clear away heat.

治法：滋阴清热。

Formulas and Herbs: Modified *Bone Heat-Clarifying Powder* (Qing Gu San), usually composed of *Stellariae Radix* (Yin Chai Hu), *Picrorhizae Rhizoma* (Hu Huang Lian), *Anemarrhenae Rhizoma* (Zhi Mu) and *Lycii Cortex* (Di Gu Pi) to clear osteopyrexia fever; *Artemisiae Annuae Herba* (Qing Hao) and *Gentianae Macrophyllae Radix* (Qin Jiao) to clear away hidden heat; *Trionycis Carapax* (Bie Jia) to nourish yin and subdue yang.

方药：清骨散加减。常用：银柴胡、胡黄连、知母、地骨皮清虚劳骨蒸；青蒿、秦艽清伏热；鳖甲滋阴潜阳。

Modification: For heavy night sweating, delete *Artemisiae Annuae Herba* (Qing Hao), add *Ostreae Concha* (Mu Li), *Fructus Tritici Levis* (Fu Xiao Mai) and *Radix Oryzae Glutinosae* (Nuo Dao Gen) to consolidate the exterior and arrest sweat; for insomnia, add *Ziziphi Spinosae Semen* (Suan Zao Ren), *Platycladi Semen* (Bai Zi Ren) and *Polygoni Multiflori Caulis* (Ye Jiao Teng) to nourish the heart and calm the spirits; for severe yin deficiency, add *Scrophulariae Radix* (Xuan Shen), *Rehmannia Radix* (Sheng Di Huang) and *Polygoni Multiflori Radix* Praeparata (Zhi Shou Wu) to nourish yin essence.

加减：盗汗较甚者，可去青蒿，加牡蛎、浮小麦、糯稻根固表敛汗；失眠者，加酸枣仁、柏子仁、夜交藤养心安神；阴虚较甚者，加玄参、生地黄、制首乌滋养阴精。

2.2.7 Interal-injury fever due to Yang Deficiency

2.2.7 阳虚发热

Manifestations: Fever, physical cold, aversion to cold, unwarm limbs, no desire to talk due to asthenia of qi, dizziness, favor for lying down, little intake, loose stool, waxy pale complexion; pale enlarged tongue fur or with teeth marks; moist white tongue fur; fine deep powerless pulse.

证候：发热，形寒怯冷，四肢不温，少气懒言，头晕嗜卧，纳少便溏，面色皖白，舌质淡胖或有齿痕，苔白润，脉沉细无力。

Treatment: To warm and supplement yang-qi, induce fire back to the origin.

治法:温补阳气,引火归原。

Formulas and Herbs: Modified *Golden Chamber Kidney Qi Pills* (Jin Kui Shen Qi Wan), usually composed of *Aconm Lateralis Radix Praeparata* (Fu Zi) and *Cinnamomi Cortex* (Rou Gui) to warm kidney-yang, *Corni Fructus* (Shan Zhu Yu) and *Rehmanniae Radix Praeparata* (Shu Di Huang) to nourish kidney-yin, *Dioscoreae Rhizoma* (Shan Yao), *Poria* (Fu Ling) and *Alismatis Rhizoma* (Ze Xie) to strengthen the spleen and promote diuresis.

方药:金匮肾气丸加减。常用:附子、肉桂温肾阳;山茱萸、熟地黄滋肾阴;山药、茯苓、泽泻健脾利水。

Modification: For severe short breath, add *Ginseng Radix et Rhizoma* (Ren Shen) to supplement primordial qi; for loose stool, add *Atractylodis Macrocephalae Rhizoma* (Bai Zhu) and *Zingiberis Rhizoma Praeparatum* (Pao Gan Jiang) to warm and transport zhong jiao.

加减:短气甚者,加人参补益元气;便溏腹泻者,加白术、炮干姜温运中焦。

Consumptive Disease

虚劳

Consumptive disease, is a general term of several choronic weakness diseases, which can be caused by many factors and characterized by weakening zang-fu organs, and deficiency of qi, blood, yin and yang.

虚劳又称虚损,是由多种原因造成所致的,以脏腑功能衰退,气血阴阳亏虚为主要病机的多种慢性衰弱证候的总称。

1 Etiology and Pathogenesis

1 病因病机

A couple of factors attacking the body together, cause weakening zang-fu organs and deficiency of qi, blood, yin and yang, which, if prolongs without treatment, leads to consumptive disease.

多种病因作用于人体,导致脏腑功能衰退,气血阴阳亏虚,日久不复均可导致虚劳。

1.1 Innate Deficiency

1.1 禀赋不足

Innate deficiency due to poor nourishment before birth, or deficiency of water, grain, essence and qi due to improper feeding after birth, will lead

或因胎中失养而先天精气不足,或生后喂养不当,水谷精气不充,均可导致正气

to healthy qi deficiency, which is likely to be prolonged and turn into consumptive disease.

亏虚，病后更易形成久病不复，日久而发展为虚劳。

1.2 Over Anxiety and Strain

Anxiety and strain, or injury of seven emotions will consume qi and hurt spirits, injure the heart and spleen, leading to qi and blood deficiency, which prolonged, turns intoconsumptive disease. Or indulgence in sex will consume kidney essence and kidney-qi, which, prolonged, turns into consumptive disease.

1.2 烦劳过度

或诸事烦劳，或七情内伤，可耗气伤神，损伤心脾，致气血亏虚，日久成劳。或房事不节，恣情纵欲致肾精亏虚，肾气不足，久则形成虚劳。

1.3 Improper Diet

Unscrupulous diet, irregular hunger and starvation, or favor for some types of food, such as raw, cold, spicy, greasy food, and over drink will hurt the root of later heaven of the spleen and stomach, which then fails to transform adaquent water, grain and essence and fails to supply adaquent qi and blood. Then the body is poorly nourishd, resulting in consumptive disease.

1.3 饮食不节

平时饮食不节，饥饱无常，或饮食偏嗜，如过食生冷、辛辣、油腻之品，饮酒过多等，损伤脾胃后天之本，使水谷精微化生不足，气血乏源，人体失于充养，而致虚劳。

1.4 Serious Diseases or Prolonged Illness

Chronic diseases that relapse frequently without cure, or prolonged and complicated without proper treatment will result in healthy qi deficiency that is hard to restore. Or serious disease hurts qi and blood, which lack in regulation and then injure the essence qi, leading toconsumptive disease.

1.4 大病久病

慢性疾病反复发作，经久不愈，或迁延失治，致使正气亏虚难复，而致虚损。或大病之后，伤及气血，失于调理，耗伤精气，因虚致损，而发展为虚劳。

1.5 Lack of Proper Treatment or Mistreatment

Wrong diagnosis or mistreatment will hurt healthy qi and delay the treatment of illness. And misuse of herbs will break the balance between yin and yang, consume and injure qi, blood and body fluid, weaken zang-fu organs, leading to consumptive disease in a long run.

1.5 失治误治

诊断有误，或治法不当，致正气损伤，耽误病情，加之药物使用不当之害，而使人体阴阳失衡，气血、津液耗伤，脏腑功能衰退，久则可为虚劳。

Overall, consumptive disease is either casue by

总之：本病或是因虚致

deficiency or by illness. Its pathogenesis is deficiency of qi, blood, yin and yang. It lies in the five zang-organs, in particular, the spleen and kidney. There are many causes that can result in the disease and the disease can be caused by one or several causes which interact with each other.

病，因病成劳；或是因病致虚，久虚不复而成劳。其病性主要是气血阴阳的亏虚，病位在五脏，其中脾、肾尤为重要。引起虚损的多种病因，不是孤立的，既可一种病因致病，又可几种病因互相影响，同时致病。

2 Syndrome Differentiation and Treatment

2 辨证论治

2.1 Key Points of Syndrome Differentiation

2.1 辨治要点

First, identify the difference among deficiency of qi, blood, yin and yang. Pattern identificaition of consumptive disease should abide by the guideline of theories of qi, blood, yin, yang, and the five zang-organs. At the same time, pay attention to the existence of complicating diseases. For example, does the original disease still exist? Is there any manifestation of deficiency leading to excess? Are there any exogenous pathogenic factors? The treatment should follow the basic principle of supplementation and invigoration, especially to the spleen and kidney. Try to eliminate the causes of deficiency. If consumptive disease lasts long with multiple factors, it is better to combine dietary and life habit change with medicinal treatment.

虚劳当首辨气血阴阳亏虚不同。虚劳的辨证应以气、血、阴、阳为纲，五脏虚候为目，同时还应注意有无兼见病证，例如原有疾病是否还继续存在，有无因虚致实的表现，是否兼感外邪。治当以补益为基本原则，重视补益脾肾，尽可能解除导致虚损的原因。虚劳病程较长，影响因素较多，要将药物治疗与饮食调养及生活调摄密切结合起来。

2.2 Therapeutic Methods for Different Patterns

2.2 分型论治

2.2.1 Qi Deficiency

2.2.1 气虚

2.2.1.1 Lung-qi Deficiency

2.2.1.1 肺气虚

Manifestations: Short breath, low timid voice, spontaneous sweating, cold and heat from time to time, prone to cold, pale complexion; pale tongue; weak pulse.

证候：短气，声音低怯，自汗，时寒时热，易于感冒，面白。舌淡，脉弱。

Treatment: To supplement and boost lung-qi.

治法：补益肺气。

Formulas and Herbs: *Lung-Supplementing Decoction* (Bu Fei Tang) and modified *Jade screen Powder* (Yu Ping Feng San), usually composed of *Astragali Radix* (Huang Qi), *Codonopsis Radix* (Dang Shen), *Atractylodis Macrocephalae Rhizoma* (Bai Zhu) and *Rehmanniae Radix Praeparata* (Shu Di Huang) to boost lung-qi and consolidate exterior, *Saposhnikoviae Radix* (Fang Feng) to expel wind; *Aster Radix et Rhizoma* (Zi Yuan) and *Schisandrae Chinensis Fructus* (Wu Wei Zi) to descend qi and stop coughing; *Mori Cortex* (Sang Bai Pi) to cleanse the lung.

方药: 补肺汤合玉屏风散加减。常用:黄芪、党参、白术、熟地益气补肺固表;防风祛风;紫菀、五味子降气止咳;桑白皮清肺。

Modification: For quite serious spontaneous sweating, add *Ostreae Concha* (Duan Mu Li) and *Ephedrae Herba* (Ma Huang) to secure the exterior and astringe sweating; for accompanying feverish sensation and nigh sweating, add *Trionycis Carapax* (Bie Jia), *Lycii Cortex* (Di Gu Pi) and *Gentianae Macrophyllae Radix* (Qin Jiao) to nourish yin and clear away heat.

加减: 自汗较多者,加煅牡蛎、麻黄根固表敛汗;兼见潮热、盗汗,加鳖甲、地骨皮、秦艽养阴清热。

2.2.1.2　Spleen-qi Deficiency

2.2.1.2　脾气虚

Manifestations: Decreasing intake, discomfort in the stomach, loose stool, fatigue, sallow yellow complexion; pale tongue; weak pulse.

证候: 饮食减少,胃脘不舒,大便溏薄,倦怠乏力,面色萎黄。舌淡,脉弱。

Treatment: To strengthen the spleen and boost qi.

治法: 健脾益气。

Formulas and Herbs: Modified *Four Nobles Decoction* (Si Jun Zi Tang), usually composed of *Ginseng Radix et Rhizoma* (Ren Shen) or *Codonopsis Radix* (Dang Shen) and *Astragali Radix* (Huang Qi) to boost qi; *Poria* (Fu Ling), *Atractylodis Macrocephalae Rhizoma* (Bai Zhu) and *Lablab Semen Album* Frictum (Chao Bian Dou) to strengthen the spleen; *Glycyrrhizae Radix et Rhizoma* (Gan Cao)

方药: 加味四君子汤加味。常以人参(党参)、黄芪益气,茯苓、白术、炒扁豆健脾,甘草益气和中。

to boost qi and harmonize zhong jiao.

Modification: For distention and fullness in the stomach and burping, add *Citri Reticulatae Pericarpium* (Chen Pi), *Pinelliae Rhizoma* (Ban Xia) and *Perillae Caulis* (Su Geng) to harmonize the stomach, regulate qi and lower reversal flow; for chest oppression, abdominal distention, burping sour, greasy tongue fur, add *Massa Fermentata Medicinalis* (Shen Qu), *Setariae Fructus Germinatus Fermentata* (Chao Gu Ya), *Crataegi Fructus* Fermentata (Chao Shan Zha), *Galli Gigerii Endothelium Corneum* (Ji Nei Jin) to digest food and invigorate the stomach; for unwarm hands and feet, abdominal pain with diarrhea, add *Cinnamomi Cortex* (Rou Gui) and *Zingiberis Rhizoma Praeparatum* (Pao Jiang) to warm the middle and expel cold.

加减：兼胃脘胀满呕吐嗳气，加陈皮、半夏、苏梗和胃理气降逆；兼脘闷腹胀、嗳气酸腐、苔腻，加神曲、炒谷芽、炒山楂、鸡内金消食健胃；兼手足欠温、腹痛即泻，加肉桂、炮姜温中散寒。

2.2.1.3 Heart-qi Deficiency

2.2.1.3 心气虚

Manifestations: Palpitation, short breath that worsens at movement, spontaneous sweating, lassitude and physical fatigue, waxy pale complexion; pale tongue; weak pulse.

证候：心悸，气短，活动时加重，自汗，神疲体倦，面色晄白。舌质淡，脉弱。

Treatment: To boost qi and nourish the heart.

治法：益气养心。

Formulas and Herbs: Modified *Seven Blessed Decoction* (Qi Fu Yin), usually composed of *Ginseng Radix et Rhizoma* (Ren Shen) and *Atractylodis Macrocephalae Rhizoma* (Bai Zhu) to boost qi; *Angelicae Sinensis Radix* (Dang Gui) and *Rehmanniae Radix Praeparata* (Shu Di Huang), to nourish blood; *Ziziphi Spinosae Semen* (Suan Zao Ren) and *Polygalae Radix* (Yuan Zhi) to calm the spirits.

方药：七福饮加减。常以人参、白术益气，当归、熟地养血，枣仁、远志安神。

Modification: For heavy spontaneous sweating, add *Astragali Radix* (Huang Qi), *Ostreae Concha* (Duan Mu Li) and *Schisandrae Chinensis Fructus* (Wu Wei Zi) to boost qi and consolidate the kid-

加减：自汗多者，加黄芪、煅牡蛎、五味子益气固摄；食少纳呆者，加砂仁、炒山楂、茯苓开胃健脾。

ney; for little food intake, add *Amomi Fructus* (Sha Ren), *Crataegi Fructus Fermentata* (Chao Shan Zha) and *Poria* (Fu Ling) to improve appetite and strengthen the spleen.

2.2.1.4　Kidney-qi Deficiency

Manifestations: Lassitude and fatigue, sorenss in the waist and knees, frequent clear away urine or urine incontinence, vaginal discharge and innate abortion; pale tongue; weak pulse.

Treatment: To supplement the kidney and nourish the origin.

Formulas and Herbs: Modified *Major Yuan (Primary) Qi-Reinforcing Decoction* (Da Bu Yuan Jian), usually composed of *Ginseng Radix et Rhizoma* (Ren Shen), *Dioscoreae Rhizoma* (Shan Yao) and *Glycyrrhizae Radix et Rhizoma* Praeparata (Zhi Gan Cao) to boost qi; *Eucommiae Cortex* (Du Zhong) to supplement kidney-yang; *Rehmanniae Radix Praeparata* (Shu Di Huang), *Lycii Fructus* (Gou Qi Zi), *Corni Fructus* (Shan Zhu Yu) to nourish kidney-yin.

Modification: For remarkable lassitude and fatigue, add *Astragali Radix* (Huang Qi) to boost qi; for frequent urine even incontinence, add *Cuscutae Semen* (Tu Si Zi), *Fructus Rosae Laevigatae* (Jin Yin Zi) and *Alpiniae Oxyphyllae Fructus* (Yi Zhi Ren) to supplement and consolidate the kidney; for loose stool, subtract *Rehmanniae Radix Praeparata* (Shu Di Huang) and *Angelicae Sinensis Radix* (Dang Gui), add *Myristicae Semen* (Rou Dou Kou), *Psoraleae Fructus* (Bu Gu Zhi) and *Schisandrae Chinensis Fructus* (Wu Wei Zi) to warm and supplement the kidney to consolidate.

2.2.1.4　肾气虚

证候: 神疲乏力,腰膝酸软,小便频数而清,或尿失禁,带下滑脱。舌质淡,脉弱。

治法: 补肾培元。

方药: 大补元煎加减。常以人参、山药、炙甘草益气,杜仲补肾阳,熟地、枸杞子、山茱萸滋肾阴。

加减: 神疲乏力甚者,加黄芪益气;尿频较甚或小便失禁者,加菟丝子、金樱子、益智仁补肾固摄;大便溏薄者,去熟地黄、当归,加肉豆蔻、补骨脂、五味子温补固涩。

2.2.2 Blood Deficiency

2.2.2.1 Heart-blood Deficiency

Manifestations: Anxiety, severe palpitation, forgetfulness, insomnia, dreaminess, lusterless face; pale tongue; fine or knot or intermittern pulse.

Treatment: To nourish blood and calm the heart.

Formulas and Herbs: Modified *Angelica Splenic Decoction* (Gui Pi Tang), usually composed of *Ginseng Radix et Rhizoma* (Ren Shen), *Scutellariae Radix* (Huang Qin) and *Angelicae Sinensis Radix* (Dang Gui) to boost qi and nourish blood; *Atractylodis Macrocephalae Rhizoma* (Bai Zhu), *Poria* (Fu Ling) to strengthen the spleen; *Polygalae Radix* (Yuan Zhi) and *Longan Arillus* (Long Yan Rou) to nourish the heart and calm the spirits.

Modification: For insomnia and dreaminess, add *Albiziae Flos* (He Huan Hua) and *Polygoni Multiflori Caulis* (Ye Jiao Teng) to nourish the heart and calm the spirits; for severe palpitation, add moderately *Ostreae Concha* (Mu Li) and *Os Draconis* (Long Gu) to settle the heart and calm the spirits.

2.2.2.2 Liver-blood Deficiency

Manifestations: Dizziness, vertigo, lusterless face, hypochondriac pain, numb limbs, muscular spasm, peristalsis of muscle, irregular menstruation, menopause; pale tongue, fine stringy pulse or fine uneven pulse.

Treatment: To supplement blood and nourish the liver.

Formuals and Herbs: Modified *Four Agents Decoction* (Si Wu Tang) and *An Ever Effective*

2.2.2 血虚

2.2.2.1 心血虚

证候: 心急,怔忡,健忘,失眠,多梦,面色不华。舌质淡,脉细或结或代。

治法: 养血宁心。

方药: 归脾汤加减。常以人参、黄芪、当归益气养血,白术、茯苓健脾,远志、龙眼肉养心安神。

加减: 失眠、多梦较甚者,加合欢花、夜交藤养心安神;心悸较甚者,酌加牡蛎、龙骨镇心安神。

2.2.2.2 肝血虚

证候: 头晕目眩,面色不华,胁痛,肢体麻木,经脉拘急,肌肉瞤动,月经不调或闭经。舌质淡,脉弦细或细涩。

治法: 补血养肝。

方药: 四物汤合一贯煎加味。常用:当归、熟地养

Decoction for Nourishing Liver and Kidney (Yi Guan Jian), usually composed of *Angelicae Sinensis Radix* (Dang Gui) and *Rehmanniae Radix Praeparata* (Shu Di Huang) to nourish blood; *Paeoniae Radix Alba* (Bai Shao Yao), *Lycii Fructus* (Gou Qi Zi) and *Ophiopogonis Radix* (Mai Men Dong) to nurrish yin and soften the liver; *Chuanxiong Rhizoma* (Chuan Xiong) to promote qi flow and *Toosendan Fructus* (Chuan Lian Zi) to disperse the liver.

血;白芍药、枸杞子、麦门冬养阴柔肝;川芎行血;川楝子疏肝。

Modification: For serious blood deficiency, add *Polygoni Multiflori Radix* Praeparata (Zhi Shou Wu), *Lycii Fructus* (Gou Qi Zi) and *Spatholobi Caulis* (Ji Xue Teng) to help to supplement kidney and nourish the liver; for hypochondriac pain, add *Luffae Fructus Retinervus* (Si Gua Luo), *Curcumae Radix* (Yu Jin) and *Cyperi Rhizoma* (Xiang Fu) to regulate qi and free colleterals; for dim sight, add *Broussone Tiaefructus* (Chu Shi Zi), *Cassiae Semen* (Jue Ming Zi) and *Lycii Fructus* (Gou Qi Zi) to nourish the liver and improve eye sight.

加减: 血虚甚者,加制首乌、枸杞子、鸡血藤补肾养肝;胁痛者,加丝瓜络、郁金、香附理气通络;视物模糊者,加楮实子、决明子、枸杞子养肝明目。

2.2.3　Yin Deficiency

2.2.3　阴虚

2.2.3.1　Lung-yin Deficiency

2.2.3.1　肺阴虚

Manifestations: Dry cough, coughing blood, dry throat, loss of voice, feverish sensation; red cheeks, night sweating; red tongue with little fluid; fine rapid pulse.

证候: 干咳,咳血,咽喉干燥,失音,潮热,面色潮红,盗汗。舌质红、少津,脉细数。

Treatment: To nourish yin and moisten the lung.

治法: 养阴润肺。

Formulas and Herbs: Modified *Glehnia and Ophiopogonis Radix* Decoction (Sha Shen Mai Dong Tang), usually composed of *Adenophorae Radix* seu Glehniae (Sha Shen), *Polygonati Odorati Rhizoma* (Yu Zhu), *Ophiopogonis Radix* (Mai Men Dong) and *Trichosanthis Radix* (Tian Hua Fen) to nourish

方药: 沙参麦冬汤加减。常以沙参、玉竹、麦门冬、花粉养阴润肺,桑叶清肺止咳。

yin and moisten the lung; *Mori Folium* (Sang Ye) to cleanse the lung and stop coughing.

Modification: For bad cough, add *Stemonae Radix* (Bai Bu) and *Farfarae Flos* (Kuan Dong Hua) to disperse the lung and stop coughing; for coughing blood, add *Bletillae Rhizoma* (Bai Ji), *Agrimoniae Herba* (Xian He Cao) and *Cirsii Herba* (Xiao Ji) to cool blood and stop bleeding; for feverish sensations, add *Lycii Cortex* (Di Gu Pi), *Gentianae Macrophyllae Radix* (Qin Jiao), *Stellariae Radix* (Yin Chai Hu) and *Trionycis Carapax* (Bie Jia) to nourish yin and clear away heat; for uncomfortable throat, add *Oroxyli Semen* (Mu Hu Die) and *Platycodi Radix*(Jie Geng).

加减: 咳嗽甚者,加百部、款冬花肃肺止咳;咳血者,加白及、仙鹤草、小蓟凉血止血;潮热者,加地骨皮、牡丹皮、秦艽、银柴胡、鳖甲养阴清热;咽喉不利者,加木蝴蝶、桔梗。

2.2.3.2 Heart-yin Deficiency

Manifestations: Palpitation, insomnia, irritation, sores in the mouth and on the tongue; red cheeks, night sweating, fine rapid pulse.

Treatment: To nourish yin and nourish the heart.

Formulas and Herbs: Modified *Celestial Emperor Heart-Supplementing Elixir* (Tian Wang Bu Xin Dan), usually composed of *Asparagi Radix* (Tian Dong), *Ophiopogonis Radix* (Mai Men Dong), *Rehmannia Radix* (Sheng Di Huang) and *Scrophulariae Radix* (Xuan Shen) to nourish yin and cleanse the heart; *Salviae Miltiorrhizae Radix et Rhizoma Radix* (Dan Shen), *Angelicae Sinensis Radix* (Dang Gui), *Platycladi Semen* (Bai Zi Ren), *Ziziphi Spinosae Semen* (Suan Zao Ren) and *Polygalae Radix* (Yuan Zhi) to nourish blood and calm the spirits.

Modification: For irritation and restlessness, soreness in the mouth and on the tongue (excessive heart-fire), subtract *Angelicae Sinensis Radix* (Dang

2.2.3.2 心阴虚

证候: 心悸,失眠,烦躁,口舌生疮,面色潮红,盗汗。舌红少津,脉细数。

治法: 滋阴养心。

方药: 天王补心丹加减。常用:天门冬、麦门冬、生地黄、玄参养阴清心;丹参、当归、柏子仁、酸枣仁、远志养血安神。

加减: 烦躁不安、口舌生疮者,去当归、远志,加黄连、川木通、淡竹叶清心泄火、导

Gui) and *Polygalae Radix* (Yuan Zhi), add *Coptidis Rhizoma* (Huang Lian), *Clematidis Armandii Caulis* (Chuan Mu Tong) and *Lophatheri Herba* (Dan Zhu Ye) to cleanse the heart and purge fire, and induce heat downward; for feverish sensation, add *Lycii Cortex* (Di Gu Pi), *Gentianae Macrophyllae Radix* (Qin Jiao) and *Stellariae Radix* (Yin Chai Hu) to clear away and retreat deficiency heat; for night sweating, add *Ostreae Concha* (Duan Mu Li) and *Fructus Tritici Levis* (Fu Xiao Mai) to consolidate the exterior and arrest sweat.

热下行；潮热者，加地骨皮、银柴胡、秦艽清退虚热；盗汗者，加煅牡蛎、浮小麦固表敛汗。

2.2.3.3 Spleen-and-Stomach-yin Deficiency

2.2.3.3 脾胃阴虚

Manifestations: No desire for food and drink, dry mouth and lips, dry stool, dry vomiting, red cheeks; red tongue with little tongue fur; fine rapid pulse.

证候：不思饮食，口干舌燥，大便干结，干呕，面潮红。舌红、少苔，脉细数。

Treatment: To nourish yin and harmonize the stomach.

治法：养阴和胃。

Formulas and Herbs: Modified *Stomach-Benefiting Decoction* (Yi Wei Tang), usually composed of *Adenophorae Radix* (Sha Shen), *Ophiopogonis Radix* (Mai Men Dong), and *Polygonati Odorati Rhizoma* (Yu Zhu) to invigorate the stomach and nourish yin; *Rehmannia Radix* (Sheng Di Huang) to nourish yin and clear away heat.

方药：益胃汤加减。常以沙参、麦门冬、玉竹益胃养阴，生地黄滋阴清热。

Modification: For serious dry mouth and lips, add *Dendrobii Caulis* (Shi Hu) and *Trichosanthis Radix* (Tian Hua Fen) to nourish and nourish stomach-yin; for no desire for food and drink, add *Hordei Fructus Germinatus* (Mai Ya), *Lablab Semen Album* (Bian Dou) and *Dioscoreae Rhizoma* (Shan Yao) to invigorate the stomach and strengthen the spleen; for hiccup, add Semen Canavaliae (Dao Dou), *Kaki Calyx* (Shi Di) and *Bambusae Caulis in*

加减：口干唇燥甚者，加石斛、花粉滋养胃阴；不思饮食甚者，加麦芽、扁豆、山药益胃健脾；呃逆者，加刀豆、柿蒂、竹茹降逆止呃。

Taenias (Zhu Ru) to stop reversal hiccup.

2.2.3.4 Liver-yin Deficiency

Manifestations: Vertigo, headache, tinnutis, aversion to light, dry eyes, dim sight, numb limbs, muscular shivering, feverish red complexion; red tongue with little fluid; stringy fine rapid pulse.

Treatment: To nourish liver-yin.

Formulas and Herbs: Modified *Liver-Supplementing Decoction* (Bu Gan Tang), usually composed of *Four Agents Decoction* (Si Wu Tang) to nourish yin-blood; *Ziziphi Spinosae Semen* (Suan Zao Ren), *Chaenomelis Fructus* (Mu Gua) and *Glycyrrhizae Radix et Rhizoma* (Gan Cao) to soften the liver and relax sinews.

Modification: For severe headache, vertigo and tinnitus, or muscular shivering, add *Haliotidis Concha* (Shi Jue Ming), *Chrysanthemi Flos* (Ju Hua), *Uncariae Ramulus cum Uncis* (Gou Teng) and *Tribuli Fructus* (Ji Li) to calm the liver and subdue yang; for dry eyes and aversion to light, or dim eyesight, add *Lycii Fructus* (Gou Qi Zi), *Ligustri Lucidi Fructus* (Nü Zhen Zi) and *Cassiae Semen* (Jue Ming Zi) to nourish the liver and improve eyesight; for irritation and easy anger, reddish urine and constipation, red tongue with rapid pulse, add *Gentianae Radix et Rhizom* (Long Dan Cao), *Scutellariae Radix* (Huang Qin) and *Gardeniae Fructus* (Zhi Zi) to cleanse the liver and purge fire.

2.2.3.5 Kidney-yin Deficiency

Manifestations: Weakness and powerlessness in the waist, knees and feet, vertigo, tinnitus, spermatorrhea; red tongue with little fluid; fine deep pulse.

Treatment: To nourish kidney-yin.

2.2.3.4 肝阴虚

证候：眩晕，头痛耳鸣，目干畏光，视物不明，肢体麻木，筋惕肉瞤，面色潮红。舌红少津，脉弦细数。

治法：滋养肝阴。

方药：补肝汤加减。常用：四物汤滋养阴血；酸枣仁、木瓜、甘草酸甘化阴以柔肝舒筋。

加减：头痛、眩晕、耳鸣较甚，或筋惕肉瞤者，加石决明、菊花、钩藤、刺蒺藜平肝潜阳；目干涩畏光，或视物不明者，加枸杞子、女贞子、决明子养肝明目；急躁易怒，尿赤便秘，舌红脉数者，加龙胆草、黄芩、栀子清肝泻火。

2.2.3.5 肾阴虚

证候：腰膝、两足痿弱，眩晕，耳鸣，遗精。舌红、少津，脉沉细。

治法：滋补肾阴。

Formulas and Herbs: Modified *Kidney Pills* (Zuo Gui Wan), usually composed of *Rehmanniae Radix Praeparata* (Shu Di Huang), *Corni Fructus* (Shan Zhu Yu), *Lycii Fructus* (Gou Qi Zi) and *Testudinis Carapacis et Plastri Colla* (Gui Ban Jiao) to nourish the kidney and nourish yin; *Cuscutae Semen*(Tu Si Zi), *Achyranthis Bidentatae Radix* (Niu Xi) and *Cervi Cornus Colla* (Lu Jiao Jiao) to supplement the kidney and strengthen the waist, meaning obtaining yin from yang, *Dioscoreae Rhizoma* (Shan Yao) to boost qi.

方药: 左归丸加减。常用:熟地黄、山茱萸、枸杞、龟版胶滋肾养阴;菟丝子、牛膝、鹿角胶补肾强腰,阳中求阴;山药益气。

Modification: For spermatorrhea, add *Ostreae Concha* (Mu Li), *Fructus Rosae Laevigatae* (Jin Yin Zi), *Euryales Semen* (Qian Shi) and *Nelumbinis Stamen* (Lian Xu) to secure the kidney and astringe essence; for feverish sensation, dry mouth, sore throat, rapid pulse, add *Anemarrhenae Rhizoma* (Zhi Mu), *Phellodendri Chinensis Cortex* (Huang Bo) and *Lycii Cortex* (Di Gu Pi) to nourish yin and purge fire. *Anemarrhena, Phellodendron, and Rehmannia Pills* (Zhi Bai Di Huang Wan) can be also used.

加减: 遗精者,加牡蛎、金樱子、芡实、莲须固肾涩精;潮热、口干、咽痛、脉数者,加知母、黄柏、地骨皮滋阴泻火,亦可选知柏地黄丸。

2.2.4 Yang Deficiency

2.2.4 阳虚

2.2.4.1 Heart-Yang Deficiency

2.2.4.1 心阳虚

Manifestations: Palpitation, spontaneous, spiritual fatigue and favor for lying down, physical cold and cold limbs, chest oppression and pain, pale complexion, pale dark purple tongue; fin weak or deep retarded pulse.

证候: 心悸,自汗,神倦嗜卧,形寒肢冷,心胸憋闷疼痛。舌质紫黯,面色苍白,舌淡,脉细弱或沉迟。

Treatment: To warm heart-yang.

治法: 温通心阳。

Formulas and Herbs: Modified *Trichosanthis, Allii Macrostemonis Bulbus and Pinelliae Decoction* (Gua Lou Xie Bai Ban Xia Tang), usually composed

方药: 瓜蒌薤白半夏汤加味。常用:瓜蒌宽胸理气;薤白、半夏温阳散结;黄芪、

of *Trichosanthis Fructus* (Gua lou) to broaden the chest and regulate qi, *Allii Macrostemonis Bulbus* (Xie Bai) and *Pinelliae Rhizoma* (Ban Xia) to warm yang and dissipate stagnation, *Codonopsis Radix* (Dang Shen), *Astragali Radix* (Huang Qi) to boost qi and warm yang; *Zingiberis Rhizoma* (Gan Jiang), *Cinnamomi Ramulus* (Gui Zhi) and *Aconm Lateralis Radix Praeparata* (Fu Zi) to activate yang and disperse cold.

党参益气温阳;干姜、桂枝、附子等以通阳散寒。

Modification: For bad pain in the chest, add moderately *Curcumae Radix* (Yu Jin), *Chuanxiong Rhizoma* (Chuan Xiong), *Salviae Miltiorrhizae Radix et Rhizoma Radix* (Dan Shen) and *Notoginseng Radix et Rhizoma* (San Qi) to activate blood and stop pain; for physical cold and cold limbs, retarded pulse, add moderately *Aconm Lateralis Radix Praeparata* (Fu Zi), *Morindae Officinalis Radix* (Ba Ji Tian), *Curculiginis Rhizoma* (Xian Mao), *Epimedii Folium* (Yin Yang Huo) and *Cervi Cornu Pantotrichum* (Lu Rong) to warm and supplement yang-qi.

加减: 心胸疼痛者,酌加郁金、川芎、丹参、三七活血定痛;形寒肢冷、脉迟者,酌加附子、巴戟天、仙茅、淫羊藿、鹿茸温补阳气。

2.2.4.2 Spleen-yang Deficiency

2.2.4.2 脾阳虚

Manifestations: Little intake, lassitude and fatigue, no desire to speak due to asthenia of qi, physical cold, rumbling noise in the intestines, loose stool and even diarrhea, sallow yellow complexion; pale tongue.

证候: 食少,神倦乏力,少气懒言,形寒,肠鸣腹痛,大便溏泄,面色萎黄,舌淡。

Treatment: To warm the middle and strengthen the spleen.

治法: 温中健脾。

Formulas and Herbs: Modified *Aconiti Praeparata-Regulating Zhong jiao Decoction* (Fu Zi Li Zhong Tang), usually composed of *Ginseng Radix et Rhizoma* (Ren Shen) and *Atractylodis Macrocephalae Rhizoma* (Bai Zhu) to strengthen the

方药: 附子理中汤加味。常以人参、白术健脾益气,干姜、附子温中散寒。

spleen and boost qi; *Zingiberis Rhizoma* (Gan Jiang) and *Aconm Lateralis Radix Praeparata* (Fu Zi) to warm the middle and disperse cold.

Modification: For bad abdominal cold pain, add *Alpiniae Officinarum Rhizoma* (Gao Liang Jiang) and *Cyperi Rhizoma* (Xiang Fu) or *Caryophylli Flos* (Ding Xiang), *Euodiae Fructus* (Wu Zhu Yu) to warm the middle and disperse cold, regulate qi and stop pain; for distention after meal and hiccup, add *Amomi Fructus* (Sha Ren), *Pinelliae Rhizoma* (Ban Xia), *Citri Reticulatae Pericarpium* (Chen Pi) to warm the middle, harmonize the stomach and descend adverse flow of qi; for severe diarrhea, add *Myristicae Semen* (Rou Dou Kou), *Psoraleae Fructus* (Bu Gu Zhi) and *Schisandrae Chinensis Fructus* (Wu Wei Zi) to warm and supplement the kidney and spleen, astringe the intestines and stop dirrehea.

加减：腹中冷痛较甚者，加高良姜、香附或丁香、吴茱萸温中散寒，理气止痛；食后腹胀及呕逆者，加砂仁、半夏、陈皮温中和胃降逆；腹泻较甚者，加肉豆蔻、补骨脂、五味子温补脾肾，涩肠止泻。

2.2.4.3　Kidney-yang Deficiency

2.2.4.3　肾阳虚

Manifestations: Soreness in the waist and back, aversion to cold and cold limbs, spermatorrhea, impotence, urine in great amount or incontinence, diarrhoea with undigested food in the stool or diarrhea in the early morning, pale complexion; pale enlarged pale tongue with teeth marks; deep retarded pulse.

证候：腰背酸痛，畏寒肢冷，遗精、阳痿，多尿或小便失禁，下利清谷或五更泄泻，面色苍白。舌淡胖有齿痕，脉沉迟。

Treatment: To warm and supplement kidney-yang.

治法：温补肾阳。

Formulas and Herbs: Modified *Vital Gate Pills* (You Gui Wan), usually composed of *Aconm Lateralis Radix Praeparata* (Fu Zi), *Cinnamomi Cortex* (Rou Gui), *Eucommiae Cortex* (Du Zhong) and *Cuscutae Semen* (Tu Si Zi) to warm yang and supplement the kidney; *Dioscoreae Rhizoma* (Shan

方药：右归丸加减。常用：附子、肉桂、杜仲、菟丝子温阳补肾；山药、炙甘草益气；枸杞子、熟地黄、当归滋肾以阴中求阳。

Yao) and *Glycyrrhizae Radix et Rhizoma Praeparata* (Zhi Gan Cao) to boost qi; *Lycii Fructus* (Gou Qi Zi), *Rehmanniae Radix Praeparata* (Shu Di Huang) and *Angelicae Sinensis Radix* (Dang Gui) to nourish the kidney, meaning obtaining yang from yin.

Modification: Spermatorrhea, add *Fructus Rosae Laevigatae* (Jin Yin Zi), *Mantidis Ootheca* (Sang Piao Xiao) and *Nelumbinis Stamen* (Lian Xu), or along with *Golden Lock Essence-Securing Pill* (Jin Suo Gu Jing Wan) to arrest essence; for diarrhoea with undigested food in the stool, delete moistening and greasy herbs like *Rehmanniae Radix Praeparata* (Shu Di Huang) and *Angelicae Sinensis Radix* (Dang Gui), add *Codonopsis Radix* (Dang Shen), *Atractylodis Macrocephalae Rhizoma* (Bai Zhu) and *Coicis Semen* (Yi Yi Ren) to boost qi and strengthen the spleen, eliminate dampness to stop diarrhea; for diarrhea in early mornings, add *Four Divinities Pills* (Si Shen Wan) to warm the spleen and kidney, consolidate the intestines and stop diarrhea.

加减：遗精者，加金樱子、桑螵蛸、莲须，或合金锁固精丸以收涩固精；下利清谷者，减去熟地黄、当归等滋润滑腻之品，加党参、白术、薏苡仁益气健脾，渗湿止泻；五更泄泻者，合四神丸温脾暖肾，固肠止泻。

Chatper 7 Diseases of Body Parts and Meridians

第 7 章 肢体经络病证

Bi Syndrome

痹 证

Bi Syndrome is caused by obstruction of meridians and collaterals block, unsmooth flow of qi and blood due to exogenous pathogenic factors of wind, cold, dampness and heat, which is characterized by pain, soreness, numbness, heaviness, difficult bending and stretching of limb sinews and bones, joints and muscles, even swelling and enlarged joints.

痹证主要因风、寒、湿、热等外邪侵袭人体，闭阻经络，气血运行不畅所导致的，以肢体筋骨、关节、肌肉发生疼痛、酸楚、麻木、重着、屈伸不利，甚则关节肿大变形为主要症状的病证。

1 Etiology and Pathogenesis

1 病因病机

Bi Syndrome is mainly caused by constitutional factors, climatical conditions, living circumstances and diet. Pathogenic qi stagnation of wind, cold, dampness and heat remain in the limb sinews and vessels, joints, muscles, meridians and collaterals, leading to obstruction of qi and blood flow. Obstruction leads to pain. Deficiency of healthy qi, looseness of striae of the skin and weakened defensive qi are the internal causes for the disease while exogeneous pathogenic factors of wind, cold, heat and dampness are the external causes.

痹证的发生主要是由于体质因素、气候条件、生活环境及饮食等因素，导致风寒湿热痰瘀等邪气滞留于肢体筋脉、关节、肌肉，经脉、气血痹阻不通，不通则痛。正气偏虚，腠理不密，卫外不固是引起痹证的内在因素，风寒湿热等外邪侵袭是发病的外在条件。

1.1 Affection Pathogenic Factors Due to Weak Constitution

1.1 体虚感邪

Innate deficiency and deficiency of healthy qi

患者素体正气亏虚，气

will lead to deficiency of qi and blood, and looseness of striae of skin, which allows for invasion of exogeneous pathogenic factors, and whereafter, the body has no power to expel pathogenic factors, which then make way deep and remain in sinews, bones and blood vessels, leading to Bi Syndrome.

血不足,腠理空疏,故外邪易于入侵,既病之后又无力驱邪外出,以致风寒湿热之邪深入,留连于筋骨血脉而为痹证。

1.2 Invasion of Cold-dampness

Damp habitation, being severely frozen, sleepingoutside, wind blowing when asleep, immersion in heavy rain, working in water or entering water after sweating will make it easy to be affected by pathogenic wind, cold and dampness. Those exogenous pathogenic factors penetrate into the muscles, striae of the skin, meridians and collaterals and remains in joints, leading to obstruction of qi and blood, causing wind-cold-damp obstruction.

1.2 寒湿侵袭人体

久居湿地,严寒冻伤,贪凉露宿,睡卧当风,暴雨浇淋,水中作业或汗出入水等,感受风寒湿邪,外邪留注于肌腠经络,滞留于关节,导致气血痹阻而发为风寒湿痹。

1.3 Pathogenic Factors of Wind, Dampness and Heat Attack or Heat Due to Stagnation of Wind-cold-dampness

Living in hot and damp places for long will make it easy to be affected by wind, dampness and heat, which attack thestriae of the skin, obstruct meridians and collaterals, block qi, blood, meridian vessels, and remain in joints, sinews and bones, leading to wind-damp-heat Bi syndrome.

1.3 感受风湿热邪或风寒湿痹郁而化热

久居炎热潮湿之地,外感风湿热邪袭于肌腠,壅于经络,痹阻气血经脉,滞留于关节筋骨,发为风湿热痹。此外,风寒湿邪内郁日久,风变为火,寒变为热,湿变为痰,亦可发为热痹。

1.4 Blockage of Meridians and Colleterals Due to Intermingled Phlegm and Stasis

Prolonged Bi Syndrome will consume qi and injure blood, damage yin and fluid, causing unsmooth flow of qi and blood. That is, blood retention leads to stasis while dampness congealing leads to phlegm. Phlegm and stasis along with exogenous pathogenic factors block meridians and collaterals, making way

1.4 痰瘀交结,痹阻经络

痹证日久耗气伤血,损阴劫津致气血运行不畅,而致"血停为瘀,湿凝为痰"。痰瘀交结亦可同外邪相合,阻痹经络,深入骨骱,出现关节肿大,甚至强直畸形,屈伸

deep into bones and joints, causing enlarged joints, even malformation, difficult bending and stretching together with manifestations of qi and blood deficiency of different intensity.

不利等症状，同时有不同程度的气血亏虚的表现。

The pathogenesis of Bi Syndrome is pathogenic factors blocking meridians and collaterals. That is, pathogenic factors of wind, dampness, heat, phlegm and stasis remains in sinews, vessels, joints, muscles, meridians and collaterals. Blockage of qi and blood leads to pain. Innate deficiency of yang-qi and yin-essence is the internal cause and pathogenic factors are external causes. Prolonged Bi Syndrome will affect zang-fu organs via meridians and collaterals, which will have pathological changes, heart impediemtn in particular. Or intermingled phlegm and stasis blocks meridians and collaterals and joints which prolonges the illness. Or consumption and damage of qi and blood, liver and kidney will cause deficiency of healthy qi and retention of pathogenic factors, leading to complication of deficiency and excess, becoming chronic disease.

痹证病机根本为邪气痹阻经脉，即风寒湿热痰瘀等邪气滞留于肢体筋脉、关节、肌肉，经脉、气血痹阻不通，不通则痛。素体阳气阴精不足为内因，风寒湿热之邪入侵为外因。痹证日久，可由经络累及脏腑，出现相应的脏腑病变，其中以心痹较多见。也可因痰浊瘀血交阻经络、关节，使疾病迁延难愈，或因气血耗伤，肝肾亏损而致正虚邪恋，虚实夹杂，而成顽疾。

2 Syndrome Differentiation and Treatment

2 辨证论治

2.1 Key Points of Syndrome Differentiation

2.1 辨治要点

Pattern identification of Bi Syndrome should first identify the predominance of the pathogenic qi and then identify deficiency and excess, finally constitution. Bi Syndrome clinically has different types. Migratory Bi refers to impediment with no fixed spots, which is due to predominance of pathogenic wind. Heavy pain in fixed spots that aggravates with cold is known as painful Bi, which is due to predominance of pathogenic cold. Soreness and heaviness in joints, heaviness and swelling belongs

痹证的辨证，一是要辨邪气的偏盛，二是要辨别虚实，三是辨体质。痹痛游走不定者为行痹，属风邪盛；痛势较甚，痛有定处，遇寒加重者为痛痹，属寒邪盛；关节酸痛、重着、漫肿者为着痹，属湿邪盛；关节肿胀，肌肤焮红，灼热疼痛为热痹，属热邪盛。关节疼痛日久，肿胀局

to fixed Bi, which is due to predominance of pathogenic dampness while swollen joints, hot skin, burning pain belongs to heat Bi, which is due to predominance of pathogenic heat. Prolonged joint, partial enlargement or clots under the skin is due to phlegm while swollen stiff joints, fixed pain spots, purple dark complexion or stasis macules are due to stasis. Generally speaking, newly developed impediment, which is obviously caused by pathogenic attacks, belongs to excess type while Bi of deficiency type is due to prolonged impediment which consumes qi and blood, damages zang-fu organs, leading to weak liver and spleen. Long duration without cure is usually due to intermingled phlegm and stasis, which belongs to complication of deficiency and excess. Those who are of innate yang excess or yin deficiency with heat are prone to exogenous pathogenic factors, which may be transformed into heat. That is heat Bi. Those who are of innate yang deficiency are prone to pathogenic factors, which then will be turned into cold. That is cold Bi. The treatment should follow the principle of eliminating pathogenic factors and freeing collaterals. In light of predominance of pathogenic qi, give respective treatments of dispelling wind, dispersing cold, eliminating dampness, clear awaying away heat, resolving phlegm and removing stasis. Give both attention to "eliminating blockage" and "dredging collaterals". In addition, pay attention to nurturing and activating blood. Treat cold along with warming yang and supplementing fire. Treat dampness along with strengthening the spleen and boosting qi. For prolonged blockage with deficiency of healthy qi, doctors should fous on strengthening healthy qi,

限,或见皮下结节者为痰;关节肿胀,僵硬,疼痛不移,肌肤紫暗或瘀斑等为瘀。一般说来:痹证新发,风、寒、湿、热之邪明显者为实;痹证日久,耗伤气血,损及脏腑,肝肾不足为虚;病程缠绵,日久不愈,常为痰瘀互结,肝肾亏虚之虚实夹杂证。素体阳盛或阴虚有热者,感受外邪易从热化,多属热痹;素体阳虚者,感受外邪易从寒化,多属寒痹。治疗应以祛邪通络为基本原则,根据邪气的偏盛,分别予以祛风、散寒、除湿、清热、化痰、行瘀,兼顾"宣痹通络"。同时治风还宜重视养血活血,治寒宜结合温阳补火,治湿宜结合健脾益气。久痹正虚者,应重视扶正、补肝肾、益气血。

supplementing the liver and kidney, and boosting qi and blood.

2.2 Therapeutic Methods for Different Types

2.2.1 Migratory Bi Syndrome

Manifestations: Soreness in limb joints in unfixed spots, difficult bending and stretching, or aversion to wind and fever; white thin tongue fur; floating pulse.

Treatment: To dispel wind and dredge collaterals; disperse cold and eliminate dampness.

Formulas and Herbs: *Ledebouriellae Decoction* (Fang Feng Tang), usually composed of *Saposhnikoviae Radix* (Fang Feng) and *Gentianae Macrophyllae Radix* (Qin Jiao) to dispel wind and eliminate dampness, dredge colalterals and stop pain; *Ephedrae Herba* (Ma Huang) and *Armeniacae Semen Amaru* (Ku Xing Ren) to expel cold and disperse the lung to eliminate pathogenic factors; *Puerariae Lobatae Radix* (Ge Gen) to relieve muscle and eliminate pathongenic factors; *Poria* (Fu Ling) to eliminate dampness with their bland nature; *Angelicae Sinensis Radix* (Dang Gui) to nourish and activate blood, relax colleterals and soften sinews; *Zingiberis Rhizoma Recens* (Sheng Jiang), *Glycyrrhizae Radix et Rhizoma* (Gan Cao) and *Jujubae Fructus* (Da Zao) to harmonize zhong jiao and regulate Ying (Nutrient) Phase.

Modification: For soreness and pain in the upper limbs such as shoulders and elbows, use *Notopterygii Rhizoma et Radix* (Qiang Huo), *Cinnamomi Ramulus* (Gui Zhi), *Angelicae Dahuricae Radix* (Bai Zhi), *Clematidis Radix et Rhizoma* (Wei Ling Xian) and *Chuanxiong Rhizoma* (Chuan Xiong) to dispel wind, dredge collaterals and stop pain; for

2.2 分型论治

2.2.1 行痹

证候：肢体关节酸痛，游走不定，关节屈伸不利，或见恶风、发热等表证。苔薄白，脉浮。

治法：祛风通络，散寒除湿。

方药：防风汤。常用：防风、秦艽祛风除湿，通络止痛；麻黄、杏仁散寒宣肺，达邪外出；葛根解肌祛邪；赤茯苓淡渗湿邪；当归能养血活血，舒络柔筋；生姜、甘草、大枣和中调营。

加减：酸痛以肩肘等上肢为主者，可选用羌活、桂枝、白芷、威灵仙、川芎祛风通络止痛；酸痛以膝踝等下肢关节为主者，选加独活、川牛膝、木瓜、萆薢通经活络，祛湿止痛；酸痛以腰背关节

soreness and pain in the lower limbs such as knees and ankles, add *Angelicae Pubescentis Radix* (Du Huo), *Cyathulae Radix* (Chuan Niu Xi), *Chaenomelis Fructus* (Mu Gua) and *Dioscoreae Hypoglaucae Rhizoma* (Bi Xie) to dredge meridian; *Cibotii Rhizoma* (Gou Ji), and activate collatrals, eliminate dampness and stop pain; for soreness and pain mainly in the waist, back and joints due to kidney-qi deficiency, add moderately *Cibotii Rhizoma* (Gou Ji), *Eucommiae Cortex* (Du Zhong), *Epimedii Folium* (Yin Yang Huo), *Morindae Officinalis Radix* (Ba Ji Tian) and *Dipsaci Radix* (Xu Duan) to warm and supplement kidney-qi; for swollen joints, aversion to wind, thin yellow tongue fur, which stands for heat transformation and complication of cold and heat, use *Cinnamon Twig, Peony, and Anemarrhena Decoction* (Gui Zhi Shao Yao Zhi Mu Tang) as the basis to warm and cool at the same time.

为主者，多为肾气虚，酌加狗脊、杜仲、淫羊藿、巴戟天、续断等温补肾气；若见关节肿大、怕冷畏风、苔薄黄，为邪有化热之象，寒热错杂，治当温凉并用，桂枝芍药知母汤主之。

2.2.2 Painful Bi Syndrome

Manifestations: Pain in joints in fixed spots, sharp pain that aggravates with cold and that is relieved with warmth, difficult bending and stretching, no redness and hotness in the pain spots but coldness; thin white tongue fur; stringy taut pulse or deep retarded stringy pulse.

Treatment: To warm the meridians to dispel cold, expel wind and eliminate dampness.

Formulas and Herbs: *Aconite Main Tuber Decoction* (Wu Tou Tang), usually composed of *Aconiti Radix* (Chuan Wu) to expel pathogenic cold and stop pain with its remarkable acrid and heat nature, *Ephedrae Herba* (Ma Huang) to disperse and expel exterior pathogenic cold; *Paeoniae Radix Alba*

2.2.2 痛痹

证候：肢体关节疼痛，痛有定处，疼痛剧烈，遇寒痛增，得温痛减，关节不可屈伸，痛处不红不热，常有冷感，舌苔薄白，脉弦紧或沉迟而弦。

治法：温经散寒，祛风除湿。

方药：乌头汤。常用：川乌大辛大热，驱寒邪、止痹痛；麻黄发散驱逐偏于在表之寒邪；白芍药、甘草缓急止痛；黄芪益气固卫，并能利血通痹。

(Bai Shao Yao) and *Glycyrrhizae Radix et Rhizoma* (Gan Cao) to relieve urgent pain; *Astragali Radix* (Huang Qi) to bloost qi and consolidate Wei (Defense) Phase as well as activate blood and remove blockage.

Modification: For cool joints and sharp pain, add *Aconm Lateralis Radix Praeparata* (Fu Zi), *Zingiberis Rhizoma* (Gan Jiang), *Cinnamomi Ramulus* (Gui Zhi) and *Asari Radix et Rhizoma* (Xi Xin) to warm meridians, disperse cold and stop pain; for cold obstructing and phlegm congealing with the symptoms of numbness, add *Pinelliae Rhizoma* (Ban Xia), *Cinnamomi Ramulus* (Gui Zhi) and *Arisaema cum Bile* (Dan Nan Xing).

加减: 若关节发凉,疼痛剧烈,可加附子、细辛、桂枝、干姜温经散寒止痛;若寒阻痰凝,兼见麻木,配半夏、桂枝、胆南星。

2. 2. 3　Fixed Bi Syndrome

2. 2. 3　着痹

Manifestations: Soreness and pain in the limb joints, heaviness, or swollen in the affected area, heavy hands and feet, inhibited movement, numbness; white greasy tongue fur; soft slow pulse.

证候: 肢体关节酸痛、重着,或见患处肿胀,手足沉重,活动不利,肌肤麻木不仁。苔白腻,脉濡缓。

Treatment: To eliminate dampness and dredge colleterals; dispel wind and disperse cold.

治法: 除湿通络,祛风散寒。

Formulas and Herbs: Coicis Decoction (Yi Yi Ren Tang), usually composed of *Coicis Semen* (Yi Yi Ren) to eliminate dampness with its sweet and bland nature, relax sinews and harmonize vessels; *Notopterygii Rhizoma et Radix* (Qiang Huo), *Angelicae Pubescentis Radix* (Du Huo) and *Saposhnikoviae Radix*(Fang Feng) to expel wind to eliminate dampness; *Atractylodis Rhizoma* (Cang Zhu) to strengthen the spleen to eliminate dampness; *Ephedrae Herba* (Ma Huang), *Cinnamomi Ramulus* (Gui Zhi) and *Aconiti Radix* Praeperata (Zhi Chuan Wu) to warm meridians and eliminate cold, dispel dampness and stop pain; *Angelicae Sinensis Radix*

方药: 薏苡仁汤。常用:薏苡仁甘淡利湿、疏筋和脉;羌活、独活、防风祛风胜湿;苍术健脾除湿;麻黄、桂枝、制川乌温经散寒,祛湿止痛;当归、川芎养血活血;生姜、甘草健脾和中。

(Dang Gui) and *Chuanxiong Rhizoma* (Chuan Xiong) to nourish and activate blood; *Zingiberis Rhizoma Recens* (Sheng Jiang) and *Glycyrrhizae Radix et Rhizoma* (Gan Cao) to strengthen the spleen and harmonize zhong jiao.

Modification: For aversion to cold, fever, restlessness and pain in the body due to exterior pathogenic wind and dampness, subtract *Aconiti Radix* (Chuan Wu) and *Angelicae Sinensis Radix* (Dang Gui), add *Angelicae Dahuricae Radix* (Bai Zhi) and *Pogostemonis Herba* (Huo Xiang) to relieve exterior symptoms and resolve dampness; for numbness, add *Liquidambaris Fructus* (Lu Lu Tong) and *Siegesbeckiae Herba* (Xi Xian Cao); for swollen joints, add *Piperis Kadsurae Caulis* (Hai Feng Teng), *Dioscoreae Hypoglaucae Rhizoma* (Bi Xie) and *Akebiae Caulis* (Mu Tong); for difficult in urination, add *Alismatis Rhizoma* (Ze Xie) and *Plantaginis Semen* (Che Qian Zi); for prolonged blockage without remarkable wind-damp-cold, use *Impediment-Alleviating Decoction* (Juan Bi Tang), a fundamental formula for wind-cold-damp impediment.

加减：若恶寒发热、身烦痛为风湿在表，可去川乌、当归，加白芷、藿香解表化湿；若肌肤麻木不仁，加路路通、豨莶草；若关节肿胀加海风藤、萆薢、木通；若小便不利加泽泻、车前子；若患者久痹风湿寒偏盛不明显，可用蠲痹汤作为风寒湿痹通用的基础方。

2.2.4 Bi Syndrome Due to Wind-damp-heat

2.2.4 风湿热痹

Manifestations: Pain in limb joints, redness and buring pain in painful area, swelling, sharp pain which alleviates with cold and refuses touch, spasm of muscles and vessels which is light at daytime and serious at night, along with fever, thirst, irritiation; red tongue with yellow tongue fur; rolling rapid pulse.

证候：肢体关节疼痛，痛处焮红灼热、肿胀，疼痛剧烈，得冷稍舒，痛不可触，筋脉拘急，日轻夜重，兼有发热、口渴、心烦等全身症状，舌红，苔黄，脉滑数。

Treatment: To clear away heat and eliminate dampness, eliminate blockage and dredge collaterals.

治法：清热除湿，宣痹通络。

Formulas and Herbs: *White Tiger Decoction*

方药：白虎加桂枝汤或

(Bai Hu Tang) and *Cinnamon-Twig Decoction* (Gui Zhi Tang) or *Impediment-Dispersing Decoction* (Xuan Bi Tang), usually composed of *Gypsum Fibrosum Fibrosum* (Shi Gao) and *Anemarrhenae Rhizoma* (Zhi Mu) to clear away heat and resolve irritation, *Cinnamomi Ramulus* (Gui Zhi) to disperse wind, relieve muscles and dredge collaterals; *Stephaniae Tetrandrae Radix* (Fang Ji), *Armeniacae Semen Amaru* (Ku Xing Ren), *Coicis Semen* (Yi Yi Ren), *Talcum* (Hua Shi), rice bean, *Pinelliae Rhizoma* (Ban Xia) and *Faeces Bombycis* (Can Sha) to clear away heat and promote diuresis, dredge collaterals and eliminate blockage; *Forsythiae Fructus* (Lian Qiao) and *Gardeniae Fructus* (Zhi Zi) to clear away heat and eliminate dampness.

宣痹汤。常用石膏、知母清热除烦；桂枝疏风解肌通络；防己、杏仁、薏苡仁、滑石、赤小豆、半夏、蚕砂清利湿热，通络宣痹；连翘、山栀清热利湿。

Modification: For heat excess consuming yin with thirst and dry mouth, add *Scrophulariae Radix* (Yuan Shen), *Ophiopogonis Radix* (Mai Men Dong) and *Rehmannia Radix* (Sheng Di Huang) to clear away heat, nourish yin and engender fluid; for predominace of heat over dampness, add *Dioscoreae Hypoglaucae Rhizoma* (Bi Xie) and *Phellodendri Chinensis Cortex* (Huang Bo); for red and swollen joints, sharp pain, spasm of muscles that gets worse at night, excessive heat, irritation, thirst, red tongue with little fluid, stringy rapid pulse which means heat-toxin has made way deep into sinews and bones, use *Cornu Rhinoceri Asiatici Powder* (Xi Jiao San) to clear away heat to detoxify and cool blood to stop bleeding; for as heat blockage due to invasion of pathongenic wind-cold-dampness which, adepressed for long, has been turned into heat, therefore when pathogenic factors has just turned into heat along with wind-cold-damp, use *modified*

加减：热盛伤阴，症见口渴心烦者，加玄参、麦门冬、生地黄以清热滋阴生津；热重于湿者，可加萆薢、黄柏；若见关节红肿，疼痛剧烈，筋脉拘急，入夜尤甚，壮热烦渴，舌红少津，脉弦数者为热毒化火深入筋骨，用犀角散清热解毒，凉血止痛；热痹亦可由风寒湿邪内侵，郁久化热而成，若邪初化热仍兼有风寒湿邪，可用麻黄连翘赤小豆汤加味。

Ephedra, Forsythia, and Rice Bean Decoction (Ma Huang Lian Qiao Chi Xiao Dou Tang).

2.2.5 Bi Syndrome Due to Phlegm and Stasis

Manifestations: Prolonged Bi Syndrome, stabbing pain in muscles and joints in unfixed spots, or purple dark skin joints and arthrocele, even joints stiffness with malformation, difficult bending and stretching with hard noids and macules; dark purple tongue with white greasy tongue fur; fine uneven pulse.

Treatment: To resolve phlegm and remove stasis; eliminate blockage and dredge collaterals.

Formulas and Herbs: *Peach Pit and Safflower Decoction* (Tao Hong Yin), usually composed of *Persicae Semen* (Tao Ren) and *Carthami Flos* (Hong Hua) to activate blood and remove stasis, free colleterals and stop pain; *Angelicae Sinensis Radix* (Dang Gui) and *Chuanxiong Rhizoma* (Chuan Xiong) to help to remove stasis and dredge collaterals; *Clematidis Radix et Rhizoma* (Wei Ling Xian) to eliminate dampness, dredge collaterals and remove blockage.

Modification: For phlegm-stasis turning into heat with thirst and dark urine, add *Forsythiae Fructus* (Lian Qiao) and *Moutan Cortex* (Mu Dan Pi); for excessive phlegm-turbid, add *Pinelliae Rhizoma* (Ban Xia) and *Arisaema cum Bile* (Dan Nan Xing) to expel phlegm, break up clots and strengthen resolving of phlegm; for remarkable blood stasis and congealing, add moderately some expelling herbs of insects, such as *Zaocys* (Wu Shao She) and *Scorpio* (Quan Xie).

2.2.6 Bi Syndrome Due to Deficiency of Qi and Blood

Maninfestations: Prolonged blockage with no

2.2.5 痰瘀痹阻

证候：痹证日久，肌肉关节刺痛，固定不移，或关节肌肤紫暗、肿胀，甚则强直畸形，屈伸不利，有硬结、瘀斑。舌质紫暗，苔白腻，脉细涩。

治法：化痰行瘀，蠲痹通络。

方药：桃红饮。常用：桃仁、红花活血化瘀，通络止痛；当归、川芎化瘀加强通络之力；威灵仙祛湿通络，除痹痛。

加减：痰瘀化热伴口渴、尿赤者，加连翘、牡丹皮；痰浊偏盛者，可配半夏、胆南星祛痰散结，加强化痰之力；瘀血凝滞较重者酌加虫类搜剔药，如乌蛸蛇、全蝎等。

2.2.6 气血亏虚

证候：痹证日久不愈，时

cure, better or worse at times, soreness and pain in joints which become most tense when it comes to bending and stretching or even sinew and muscle contracture, emaciation, lassitude and fatigue; short breath, spontaneous sweating, dizziness, little intake, loose stool, dull skin; pale tongue with thin tongue fur; fine powerless pulse.

轻时重，骨节酸痛，而以屈伸时为甚，甚则筋肉挛缩，伴形瘦神疲乏力，气短，自汗，头晕，食少便溏，皮肤不仁无光泽。舌淡苔薄，脉细无力。

Treatment: To regulate and supplement qi and blood; activate blood and dredge collaterals.

治法： 调补气血，活血通络。

Formulas and Herbs: Astragal, Cinnamon and Five Agents Decoction (Huang Qi Gui Zhi Wu Wei Tang), usually composed of *Ginseng Radix et Rhizoma* (Ren Shen), *Astragali Radix* (Huang Qi) to boost qi and consolidate Wei (Defensive) Phase; *Schisandrae Chinensis Fructus* (Wu Wei Zi) and *Ophiopogonis Radix* (Mai Men Dong) to nourish yin; *Angelicae Sinensis Radix* (Dang Gui) and *Paeoniae Radix Alba* (Bai Shao Yao) and *Cinnamomi Ramulus* (Gui Zhi) to activate blood and dredge collaterals, accompanied by *Zingiberis Rhizoma Recens* (Sheng Jiang); *Jujubae Fructus* (Da Zao) to harmonize spleen and stomach; *Glycyrrhizae Radix et Rhizoma* (Gan Cao) to harmonize all the ingredients.

方药： 黄芪桂枝五物汤。常用：人参、黄芪益气固卫；麦门冬、五味子养阴；当归、白芍药、桂枝活血通络；佐以生姜、大枣调和脾胃；甘草调和诸药。

Modification: For remarable qi deficiency, use in great amounts of *Ginseng Radix et Rhizoma* (Ren Shen) and *Astragali Radix* (Huang Qi); for remarkable blood deficiency, add *Rehmanniae Radix Praeparata* (Shu Di Huang), *Spatholobi Caulis* (Ji Xue Teng) and *Chuanxiong Rhizoma* (Chuan Xiong).

加减： 偏于气虚者，可重用黄芪、人参；偏于血虚者，加熟地黄、鸡血藤、川芎。

2.2.7 Bi Syndrome Due to Deficiency of the Liver and Kidney

2.2.7 肝肾两虚

Manifestations: Prolonged Bi blockage with no cure, pain in the body and joints, difficult bending

证候： 痹证日久不愈，肢体、关节疼痛，屈伸不利，关

and stretching, enlarged and stiff joints and malformation, even muscle atrophy, sinews and vessels contracture, soreness in the waist and knees, spontaneous sweating, night sweating, irritatation, dry mouth or aversion to cold and physical cold; red or pale tongue; fine deep pulse or fine rapid pulse.

节肿大僵硬、变形，甚至肌肉萎缩，筋脉拘急，伴腰膝酸软，自汗盗汗，心烦口干，或畏寒肢冷。舌质红或淡，脉沉细或细数。

Treatment: To nourish and supplement the liver and kidney, activate blood and dredge collaterals.

治法：培补肝肾，活血通络。

Formulas and Herbs: *Pubescent Angelica and Mistletoe Decoction* (Du Huo Ji Sheng Tang), usually composed of *Angelicae Pubescentis Radix* (Du Huo) to dispel wind and dampness, *Taxilli Herba* (Sang Ji Sheng) supplement the liver and kidney, empower sinews and bones; *Saposhnikoviae Radix* (Fang Feng) and *Gentianae Macrophyllae Radix* (Qin Jiao) to dispel wind, resolve dampness and stop pain; *Cinnamomi Ramulus* (Gui Zhi) and *Asari Radix et Rhizoma* (Xi Xin) to warm meridians and dredge collaterals; *Achyranthis Bidentatae Radix* (Niu Xi) and *Eucommiae Cortex* (Du Zhong) to supplement and invigorate the liver and kidney; *Ginseng Radix et Rhizoma* (Ren Shen), *Poria* (Fu Ling) and *Glycyrrhizae Radix et Rhizoma* (Gan Cao) to invigorate the spleen and boost qi; *Angelicae Sinensis Radix* (Dang Gui), *Chuanxiong Rhizoma* (Chuan Xiong), *Rehmannia Radix* (Sheng Di Huang) and *Paeoniae Radix Alba* (Bai Shao Yao) to harmonize Ying (Nutrient) Phase and nourish blood, *Glycyrrhizae Radix et Rhizoma* (Gan Cao) to harmonize all the ingredients.

方药：独活寄生汤。常用：独活祛风湿，桑寄生补肝肾、强筋骨；防风、秦艽祛风化湿止痛；桂枝、细辛温经通络；牛膝、杜仲补益肝肾；人参、茯苓、甘草健脾益气；当归、川芎、生地黄、白芍药和营养血；甘草调和诸药。

Modification: For yin deficiency of the liver and kidney, add *Placenta Major Bollus* (He Che Da Zao Wan); for kidney-yang deficiency, add Yang-Harmonizing Decoction (Yang He Tang); for tense

加减：若肝肾偏于阴虚者，合用河车大造丸；偏于肾阳虚者，合用阳和汤；关节疼痛拘挛者加木瓜、鸡血藤、地

joints with pain, add *Chaenomelis Fructus* (Mu Gua), *Spatholobi Caulis* (Ji Xue Teng), *Pheretima* (Di Long), *Scolopendra* (Wu Gong) and *Zaocys* (Wu Shao She); for prolonged blockage hidden in the zang-fu organs, in particular, in the heart with symptoms such as palpitation, short breath which aggravates with movements, lusterless face, pale tongue, deficient rapid pulse or knot and intermitten pulse, it is better to boost qi and nourish heart, warm yang to restore vessels with modified *Honeyed Liquorice Decoction* (Zhi Gan Cao Tang).

龙、蜈蚣、乌梢蛇；痹证日久内舍于脏腑，以心痹多见，若见心悸短气、动则尤甚，面色少华，舌质淡，脉虚数或结代，治以益气养心、温阳复脉，用炙甘草汤加减。

Flaccidity Syndrome

痿　证

Flaccidity Syndrome refers to a type of diseases caused by zang-fu organ injuries and poorly nourished body, sinews and vessels, characterized by flaccidity, weakness, powerlessness or muscle atrophy.

痿证主要是因脏腑内伤，肢体筋脉失养，而致肢体筋脉弛缓，软弱无力，日久不用或伴有肌肉萎缩的一类病证。

1　Etiology and Pathogenesis

1　病因病机

Flaccidity Syndrome is mainly caused by exogenous affection of pathogenic warmth, heat and toxin, spiritual and emotional injury, gluttony, overstrain, congenital defects, indulgence in sex, falling and injury, consumption due to prolonged illness, which leads to damage of the five fu-organs, causing deficiency of qi and blood, consumption of qi and blood. Sinews and vessels in body fail to be nourished, leading to flaccidity.

痿证的发生主要是由于外感温热邪毒、内伤情志、饱食劳倦、先天不足、房室不节、跌打损伤、久病耗损，致使五脏受损，精血不足，气血亏耗，肢体筋脉失养而发病。

1.1　Consumption of Fluid Due to Lung-heat and Undistribution of Fluid

1.1　肺热津伤，津液不布

The lung is a delicate organ that favors moisture and averts dryness. It is prone tobe attacked by pathogenic factors. When the body is attacked by

肺为娇脏，喜润恶燥，不耐邪侵。肌体感受温热邪毒，高热不退或病后余热燔

pathogenic warmth, heat and toxin, it will generate high fever or even the remaining heat after recovery will injure body fluid and qi, and attack the lung. When lung is burned and scorched by heat, it fails to distribute body fluid to moisten the five zang-organs, leading to impairment of nourishment of sinews and vessels, causing flaccidity.

灼,伤津耗气,上犯于肺,每致肺热熏灼,肺热叶焦不能布散津液以润泽五脏,筋脉失其濡养而成痿证。

1.2 Unsmooth Flow of Qi and Blood Due to Spreading Dampness and Heat

Living in damp places for long, or walking in rain will affect pathogenic dampness. If it accumulates in the body for long enough to turn into heat, obstructing activity of Ying (Nutreint) qi and blood. When it prolongs, it will inhibit the flow of qi and blood, causing impairment of moisturization and nourishment of sinews and vessels that become floppy, leading to flaccidity. Or over intake of sweet greasy spicy food will damage the spleen and stomach, engender damp-heat which spreads to sinews and vessels and inhibit the flow of qi and blood, causing poor nourishment of sinews and vessel, leading to flaccidity.

1.2 湿热浸淫,气血不运

久居湿地,冒雨涉水,感受湿邪,湿邪积聚日久,郁而生热,营血运行受阻。久则气血运行不畅,筋脉失于濡养则弛缓不用,成为痿证。或过食肥甘厚味、辛辣之品,损伤脾运,湿热内生,浸淫筋脉,血行不畅,筋脉失养而为痿证。

1.3 Failure of the Spleen and Stomach to Transport Essence Due to Their Deficiency

Innate weakness of the spleen and stomach or improper diet that hurts the spleen and stomach, or deficiency and damage of middle-qi due to prolonged illness can lead to dysfunction of the spleen and stomach to accept, transfer and transport, causing inadequent sources of qi and blood transformation, which fails to moisturize the five organs and support qi and blood flow. Then poor nourishment of sinews and vessels results in flaccidity.

1.3 脾胃虚弱,精微不输

素体脾胃虚弱或饮食不节伤及脾胃,或久病成虚,中气受损导致脾胃受纳运化功能失常,气血生化之源不足,无以濡养五脏,运行气血以致筋脉失养而成痿证。

1.4 Withered Marrow and Flaccid Sinews Due to Deficiency of the Liver and Kidney

Innate deficiency of the liver and kidney or indulgence in sex will lead to consumption and damage of the essence and blood, causing the sinews and bones lacking in moisturization and nourishement, leading to flaccidity.

1.4 肝肾亏虚，髓枯筋痿

若平素肾虚或房劳太过，久病导致精血亏损，筋脉失其濡养而产生痿证。

1.5 Obstruction of Collaterals and Blood Flow Due to Blood Stasis

Falling and injury, or postpartum discharge that remains and goes downward into the waist and knees, or prolonged illness invading deep into collaterals which lead to stagnation of blood and qi, resulting in unsmooth flow of blood, can make the sinews and vessels of the limbs lacking in moisturization and nourishment, leading to flaccidity.

1.5 瘀血阻络，血行不畅

跌仆损伤；或产后恶露未尽，留于腰膝；或久病入络，气血瘀阻，血液运行不畅，四肢筋脉失其濡养而发为痿证。

Flaccidity lies in the sinews, vessels and muscles, and involves the lung, stomach, liver and kidney. Deficiency of the liver is the primary while lung heat is the secondary. Internal injury takes up the mojortity. Heat type is more than cold type. During the onset stage, affection of exogenous pathogenic warmth and damp-heat without remarkable damage and consumption of the yin-fluid belongs to excess type. Consumption of fluid due to prolonged illness that leads to damage of yin-blood of the liver and kidney belongs to deficiency type transformed from excess or complication of both types. If internal injuries are due to weakness of the spleen and stomach, deficiency of the liver and kidney, injury and deficiency of qi, blood and fluid, then it is mostly of deficiency type, which along with phlegm and stasis, can show up as primary deficiency and secondary excess.

痿证病位在筋脉、肌肉，涉及脏腑以肺胃肝肾为主。本病以肾虚为本，肺热为标，内伤为多，热多寒少。初起外感温邪，湿热所致者，阴津亏耗不甚，以邪热偏重故属实证；病久津亏液伤，肝肾阴血耗损，则由实转虚，或虚实夹杂。若为内伤致病多由脾胃虚弱，肝肾亏虚，气血津液虚损引起，临床则以虚证为主，但可夹痰、夹瘀，表现本虚标实证。

2 Syndrome Differentiation and Treatment

2.1 Key Points of Syndrome Differentiation

For pattern identification of flaccidity, it is very important to identify the organ. Fever, dry throat, choking and coughing or wilted limbs after fever is due to the lung. Wiltled limbs, little intake, loose stool is due to the stomach. Wilted lower limbs, soreness in the waist and knees, dizziness, tinnitus or irregular menstruation, premature ejaculation and spermatorrhea is due to the liver and kidney. Then examine the primary deficiency and secondary excess. Affection of pathogenic warmth, heat and toxin or spreading damp-heat, sudden attack and other exogenous affection symptoms such as fever are more likely to be excess. However, as pathogenic heat can consume fluid and injure qi, therefore, during the onset stage, it might be complication of deficiency and excess. Insidious attack, prolonged illness without cure due to innate weakness. Yin-deficiency of the liver and kidney, hereditary factors or indulgence in sex, or innate weak spleen and stomach are likely to be deficiency type. However, if there are accompanying phlegm, stasis and heat, it is excess in deficiency and complication of both types. As for the treatment, for deficiency type, strengthen healthy qi and supplement deficiency. For liver-and-kidney deficiency, nourish the liver and kidney. For weak spleen and stomach, boost qi and strengthen the spleen. For excess type, dispel pathogenic factors and harmonize the collaterals. For lung-heat injuring fluid, clear away heat and moisten dryness. For spreading damp-heat, clear away heat and eliminate dampness. For stasis

2 辨证论治

2.1 辨治要点

痿证辨证，重在辨脏腑病位。凡病起发热、咽干、呛咳或热病后出现肢体痿软不用，病变多在肺；若四肢痿弱无力、食少、便溏，脏腑病位多在脾胃；若下肢痿软无力，伴腰膝酸软、头晕、耳鸣或月经不调、早泄、遗精者，病位多在肝肾。其次当审标本虚实，感受温热毒邪或湿热浸淫者，大多起病急，病起可伴见发热等外感症状，多属实证，但热邪易耗津伤气，疾病早期亦可见虚实夹杂。若起病隐袭，经久不愈，主要病因为先天不足，遗传因素或房劳过度导致肝肾阴虚或素体脾胃虚弱，多属虚证，但多又夹痰、夹瘀、夹热，出现虚中有实，虚实错杂之证。治疗虚证以扶正补虚为主，肝肾亏虚者宜滋养肝肾，脾胃虚弱者宜益气健脾。实证宜祛邪和络、肺热伤津者宜清热润燥，湿热浸淫者宜清热利湿，瘀阻脉络者宜活血行瘀，虚实兼夹者当兼顾之。

obstructing vessels and collaterals, activate blood and remove stasis. For complication, treat both.

2.2 Therapeutic Methods for Different Types

2.2.1 Injury of Fluid Due to Lung-heat

Manifestations: Fever at the beginning or wilted limbs right after heat diseases, dry skin, chocking cough with little phlegm, irritatation, thirst, discomfort and dry throat, dark short urine, constipation; red tongue with yellow tongue fur; fine rapid pulse.

Treatment: To clear away heat and moisten dryness, nourish yin and moisten sinews.

Formulas and Herbs: *Dryness-Eliminating and Lung-Rescuing Decoction* (Qing Zao Jiu Fei Tang), usually composed of *Gypsum Fibrosum Fibrosum* (Shi Gao) to clear away dryness and heat of lung, *Mori Folium* (Sang Ye) to clear away and disperse the lung-heat; *Ophiopogonis Radix* (Mai Men Dong), *Asini Corii Colla* (E Jiao) and *Cannabis Fructus* (Huo Ma Ren) to moisten the lung and nourish yin in case dry-heat consumes fluid and injuries yin; *Armeniacae Semen Amaru* (Ku Xing Ren) and *Eriobotryae Folium* (Pi Pa Ye) to disperse the lung and activate qi and distribute fluid over the body; *Ginseng Radix et Rhizoma* (Ren Shen), *Glycyrrhizae Radix et Rhizoma* (Gan Cao) to boost lung qi.

Modification: For blood in phlegm, add *Lilii Bulbus* (Bai He), Fresh Rehmannia Decoction (Sheng Di Huang Tang) and *Scrophulariae Radix* (Xuan Shen); for fever retreated, poor appetite and remarkable dry mouth and throat that stands for yin injury of the lung and stomach, use *Stomach-Benefiting Decoction* (Yi Wei Tang) and add

2.2 分型论治

2.2.1 肺热伤津

证候：病起发热，或温热病后突然出现肢体软弱无力，皮肤枯燥，呛咳少痰，心烦口渴，咽干不利，小便短赤，大便秘结。舌质红，苔黄，脉细数。

治法：清热润燥，养阴濡筋。

方药：清燥救肺汤。常用：石膏清肺金燥热；桑叶清宣肺热；麦门冬、阿胶、火麻仁润肺养阴，以防燥热耗津伤阴；杏仁、枇杷叶宣肺利气，布津于周身；人参、甘草益肺气。

加减：若痰中带血者加百合、生地黄、玄参；若身热已退、食欲欠佳、口燥咽干较甚者，证属肺胃阴伤，宜用益胃汤加薏苡仁、谷芽、石斛；若高热、口渴、汗多为热蒸气分加金银花、连翘，重用石

Coicis Semen (Yi Yi Ren), *Setariae Fructus Germinatus* (Gu Ya) and *Dendrobii Caulis* (Shi Hu); for high fever, thirst and sweating due to steaming heat, add *Lonicerae Japonicae Flos* (Jin Yin Hua), *Forsythiae Fructus* (Lian Qiao) and use *Gypsum Fibrosum Fibrosum* (Shi Gao) in great amount; for choking cough with little phlegm, add *Trichosanthis Fructus* (Gua Lou) and *Fritillariae Cirrhosae Bulbus* (Bei Mu) to cleanse, moisten and disperse the lung; for epidemic pathogenic factors injuring the lung, leading to flaccidity, use *Rhinoceros Horn and Platycodi Decoction* (Xi Jiao Jie Geng Tang).

膏;若呛咳少痰加全瓜蒌、川贝清润肃肺;若疫毒伤肺致痿者,可用犀角桔梗汤。

2. 2. 2 Damp-heat Spreading

Manifestations: Wilted limbs, general heaviness, fatigue or numbness, slight edema particualarly in lower limbs, or steaming heat at ankles, or fever, stomach oppression, dark urine and rought hot pain during urination; white greasy tongue fur; soft rapid pulse.

Treatment: To clear away heat and eliminate dampness, dredge sinews and vessels.

Formulas and Herbs: Modified *Two Wonderful Drugs Powder* (Er Miao San), usually composed of *Phellodendri Chinensis Cortex* (Huang Bo) to clear away heat; *Atractylodis Rhizoma* (Cang Zhu) to dry dampness, clear away damp-heat in xia jiao without consuming yin; *Achyranthis Bidentatae Radix* (Niu Xi), *Dioscoreae Hypoglaucae Rhizoma* (Bi Xie) and *Stephaniae Tetrandrae Radix* Tetrandrae (Fang Ji) to induce damp-heat downward, *Angelicae Sinensis Radix* (Dang Gui) to activate blood and nourish blood, *Testudinis Carapax et Plastrum* (Gui Jia) to nourish yin and subjugate yang, supplement blood and strengthen bones.

2. 2. 2 湿热浸淫

证候: 肢体痿软,身体重着、倦怠或肢体麻木、微肿,以下肢多见,或足胫热蒸,或有发热、脘闷、小便赤涩热痛。苔白腻,脉濡数。

治法: 清热利湿,通利筋脉。

方药: 加味二妙散。常用:黄柏清热,苍术燥湿,共奏清化下焦湿热,而又不伤阴之效;牛膝、萆薢、防己导湿热下行;当归活血养血;龟甲滋阴潜阳,补血健骨。

Modification: For dampness excess, oppression and discomfort in the chest and stomach, heavy body, add *Magnoliae Officinalis Cortex* (Hou Pu), *Coicis Semen* (Yi Yi Ren) and *Citri Reticulatae Pericarpium* (Chen Pi) to regulate qi and resolve dampness; for summer and rain season, add moderately *Pogostemonis Herba* (Huo Xiang) and *Eupatorii Herba* (Pei Lan) to resolve turbidity with aromatizatin, stenghten the spleen and expel dampness; for emaciation, extreme heat in the soles, irritation, reddish tongue tips and sides or peeled tongue fur in the middle, fine rapid pulse, which means damp-heat consuming yin, subtract *Atractylodis Rhizoma* (Cang Zhu) and add *Dioscoreae Rhizoma* (Shan Yao), *Coicis Semen* (Yi Yi Ren), *Rehmannia Radix* (Sheng Di Huang) and *Ophiopogonis Radix* (Mai Men Dong) to clear away heat and nourish yin.

加减：若湿盛，胸脘痞闷，肢体困重者，可加厚朴、薏苡仁、陈皮理气化湿；长夏雨季酌加藿香、佩兰芳香化浊、健脾除湿；如形瘦、两足奇热、心烦、舌边尖红或中剥无苔、脉细数，此为湿热伤阴，上方去苍术加山药、薏苡仁、生地黄、麦门冬清热养阴。

2. 2. 3　Deficiency of Spleen and Stomach

Manifestations: Wilted limbs that goes worse, even barylalia, difficult to breath and swallow, floppy eyelid, innate little intake and loose stool, distention in the abdomen, short breath, lassitude; white thin tongue fur; fine pulse.

Treatment: To strengthen the spleen and nourish the stomach, boost qi and engender fluid.

Formulas and Herbs: *Ginseng, Poria and Atractylodes Powder* (Shen Ling Bai Zhu San), usually composed of *Ginseng Radix et Rhizoma* (Ren Shen), *Atractylodis Macrocephalae Rhizoma* (Bai Zhu) and *Poria* (Fu Ling) to strengthen the spleen and eliminate dampness; *Dioscoreae Rhizoma* (Shan Yao) and *Nelumbinis Semen* (Lian Zi) to strengthen the spleen, boost qi and stop diarrhea; *Lablab*

2. 2. 3　脾胃亏虚

证候：肢体痿软无力逐渐加重，甚则语言不清，呼吸吞咽困难，眼睑肌肉松弛，平素食少便溏，腹胀，气短，神疲。苔薄白，脉细。

治法：健脾养胃，益气生津。

方药：参苓白术散。常用：人参、白术、茯苓益气健脾渗湿；山药、莲子肉健脾益气止泻；扁豆、薏苡仁健脾渗湿；砂仁和胃，行气化滞；桔梗载药上行保肺；炙甘草健脾和中。

Semen Album (Bian Dou) and *Coicis Semen* (Yi Yi Ren) to invigorate the spleen and eliminate dampness; *Amomi Fructus* (Sha Ren) to harmonize the stomach, regulate qi and remove stagnation; *Platycodi Radix*(Jie Geng) to carry ingredients upward to protect the lung; *Glycyrrhizae Radix et Rhizoma Praeparata* (Zhi Gan Cao) to strengthen the spleen and harmonize zhong jiao.

Modification: For deficiency of middle qi, diarrhea for long and dropping annus, use *Center-Supplementing qi-Boosting Decoction* (Bu Zhong Yi Qi Tang) to raise yang and improve the functional activities of qi and viscera; for fat patients with much phlegm, use *Six Nobles Decoction* (Liu Jun Zi Tang) to supplement the spleen and resolve phlegm; for heat injuring the stomach and yin with symptoms such as dry mouth and throat, dry stool and hiccup, use *Jade Lady Decoction* (Yu Nü Jian) to invigorate the stomach and engender fluid; for weakness due to prolonged illness, defieciency of qi and blood, use in great amouts *Dioscoreae Rhizoma* (Shan Yao), *Atractylodis Macrocephalae Rhizoma* (Bai Zhu) and add *Astragali Radix* (Huang Qi) and *Angelicae Sinensis Radix* (Dang Gui).

加减: 若中气不足,久泻脱肛,可用补中益气汤升阳举陷;若肥人痰多可用六君子汤补脾化痰;若热伤胃阴,口燥咽干、大便干结、干呕可用玉女煎益胃生津;若久病体虚、气血亏损,重用党参、山药、白术,加黄芪、当归。

2. 2. 4 Deficiency of the Liver and Kidney

Manifestations: Slow attack, wilted lower limbs, weak and wilted knees and ankles, unable to stand long, even unable to walk, soreness in the waist and back, dizzy vision and hair loss, spermatorrhea, premature ejaculation, enuresis; red tongue with little tongue fur; fine rapid pulse.

Treatment: To supplement and nourish the liver and kidney; nourish yin and clear away heat.

Formulas and Herbs: Modified *Tiger Diving*

2. 2. 4 肝肾虚损

证候: 起病缓慢,下肢痿软无力,膝胫痿软,不能久立,甚则步履全废,腰背酸软,或伴目眩发落,遗精早泄,遗尿。舌红少苔,脉细数。

治法: 补养肝肾,滋阴清热。

方药: 虎潜丸加减。常

Pills (Hu Qian Wan), usually composed of *Os Tigris* (Hu Gu) [which can be substituted for *Os Bubali* (Shui Niu Gu)] to empower sinews and bones, *Cynomorii Herba* (Suo Yang) to supplement kidney-yang; *Phellodendri Chinensis Cortex* (Huang Bo), *Anemarrhenae Rhizoma* (Zhi Mu), *Rehmanniae Radix Praeparata* (Shu Di Huang), *Testudinis Carapax et Plastrum* (Gui Jia) to nourish yin and subdue fire, supplement yin to cultivate yang; *Angelicae Sinensis Radix* (Dang Gui) and *Paeoniae Radix Alba* (Bai Shao Yao) to nourish blood and soften the liver.

用:虎骨(牛骨代)强壮筋骨;锁阳能补肾阳;黄柏、知母、熟地黄、龟版滋阴降火,补阴配阳;当归、白芍药养血柔肝。

Modification: For remarkable heat, change for *Rehmannia Pills with Six Ingredients* (Liu Wei Di Huang Wan); for prolonged illness consuming yin, which affects yang, with symptoms like aversion to cold, impotence, clear away long urine, pale tongue and fine deep powerless pulse, add moderately Cervi Cornu Sectum (Lu Jiao Pian), *Psoraleae Fructus* (Bu Gu Zhi), *Morindae Officinalis Radix* (Ba Ji Tian), *Cinnamomi Cortex* (Rou Gui), *Aconm Lateralis Radix Praeparata* (Fu Zi) and *Epimedii Folium* (Yin Yang Huo) to supplement the kidney to assist yang, or use *Cervi Cornus Colla* Pills (Lu Jiao Jiao Wan); for lusterless face or sallow yellow complexion, dizziness and palpitation, add *Astragali Radix* (Huang Qi), *Codonopsis Radix* (Dang Shen), *Polygoni Multiflori Radix* (He Shou Wu) and *Angelicae Sinensis Radix* (Dang Gui) to supplement qi and nourish blood.

加减: 若热甚者可改用六味地黄丸;若久病阴损及阳,阴阳共虚,症见畏寒、阳痿、小便清长、舌淡、脉沉细无力,可酌加鹿角片、补骨脂、巴戟天、肉桂、附子、淫羊藿补肾助阳,或用鹿角胶丸;若面色无华或萎黄、头晕心悸,加黄芪、党参、首乌、当归以补气养血。

2.2.5 Stasis Obstructs Vessels and Collaterals

Manifestations: Wilted limbs, numbness, coarse skin, tense and pain sometimes; purple dark tongue with macules, white thin tongue fur; fine uneven

2.2.5 瘀阻脉络

证候: 四肢痿软,麻木不仁,肌肤甲错,时有拘挛痛感,舌质紫暗有瘀斑。苔薄

pulse.

Treatment: To boost qi and nourish ying; activate blood and remove stasis.

Formulas and Herbs: Modified *Yang-Supplementing and Five-Restoring Decoction* (Bu Yang Huan Wu Tang) and *Holy Cure Decoction* (Sheng Yu Tang), usually composed of *Ginseng Radix et Rhizoma* (Ren Shen) and *Astragali Radix* (Huang Qi) to boost qi, *Angelicae Sinensis Radix* (Dang Gui), *Paeoniae Radix Rubra* (Chi Shao Yao), *Rehmanniae Radix Praeparata* (Shu Di Huang) and *Pheretima* (Di Long) to nourish and activate blood and remove stasis, *Persicae Semen* (Tao Ren) and *Carthami Flos* (Hong Hua) to activate blood and remove stasis.

Modification: For remarkable coarse skin and emaciation, add *Rhubarb and Ground Beetle Pills* (Da Huang Zhe Chong Wan); for wilted lower limbs, add *Eucommiae Cortex* (Du Zhong), *Cynomorii Herba* (Suo Yang) and *Taxilli Herba* (Sang Ji Sheng).

白，脉细涩。

治法：益气养营，活血行瘀。

方药：补阳还五汤合圣愈汤加减。常用人参、黄芪补气，当归、熟地黄、赤芍药、地龙养血活血化瘀，桃仁、红花活血行瘀。

加减：肌肤甲错明显、形体消瘦者加大黄䗪虫丸补虚活血；下肢萎软无力，加杜仲、锁阳、桑寄生。

Tremor

Tremor is a type of disease caused by poor nourishment of the sinews and collaterals, and stirring of liver-wind, characterized by head or body shaking and trembling which cannot be controlled consciously.

1 Etiology and Pathogenesis

Themajor causes oftremor are weak constitution due to aging, emotional stress, improper diet and proloned illness without proper nourishment. Its

颤证

颤证是由于各种原因导致筋脉失养，肝风内动，临床以头部或肢体摇动、颤抖，不能自制为主要表现的一种病证。

1 病因病机

颤证的主要病因为年老体虚、情志过极、饮食不节、久病失养。基本病机是肝风

pathogenesis is stirring of liver-wind and poorly nourished sinews and vessels.

内动，筋脉失养。

1.1 Deficiency of Liver and Kidney Due to Weak Constitution and Aging

1.1 年老体虚，肝肾不足

Old age or overstrain will cause deficiency of blood and essence of the liver and kidney, and impairment of nourishment of sinews and collaterals. Or kidney-yang is inadaquent to warm and moisten sinews and bones. Both can lead totremor.

年老之人或劳欲过度，导致肝肾精血亏虚，筋脉失于濡养；或肾阳不足，筋骨不得温润，而成本病。

1.2 Deficiency of Blood and Qi Due to Prolonged Illness With Poor Nourishment

1.2 久病失养，气血亏虚

Prolonged illness without proper nourishment and deficiency of qi and blood leads to impairment of supporting the body, sinews and vessels, leading totremor.

久病失养，气虚血少，不能荣于肢体，筋脉失养，乃成颤证。

1.3 Injury of the Spleen and Stomach Due to Improper Diet

1.3 饮食不节，脾胃损伤

Over eating sweet and greasy food and over drinking will damage the spleen and stomach, which then fail to transform and transport. Dampness accumulates and turns into phlegm, which obstructs and stagnates movement of qi and blood, leading to poor nourishment of the sinews and vessels. Or stagnation of phlegm turns into fire. Phlegm and heat intermingles. Then heat engenders wind which interferes with sinews and vessels, leading to tremor.

过食甘肥、饮酒过度，脾胃受损，运化失司，湿聚为痰，痰浊阻滞，气血运行不畅，筋脉失养；或痰郁化火，痰热互结，热极生风，扰动筋脉，而成颤证。

1.4 Injury of the Liver and Spleen Due to Emotional and Spiritual Disharmony

1.4 情志失调，损伤肝脾

Depression and anger hurts the liver. Liver qi canbe depressed and turns into heat that engenders wind. The wind intereferes with sinews and vessels, leading to tremor.

郁怒伤肝，肝气郁结，化热生风，扰动筋脉，而成颤证。

Overall, tremor lies in sinews and vessels but is closely related to the live, spleen and kidney. The

综上所述颤证的病位在筋脉，与肝、肾、脾等脏关系

pathological factors are wind, fire, phlegm and stasis. Its nature genrally is primary deficiency and secondary excess. The primary is deficiency of qi, blood, yin and yang, among which deficiency of yin fluid and blood essence is the major one. The secondary is wind, fire, phlegm and stasis. The primary and secondary symptoms are closely related. If the pattern lasts long, deficiency and excess, cold and heat are interchangeable, leading to complicationg of both.

密切。病理因素为风、火、痰、瘀。病理性质总属本虚标实。本为气血阴阳亏虚，其中以阴津精血亏虚为主，标为风、火、痰、瘀为患，标本之间密切联系。病久则虚实、寒热转化不定，而成寒热错杂，虚实夹杂之证。

2 Syndrome Differentiation and Treatment

2 辨证论治

2.1 Key Points of Syndrome Differentiation

2.1 辨治要点

It's critical to identify deficiency and excess, the primary and secondary symptoms. Yin deficiency of the liver and kidney, deficiency of qi and blood are the primary oftremor while wind, fire, phlegm and stasis are the secondary. Generally speaking, serious tremor, stiff limbs, irritation, agitation, chest oppression, abesity, trigged by depression and anger are manifestations of excess types while light tremor which is continuous with no cure, and accompanied with symptoms such as soreness in the waist and knees, emaciation, vertigo, aggravated by overstrain are symptoms of deficiency type. But when it prolongs, it will be complication of both types.

颤证主要是辨清标本虚实。肝肾阴虚、气血不足为病之本；风、火、痰、瘀等病理因素多为病之标。一般震颤较剧，肢体僵硬，烦躁不宁，胸闷体胖，遇郁怒而发者，多为实证；颤抖无力，缠绵难愈，腰膝酸软，体瘦眩晕，遇烦劳而加重者，多为虚证。但病久常标本虚实夹杂。

As for the treatment principles, during on the onset stage when deficiency of the primary sympotoms are not quite remarkable and but secondary excess of wind and fire stirring up each other, phlegm-heat obstruction, then focus on clearing away heat, resolving phlegm and stopping fire. As it develops and lasts, for old people and those of weak constitu-

本病的治疗原则：初期，本虚之象并不明显，常见风火相煽、痰热壅阻之标实证，治疗当以清热、化痰、息风为主；病程较长，年老体弱，其肝肾亏虚、气血不足等本虚之象逐渐突出，治疗当滋补

tion, primary deficiency will come up, then focus on nourishing and supplementing the liver and kidney, boosting qi and nurturing blood, regulating and nourishing yin and yang as well as stopping wind and dredging collaterals. Since tremor are more likely to happen to old people and primary deficiency are likely to lead to secondary excess, therefore, the treatment should be focused more on supplementing and invigorating the liver and kidney, to treat the primary.

肝肾，益气养血，调补阴阳为主，兼以息风通络。由于本病多发于中老年人，多在本虚的基础上导致标实，因此治疗更应重视补益肝肾，治病求本。

2.2 Therapeutic Methods for Different Types

2.2.1 Stirring of Wind-yang

Manifestations: Serious tremor of the limbs that cannot be controlled, dizziness, vertigo, red cheeks, irritiation, agitation, aggravating tremor with nervousness with accompanied numbness, bitter and dry mouth, slow speech, drooling, dark urine and dry stool; red tongue with greasy tongue fur; stringy pulse.

Treatment: To calm the liver and stop wind; relax sinews and stop tremor.

Formulas and Herbs: *Gastrodia and Uncaria Decoction* (Tian Ma Gou Teng Yin) and *Liver-Sedating and Wind-Eliminating Decoction* (Zhen Gan Xi Feng Tang), usually composed of *Gastrodiae Rhizoma* (Tian Ma) and *Uncariae Ramulus cum Uncis* (Gou Teng) to calm the liver and subdue yang; *Haliotidis Concha* (Shi Jue Ming), *Haematitum* (Zhe Shi), *Ostreae Concha* Crudus (Sheng Mu Li) to calm the liver to stop wind; *Rehmannia Radix* (Sheng Di Huang), *Paeoniae Radix Alba* (Bai Shao Yao), *Scrophulariae Radix* (Xuan Shen), *Testudinis Carapax et Plastrum* (Gui Jia), *Asparagi Radix* (Tian Dong), *Cyathulae Radix* (Chuan Niu Xi),

2.2 分型论治

2.2.1 风阳内动

证候：肢体颤动粗大，程度较重，不能自制，眩晕耳鸣，面赤烦躁，易激动，心情紧张时颤动加重，伴有肢体麻木，口苦而干，语言迟缓不清，流涎，尿赤，大便干。舌质红，苔黄，脉弦。

治法：镇肝息风，舒筋止颤。

方药：天麻钩藤饮合镇肝息风汤。常用：天麻、钩藤平肝潜阳；石决明、代赭石、生龙骨、生牡蛎镇肝息风；生地黄、白芍药、玄参、龟甲、天门冬、怀牛膝、杜仲、桑寄生滋肾柔肝；黄芩、山栀清肝泻火；夜交藤、茯神养心安神。

Eucommiae Cortex (Du Zhong) and *Taxilli Herba* (Sang Ji Sheng) to nourish the kidney and soften the liver; *Taxilli Herba* (Sang Ji Sheng) and *Gardeniae Fructus* (Zhi Zi) to cleanse the liver and purge fire; *Polygoni Multiflori Caulis* (Ye Jiao Teng) and Poria cum Ligno Hospite (Fu Shen) to nourish the heart and calm the spirits.

Modification: For liver-fire excess, anxiety and irritation, add *Gentianae Radix et Rhizom* (Long Dan) and *Prunellae Spica* (Xia Ku Cao); for stop-less tremor, add *Bombyx Batryticatus* (Jiang Can) and *Scorpio* (Quan Xie); for irritation and insomnia, add *Ziziphi Spinosae Semen* Frictum (Chao Zao Ren), *Platycladi Semen* (Bai Zi Ren) and *Salviae Miltiorrhizae Radix et Rhizoma Radix* (Dan Shen).

加减: 若肝火偏盛,焦虑心烦,加龙胆草、夏枯草;若颤动不止,加僵蚕、全蝎;若心烦失眠,加炒枣仁、柏子仁、丹参养血补心安神。

2.2.2 Phlegm-heat and Stirring of Wind

2.2.2 痰热风动

Manifestations: Continuous shaking head, numb and trembling limbs so much as unable to hold things, dizziness, vertigo, discomfort and oppression in the chest and stomach, bitter and sticky mouth even drooling and spitting phlegm; enlarged tongue with teeth marks, red tongue with yellow greasy tongue fur; stringy rolling rapid pulse.

证候: 头摇不止,肢麻震颤,重则手不能持物,头晕目眩,胸脘痞闷,口苦口黏,甚则口吐痰涎。舌体胖大,有齿痕,舌质红,舌苔黄腻,脉弦滑数。

Treatment: To clear away heat and resolve phlegm; calm the liver to stop wind.

治法: 清热化痰,平肝息风。

Formulas and Herbs: *Phlegm-Abducting Decoction* (Dao Tan Tang) and *Antelope Horn and Uncaria Decoction* (Ling Jiao Gou Teng Tang), usually composed of *Pinelliae Rhizoma* (Ban Xia), *Arisaema cum Bile* (Dan Nan Xing), *Bambusae Caulis in Taenias* (Zhu Ru), *Fritillariae Cirrhosae Bulbus* (Bei Mu), *Citri Exocarpium Rubrum* (Ju Hong), *Poria* (Fu Ling) and *Aurantii Fructus Immaturus* (Zhi Shi) to resolve phlegm and dredge collaterals;

方药: 导痰汤合羚角钩藤汤。常用:半夏、胆南星、竹茹、川贝母、橘红、茯苓、枳实化痰通络;羚羊角、桑叶、钩藤平肝潜阳;黄芩、菊花清泻肝火;生地黄、生白芍药滋养肝阴。

Cornu Antelopis (Ling Yang Jiao), *Mori Folium* (Sang Ye) and *Uncariae Ramulus cum Uncis* (Gou Teng) to calm the liver and subjugate yang; *Scutellariae Radix* (Huang Qin) and *Chrysanthemi Flos* (Ju Hua) to cleanse and purge liver-fire; *Rehmannia Radix* (Sheng Di Huang) and *Paeoniae Radix Alba* (Bai Shao Yao) to nourish liver-yin.

Modification: For chest oppression and stomach discomfort, add *Trichosanthis Pericarpium* (Gua Lou Pi), *Magnoliae Officinalis Cortex* (Hou Pu) and *Atractylodis Rhizoma* (Cang Zhu); for heavy tremor, add *Margaritifera Concha* (Zhen Zhu Mu), *Haliotidis Concha* (Shi Jue Ming) and *Scorpio* (Quan Xie); for limb numbness, add *Pheretima* (Di Long), *Luffae Fructus Retinervus* (Si Gua Luo) and *Succus Bambosae* (Zhu Li).

加减: 若胸闷脘痞,加瓜蒌皮、厚朴、苍术;若震颤较重,加珍珠母、生石决明、全蝎;若肌肤麻木不仁,加地龙、丝瓜络、竹沥。

2.2.3 Deficiency of Qi and Blood

Manifestations: Head and body shaking, pale complexion, indifferent facial expression, lassitude and fatigue, short breath in movements, palpitation, forgetfulness, dizziness, poor appetite; enlarged pale red tongue, white slippery thin tongue fur; deep soft powerless or deep fine pulse.

Treatment: To boost qi and nourish blood; moist and nourish sinews and vessels.

Formulas and Herbs: *Ginseng Construction-Nourishing Decoction* (Ren Shen Yang Rong Tang), usually composed of *Ginseng Radix et Rhizoma* (Ren Shen), *Astragali Radix* (Huang Qi), *Atractylodis Macrocephalae Rhizoma* (Bai Zhu), *Poria* (Fu Ling) and *Glycyrrhizae Radix et Rhizoma Praeparata* (Zhi Gan Cao) to boost qi; *Rehmanniae Radix Praeparata* (Shu Di Huang), *Angelicae Sinensis Radix* (Dang Gui) and *Paeoniae Radix Alba* (Bai

2.2.3 气血亏虚

证候: 头摇肢颤,面色淡白,表情淡漠,神疲乏力,动则气短,心悸健忘,眩晕,纳呆。舌体胖大,舌质淡红,舌苔薄白滑,脉沉濡无力或沉细弱。

治法: 益气养血,濡养筋脉。

方药: 人参养荣汤。常用:人参、黄芪、白术、茯苓、炙甘草益气;熟地黄、当归、白芍药补血;天麻、钩藤、珍珠母平肝息风;五味子、远志养心安神。

Shao Yao) to supplement blood; *Gastrodiae Rhizoma* (Tian Ma), *Uncariae Ramulus cum Uncis* (Gou Teng) and *Margaritifera Concha* (Zhen Zhu Mu) to calm the liver and stop wind; *Schisandrae Chinensis Fructus* (Wu Wei Zi) and *Polygalae Radix* (Yuan Zhi) to nourish the heart and calm the spirits.

Modification: For deficiency of qi unable to transform, accumulated dampness turning into phlegm, resolve phlegm, dredge collaterals to stop tremor with *Pinelliae Rhizoma* (Ban Xia), *Sinapis Semen* (Jie Zi) and *Arisaema cum Bile* (Dan Nan Xing); for blood deficiency unable to nourish the heart spirit, palpitation, forgetfulness and insomnia, add *Ziziphi Spinosae Semen Frictum* (Chao Zao Ren) and *Platycladi Semen* (Bai Zi Ren); for qi deficiency and blood stagnation, trembling body, pain and numbness, add *Spatholobi Caulis* (Ji Xue Teng), *Salviae Miltiorrhizae Radix et Rhizoma Radix* (Dan Shen), *Persicae Semen* (Tao Ren) and *Carthami Flos* (Hong Hua).

加减：若气虚运化无力，湿聚成痰，应化痰通络止颤，加半夏、白芥子、胆南星；若血虚心神失养，心悸、失眠、健忘，加炒枣仁、柏子仁；若气虚血滞，肢体颤抖、疼痛麻木，加鸡血藤、丹参、桃仁、红花。

2.2.4 Deficiency of Marrow Sea

Manifestations: Head shaking and body trembling as unable to hold a thing, soreness in the waist and knees, insomnia, irritation, dizziness, tinnitus, forgetfulness, and spiritual dullness, dementia with old people; red tongue with white thin tongue fur, or scarlet tongue with no tongue fur; fine rapid pulse.

Treatment: To fulfill essence and supplement marrow; nourish yin and stop wind.

Formulas and Herbs: *Plastrum-Testudinis and Cornus-Cervi Two Divines Paste* (Gui Lu Er Xian Gao), usually composed of *Testudinis Carapax et Plastrum* (Gui Jia), *Trionycis Carapax* (Bie Jia),

2.2.4 髓海不足

证候：头摇肢颤，持物不稳，腰膝酸软，失眠心烦，头晕，耳鸣，善忘，老年患者常兼有神呆、痴傻。舌质红，舌苔薄白，或红绛无苔，脉象细数。

治法：填精补髓，育阴息风。

方药：龟鹿二仙膏合大定风珠。常用：龟甲、鳖甲、鹿角、熟地黄填精补髓；鸡子黄、阿胶、枸杞子、生地黄、白

Cervi Cornu (Lu Jiao) and *Rehmanniae Radix Praeparata* (Shu Di Huang) to fulfill essence and supplement marrow; *Egg Yolk* (Ji Zi Huang), *Asini Corii Colla* (E Jiao), *Lycii Fructus* (Gou Qi Zi), *Rehmannia Radix* (Sheng Di Huang), *Paeoniae Radix Alba* (Bai Shao Yao) and *Ophiopogonis Radix* (Mai Men Dong) to nourish the kidney and nourish yin; *Ostreae Concha* Crudus (Sheng Mu Li) and *Uncariae Ramulus cum Uncis* (Gou Teng) to calm the liver and stop wind; *Ginseng Radix et Rhizoma* (Ren Shen) to supplement greatly orginal qi.

芍药、麦门冬滋肾养阴;生牡蛎、钩藤平肝息风;人参大补元气。

Modification: For heavy liver-wind, remarkable trembling body and vertigo, add *Gastrodiae Rhizoma* (Tian Ma), *Scorpio* (Quan Xie) and *Haliotidis Concha* (Shi Jue Ming); for yin deficiency and fire excess with feverish sensation in five centers, agitation, insomnia, constipation and dark urine, add *Phellodendri Chinensis Cortex* (Huang Bo), *Anemarrhenae Rhizoma* (Zhi Mu), *Moutan Cortex* (Mu Dan Pi) and *Scrophulariae Radix* (Xuan Shen); for spasm and limb numbness, add *Chaenomelis Fructus* (Mu Gua), *Bombyx Batryticatus* (Jiang Can) and *Pheretima* (Di Long), and use great amounts of *Paeoniae Radix Alba* (Bai Shao Yao) and *Glycyrrhizae Radix et Rhizoma* (Gan Cao) to relax sinews and relieve urgency.

加减: 若肝风甚,肢体颤抖、眩晕较著,加天麻、全蝎、石决明;若阴虚火旺,兼见五心烦热、躁动失眠、便秘溲赤,加黄柏、知母、牡丹皮、玄参;若肢体麻木、拘急强直,加木瓜、僵蚕、地龙,重用白芍药、甘草以舒筋缓急。

2.2.5 Decline of Yang-qi

Manifestations: Shaking head, trembling body, spasm of sinews and vessels, waxy pale complexion, aversion to cold and physical cold, limb numbness, no desire to talk due to palpitation, short breath with movements, spontaneous sweating, clear long urine or enuresis, loose stool; pale tongue with white thin tongue fur; deep retarded powerless

2.2.5 阳气虚衰

证候: 头摇肢颤,筋脉拘挛,面色㿠白,畏寒肢冷,四肢麻木,心悸懒言,动则气短,自汗,小便清长或自遗,大便溏。舌质淡,舌苔薄白,脉沉迟无力。

pulse.

Treatment: To supplement the kidney and boost yang; warm sinews and vessels.

治法：补肾助阳，温煦筋脉。

Formulas and Herbs: *Rehmannia Decoction* (Di Huang Yin Zi), usually composed of *Aconm Lateralis Radix Praeparata* (Fu Zi), *Cinnamomi Cortex* (Rou Gui), *Morindae Officinalis Radix* (Ba Ji Tian), *Cistanchis Herba* (Rou Cong Rong) and *Zingiberis Rhizoma Recens* (Sheng Jiang) to warm and supplement kidney-yang; *Rehmannia Radix* (Sheng Di Huang), *Corni Fructus* (Shan Zhu Yu), *Ophiopogonis Radix* (Mai Men Dong) and *Dendrobii Caulis* (Shi Hu) to obtain yang from yin; *Polygalae Radix* (Yuan Zhi) and *Schisandrae Chinensis Fructus* (Wu Wei Zi) to nourish the heart and calm the spirits.

方药：地黄饮子。常用：附子、肉桂、巴戟天、肉苁蓉、生姜温补肾阳；生地黄、山茱萸、麦门冬、石斛从阴引阳；远志、五味子养心安神。

Modification: For loose stool, add *Zingiberis Rhizoma* (Gan Jiang) and *Myristicae Semen* (Rou Dou Kou) to warm the middle and strengthen the spleen; for palpitation, add *Ziziphi Spinosae Semen* (Suan Zao Ren) and *Platycladi Semen* (Bai Zi Ren) to nourish the heart and calm the spirits.

加减：若大便稀溏者，加干姜、肉豆蔻温中健脾；若心悸者加酸枣仁、柏子仁养心安神。

Lumbago

腰　痛

Lumbago refers to a disease caused by exogenous affection, internal injury or wrenching of the waist that leads to inhibited qi and blood flow in the waist or lack of moisturization and nourishment, characterized by pain in the waist, spine or areas nearby the spine.

腰痛是指因外感、内伤或挫闪导致腰部气血运行不畅，或失于濡养，引起腰脊或脊旁部位疼痛为主要症状的一种病证。

1 Etiology and Pathogenesis

1 病因病机

The cause of lumbago can be caused by exoge-

腰痛病因主要是外邪侵

nous pathogeni factors, weak constitution due to old age, falling and wrenching. Its pathogenesis is obstruction of sinews and vessels that leads to poor nourishment of the lumbus.

袭、体虚年衰、跌仆闪挫，基本病机是筋脉痹阻，腰府失养。

1.1 Blockage of Meridians and Collaterals Due to Exogenous Pathogenic Factors

1.1 感受外邪，经脉闭阻

Living in damp places or affection of wind after sweating, or indulgence in coolness in summer will cause loss of protection of the lumbus house. Then the six climatic pathogenic factors of damp-heat, cold-damp and summer-heat will make way into the body, blocking meridians and collaterals, inhibit qi and blood flow and leads to lumbago.

由于居所潮湿，或劳作汗出当风，或暑夏贪凉，腰府失护，湿热、寒湿、暑热等六淫之邪侵入，致经脉受阻，气血运行不畅而发生腰痛。

1.2 Obstruction of Vessels Due to Blood Stasis Caused by Wrenching and Falling

1.2 闪挫坠堕，瘀阻脉络

Overstrains, falling and internal injuries will hurt the lumbus muscles, spine, meridians and vessels, causing unsmooth flow of qi and blood and blockage of the meridians and collaterals. Blood stasis that remains in the waist leads to pain.

过度劳累，跌仆外伤，损伤腰肌、脊柱、经脉，导致气血运行不畅，经络阻滞不通，瘀血留着腰部而发生疼痛。

1.3 Poor Nourishment of Lumbus Due to Deficiency of Kidney-essence

1.3 肾精亏虚，腰府失养

Innate deficiency, or overstrain, or prolonged illness and old age leads to consumption of kidney-essence, resulting in poor nourishment and moisturization of the sinews and vessels, finally leading to lumbago.

素体禀赋不足，或劳累太过，或年老久病体虚，以致肾精亏损，无以濡养筋脉而发生腰痛。

In a word, lumbago lies in the lumbus house, but is also related to the kidney and bladder meridian, controlling vessel, conception vessels, throughfare vessel and girdling vessel. The pathological factors are mainly dampness and stasis. Its nature is primary deficiency and secondary excess, or complication of both. Deficiency of kidney-qi is the pri-

综上所述，腰痛病位在腰府，与肾脏及膀胱经，任、督、冲、带脉等诸经脉相关。病理因素主要是湿与瘀；病理性质为本虚标实，或虚实夹杂。肾气亏虚为本，风、寒、湿、热、瘀血、气滞为标，

mary while wind, cold, dampness, heat, blood stasis and qi stagnation are the secondary. Deficiency and excess often interchanges and complicates, which is the pathological feature of lumbago.

虚实之间常互相转化与夹杂，是本病病理变化的特点。

2 Syndrome Differentiation and Treatment

2 辨证论治

2.1 Key Points of Syndrome Differentiation

2.1 辨治要点

For lumbago, first differentiate exogenous affection, internal injury and falling and wrenching injury. Exogenous affection usually attacks suddenly with remarkable pain in the waist and other symptoms of exogenous pathogenic affection such as wind, dampness, cold and heat. Cold pain and heaviness in the waist, difficulty in turning body over, and pain unrelieved after lying down are due to cold-dampness. Hot pain and heaviness in the waist which gets worse in summer heat dampness which can be relieved after exercise are due to damp-heat. Unconscious attack, soreness in the waist, long duration with deficiency and injury of zang-fu organs, kidney deficiency particularly, are due to internal injury. Endless pain, soreness and powerlessness in the waist are due to deficiency of kidney-essence. Cold pain in the waist and knees that favors warmth and pressure, which aggravates with strain and is relieved after lying down is due to deficiency of kidney-yang. Dull pain in the waist, feverish dysphoria in five centers are due to injury and exhaustion of kidney-yin. Sudden attack, pain in fixed spots with remarkable blood stasis pattern with clinical history of external injury are due to falling and wrenching.

腰痛辨证应辨外感、内伤与跌仆闪挫之外伤。外感者，多起病较急，腰痛明显，常伴有感受风、湿、寒、热等外邪症状：寒湿者，腰部冷痛重着，转侧不利，静卧病痛不减；湿热者，腰部热痛重着，暑湿天加重，活动后或可减轻。内伤者，多起病隐袭，腰部酸痛，病程缠绵，常伴有脏腑虚损症状，多见于肾虚：肾精亏虚者，腰痛缠绵，酸软无力；肾阳不足者，腰膝冷痛，喜温喜按，遇劳更甚，卧则减轻；肾阴亏损者，腰部隐痛，五心烦热。跌仆闪挫者，起病急，疼痛部位固定，瘀血症状明显，常有外伤史可鉴。

The treatment of lumbago should be in accordance with the primary and secondary symptoms, deficiency and excess. For exogenous pathogenic fac-

腰痛治疗当分标本虚实。感受外邪属实，治宜祛邪通络；外伤腰痛属实，治宜

tors, which belongs to excess, it is better to eliminate pathogenic factors and dredge collaterals. For lumbago due to external injury of excess type, activate blood and remove stasis, dredge collaterals and stop pain. For that due to internal injury, which is often deficiency type, it is advisable to supplement the kidney and consolidate the origin as well as treating the liver and spleen. For complication of both types, identify their conflicting relationship and then treat both.

活血祛瘀,通络止痛为主;内伤致病多属虚,治宜补肾固本为主.兼顾肝脾;虚实兼见者,宜辨主次轻重,标本兼顾。

2.2 Therapeutic Methods for Different Types

2.2 分型论治

2.2.1 Lumbago due to Cold-dampness

2.2.1 寒湿腰痛

Manifestations: Cold pain and heaviness in the waist, difficulty in turning body over which takes on graudully and can not be alleviated by lying down, aggravated on cold and rainy days; pale tongue with white greasy tongue fur; deep retarded slow pulse.

证候: 腰部冷痛重着,转侧不利,逐渐加重,静卧病痛不减,寒冷和阴雨天则加重。舌质淡,苔白腻,脉沉而迟缓。

Treatment: To dispel cold and eliminate dampness; warm meridians and dredge collaterals.

治法: 散寒除湿,温经通络。

Formulas and Herbs: *Zingiberis, Poria and Atractylodis Decoction* (Gan Jiang Ling Zhu Tang), usually composed of *Zingiberis Rhizoma* (Gan Jiang), *Glycyrrhizae Radix et Rhizoma* (Gan Cao) and *Caryophylli Flos* (Ding Xiang) to disperse cold and warm the middle jiao; *Atractylodis Rhizoma* (Cang Zhu), *Atractylodis Macrocephalae Rhizoma* (Bai Zhu) and *Citri Exocarpium Rubrum* (Ju Hong) to dry the spleen and eliminate dampness.

方药: 甘姜苓术汤。常用:干姜、甘草丁香散寒温中;苍术、白术、橘红燥脾除湿。

Modification: For predominance of pathogenic cold, cold pain in the waist, spasm and discomfort, add *Aconiti Radix Lateralis Praeparata Secta* (Shu Fu Pian) and *Asari Radix et Rhizoma* (Xi Xin); for predominance of pathogenic dampness with pain

加减: 寒邪偏胜,腰部冷痛、拘急不舒,可加熟附片、细辛;若湿邪偏胜,腰痛重着、苔厚腻,可加苍术、薏苡仁;久病不愈,肝肾虚损,气

and heaviness in the waist and greasy thick tongue fur, add *Atractylodis Rhizoma* (Cang Zhu) and *Coicis Semen* (Yi Yi Ren); for prolonged illness without cure, deficiency and injury of the liver and kidney, deficiency and exhaustion of qi and blood along with soreness and powerless in the waist and knees and deep weak pulse, use *Pubescent Angelica and Mistletoe Decoction* (Du Huo Ji Sheng Tang) plus *Aconm Lateralis Radix Praeparata* (Fu Zi).

血亏虚，而兼见腰膝酸软无力、脉沉弱等症，宜独活寄生汤加附子。

2.2.2 Lumbago due to Damp-heat

Manifestation: Pain in the waist with sensation of heat and heaviness which aggravates on summer rainy days and can be alleviated after exercise, general heaviness, short dark urine; yellow greasy tongue fur; soft rapid pulse or stringy rapid pule.

Treatment: To clear away heat and eliminate dampness; relax sinews and stop pain.

Formulas and Herbs: *Mysterious Four Pills* (Si Miao Wan), usually composed of *Phellodendri Chinensis Cortex* (Huang Bo) and *Atractylodis Rhizoma* (Cang Zhu) to clear away and resolve damp-heat with their acrid, bitter and dry nature; *Coicis Semen* (Yi Yi Ren) to strengthen the spleen, promote urination and help to purge damp-heat; *Achyranthis Bidentatae Radix* (Niu Xi) to induce the ingredients to the affected area.

Modification: For difficult urination with short dark urine, red tongue and stringy rapid pulse, add *Gardeniae Fructus* (Zhi Zi), *Dioscoreae Hypoglaucae Rhizoma* (Bi Xie), *Alismatis Rhizoma* (Ze Xie) and *Akebiae Caulis* (Mu Tong) to clear away and eliminate damp-heat; for accumulation of damp-heat for long consuming yin-fluid with pain in the waist, dry throat, hot palms and soles, focus on clear awa-

2.2.2 湿热腰痛

证候：腰部疼痛，重着而热，暑湿阴雨天气症状加重，活动后或可减轻，身体困重，小便短赤。苔黄腻，脉濡数或弦数

治法：清热利湿，舒筋止痛。

方药：四妙丸。常用：黄柏、苍术辛开苦燥以清化湿热；薏苡仁健脾利水，助湿热排泄；牛膝引药下行直达病所。

加减：若小便短赤不利、舌质红、脉弦数，加栀子、萆薢、泽泻、木通以助清利湿热；若湿热蕴久，耗伤阴津，腰痛，伴咽干、手足心热，治当清利湿热为主，佐以滋补肾阴，酌加生地黄、女贞子、旱莲草。

ying and inducing damp-heat along with nourishing and supplementing kidney-yin, add moderately *Rehmannia Radix* (Sheng Di Huang), *Ligustri Lucidi Fructus* (Nü Zhen Zi) and *Ecliptae Herba* (Han Lian Cao).

2.2.3 Lumbago due to Blood Stasis

Manifestations: Stabbing pain in the waist in fixed spots which refuses pressure and alleviates in daytime and aggravates at night, difficult bending and leaning backward when it is light, difficulty in turning body over when it is serious; dark puple tongue with macules; uneven pulse. Some patients might have clinical history of falling and wrenching.

Treatment: To activate blood to remove stasis; dredge collaterals and stop pain.

Formulas and Herbs: Generalized Pain Stasis-Expelling Decoction (Shen Tong Zhu Yu Tang), usually composed of *Angelicae Sinensis Radix* (Dang Gui), *Chuanxiong Rhizoma* (Chuan Xiong), *Persicae Semen* (Tao Ren), *Carthami Flos* (Hong Hua) to activate blood and remove stasis as well as dredge colleterals and meridians; *Myrrha* (Mo Yao), *Faeces Trogopterorum* (Wu Ling Zhi), *Pheretima* (Di Long) to remove stasis, eliminate swelling and stop pain; *Cyperi Rhizoma* (Xiang Fu) to regulate qi and promote blood flow; *Achyranthis Bidentatae Radix* (Niu Xi) to empower the waist and strengthen the kidney as well as induce the ingredients to the affected area.

Modification: For prolonged lumbago that relapses frequently, use herbs that can activate blood and remove stasis along with those that can catch wind and dredge collaterals, such as *Persicae Semen*

2.2.3 瘀血腰痛

证候：腰痛如刺，痛有定处，痛处拒按，日轻夜重，轻者俯仰不便，重则不能转侧。舌质暗紫，或有瘀斑，脉涩。部分患者有跌仆闪挫病史。

治法：活血化瘀，通络止痛。

方药：身痛逐瘀汤。常用：当归、川芎、桃仁、红花活血化瘀，以疏通经络；没药、五灵脂、地龙化瘀消肿止痛；香附理气行血，牛膝强腰壮肾，又引药下行直达病所。

加减：若腰痛日久，屡次复发者，可活血化瘀配合搜风通络的药物，如桃仁、红花、三七、莪术、虻虫、水蛭、

(Tao Ren), *Carthami Flos* (Hong Hua), *Notoginseng Radix et Rhizoma* (San Qi), *Curcumae Rhizoma* (E Zhu), Tabanus (Meng Chong), *Hirudo* (Shui Zhi), *Vespae Nidus* (Feng Fang), *Scorpio* (Quan Xie), *Scolopendra* (Wu Gong); for clinical history of falling, sprain and wrenching, add *Olibanum* (Ru Xiang) and *Citri Reticulatae Pericarpium Viride* (Qing Pi) to regulate qi, activate blood and stop pain; for prolonged lumbago leading to kidney deficiency, with soreness and powerlessness in the waist and knees, dizziness, tinnitus, add *Taxilli Herba* (Sang Ji Sheng), *Eucommiae Cortex* (Du Zhong), *Dipsaci Radix* (Xu Duan) and *Rehmanniae Radix Praeparata* (Shu Di Huang).

蜂房、全蝎、蜈蚣等；若有跌仆、扭伤、挫闪病史者，加乳香、青皮行气活血止痛；若腰痛日久肾虚者，兼见腰膝酸软无力、眩晕、耳鸣，加桑寄生、杜仲、续断、熟地黄。

2.2.4 Lumbago due to Kidney Deficiency

2.2.4 肾虚腰痛

2.2.4.1 Kidney-yin Deficiency

2.2.4.1 肾阴虚

Manifestations: Dull pain in the waist, soreness and powerlessness, long duration without cure, irritation, insomnia, dry mouth and throat, red cheeks, hot palms and soles; red tongue with little tongue fur; stringy fine rapid pulse.

证候：腰部隐隐作痛，酸软无力，缠绵不愈，心烦少寐，口燥咽干，面色潮红，手足心热。舌红少苔，脉弦细数。

Treatment: To nourish and supplement kidney-yin; moisten and nourish sinews and vessels.

治法：滋补肾阴，濡养筋脉。

Formulas and Herbs: *Kidney Pills* (Zuo Gui Wan), usually composed of *Rehmannia Radix* (Di Huang), *Lycii Fructus* (Gou Qi Zi), *Corni Fructus* (Shan Zhu Yu) and *Testudinis Carapacis et Plastri Colla* (Gui Jia Jiao) to fulfill and supplement kidney-yin, *Cuscutae Semen* (Tu Si Zi), *Cervi Cornus Colla* (Lu Jiao Jiao) and *Achyranthis Bidentatae Radix* (Niu Xi) to warm the kidney and strengthen the waist.

方药：左归丸。常用：地黄、枸杞子、山茱萸、龟版胶填补肾阴；菟丝子、鹿角胶、牛膝温肾壮腰。

Modification: For indulgence in sex that leads to kidney deficiency and lumbago, use *Placenta Major*

加减：若房劳过度而致肾虚腰痛者，可用血肉有情

Bollus (He Che Da Zao Wan); for prolonged lumbar pain with no cure and deficiency of both yin and yang, use *Eucommiae Pills* (Du Zhong Wan).

2.2.4.2　Kidney-yang Deficiency

Manifestations: Cold pain in the waist without cure, feeling cool in some areas that favors warmth and pressure, aggravates with strain and alleviates with lying down, frequent relapse, spasm in lower abdomen, waxy pale complexion, cold limbs and aversion to cold; pale tongue; fine deep powerless pulse.

Treatment: To supplement the kidney and strengthen yang; warm meridians and vessels.

Formulas and Herbs: *Vital Gate Pills* (You Gui Wan), usually composed of *Rehmanniae Radix Praeparata* (Shu Di Huang), *Dioscoreae Rhizoma* (Shan Yao), *Corni Fructus* (Shan Zhu Yu) and *Lycii Fructus* (Gou Qi Zi) to nourish and fulfill kidney-essence, meaning obtaining yang from yin, *Eucommiae Cortex* (Du Zhong) to empower the waist and supplement essence, *Cuscutae Semen* (Tu Si Zi) to supplement and invigorate the liver and kidney, *Angelicae Sinensis Radix* (Dang Gui) to supplement blood and promote blood flow. All combined to warm the kidney and strengthen the waist.

Modification: For kidney deficiency that affects the spleen, causing exhaustion and deficiency of spleen-qi with such symptoms as pain in the waist, fatigue, little intake, loose stool even with pendulous organs, focus on supplementing the kidney along with strengthening the spleen, boosting qi and raising clear away-yang, add *Astragali Radix* (Huang Qi), *Codonopsis Radix* (Dang Shen), *Cimicifugae Rhizoma* (Sheng Ma), *Bupleuri Radix* (Chai

之品调理，如河车大造丸；若虚劳腰痛，日久不愈，阴阳俱虚者，可选用杜仲丸。

2.2.4.2　肾阳虚

证候：腰部冷痛，缠绵不愈，局部发凉，喜温喜按，遇劳更甚，卧则减轻，常反复发作，少腹拘急，面色㿠白，肢冷畏寒。舌质淡，脉沉细无力。

治法：补肾壮阳，温煦经脉。

方药：右归丸。常用：熟地黄、山药、山茱萸、枸杞子培补肾精，是为阴中引阳；杜仲强腰益精；菟丝子补益肝肾；当归补血行血，诸药合用，共奏温肾壮腰之功。

加减：若肾虚及脾，脾气亏虚，症见腰痛乏力、食少便溏，甚或脏器下垂，应补肾为主，佐以健脾益气、升举清阳，加黄芪、党参、升麻、柴胡、白术；如无明显阴阳偏盛者，可服用青娥丸，补肾治腰痛。

Hu) and *Atractylodis Macrocephalae Rhizoma* (Bai Zhu); for unremarkable predominance of yin or yang, use *Young Maid Pill* (Qing E Wan).

Shanghai Pujiang Education Press (Former Shanghai University of Traditional Chinese Medicine Press)
1550 Haigang Ave, Shanghai, P.R.China 201306

图书在版编目(CIP)数据

中医内科学:英汉对照/余小萍主编. —上海:上海浦江教育出版社有限公司,2018.12
(精编实用中医文库/陈凯先,李其忠,何星海总主编)
ISBN 978-7-81121-589-2

Ⅰ.①中… Ⅱ.①余… Ⅲ.①中医内科学—英、汉
Ⅳ.①R25

中国版本图书馆 CIP 数据核字(2018)第300706号

上海浦江教育出版社出版
社址:上海海港大道 1550 号上海海事大学校内　　邮政编码:201306
电话:(021)38284910(12)(发行)　38284923(总编室)　38284916(传真)
E-mail: cbs@shmtu. edu. cn　URL: http://www. pujiangpress. cn
上海盛通时代印刷有限公司印装　上海浦江教育出版社发行
幅面尺寸:170 mm×240 mm　印张:25.25　字数:481 千字
2018 年 12 月第 1 版　2019 年 5 月第 1 次印刷
责任编辑:黄　健　张洁怡　封面设计:赵宏义
定价:108. 00 元